The
Keystone Perforator
Island Flap
Concept

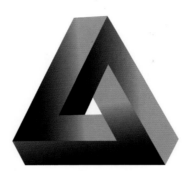

Reconstructive diversity

The limitless potential of the
keystone perforator island flap concept

The Keystone Perforator Island Flap Concept

Felix C Behan FRCS, FRACS
Associate Professor of Surgery, University of Melbourne
Plastic and Reconstructive Surgeon
Department of Surgical Oncology, Peter MacCallum Cancer Centre, Melbourne, & Western Health

Michael Findlay MBBS, PhD, FRACS (Plast)
Plastic, Reconstructive and Hand Surgeon
Department of Surgical Oncology, Peter MacCallum Cancer Centre, Melbourne
Western Health, Austin Health, Peninsula Health
Adjunct Senior Lecturer, Department of Surgery, Monash University, Melbourne

Cheng Hean Lo MBBS
Registrar, Plastic, Hand and Faciomaxillary Surgery Unit
The Alfred Hospital, Melbourne

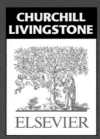

CHURCHILL
LIVINGSTONE

ELSEVIER

Sydney   Edinburgh   London   New York   Philadelphia   St Louis   Toronto

Churchill Livingstone
is an imprint of Elsevier

Elsevier Australia. ACN 001 002 357
(a division of Reed International Books Australia Pty Ltd)
Tower 1, 475 Victoria Avenue, Chatswood, NSW 2067

ELSEVIER

National Library of Australia Cataloguing-in-Publication Data

Author: Behan, Felix.

Title: The keystone perforator island flap concept /
            Felix Behan, Michael Findlay, Cheng Lo.

ISBN: 9780729539715 (hbk.)

Subjects: Flaps (Surgery)
          Surgery, Plastic.

Other Authors/Contributors: Findlay, Michael William. Lo, Cheng.

Dewey Number: 617.952

Publisher: Sophie Kaliniecki
Developmental Editor: Neli Bryant
Publishing Services Manager: Helena Klijn
Project Coordinator: Geraldine Minto
Edited by Carolyn Pike
Proofread by Kerry Brown
Illustrations by Joseph Lucia of Lucia Diagraphics
Cover, internal design and typesetting by Lamond Art & Design
Index by Forsyth Publishing Services
Printed by 1010 Printing International Ltd, China

Foreword by Wayne A Morrison

Now you see it—now you don't. Felix Behan, Michael Findley and Cheng Hean Lo fill impossible holes with local manipulations that defy immediate explanation. Leaving no secondary defect, it is difficult to surmise the design or even source of the flap. These flaps, called 'keystone' because of their arch form, are essentially fasciocutaneous islands from immediate adjacent territories designed in the axis of the dermatomes to capture underlying perforators and neurocutaneous connections. Typically, the flaps move as V–Y advancements or island transpositions but, remarkably, the secondary defect, which is often larger than the primary defect, is able to be directly closed. This involves incision of the deep fascia, the keystone double V–Y advancement shape and the redistributed circumferential tension around the newly sited flaps.

Opportunity demands auditing and recording. Felix Behan began his research observations at the Royal College of Surgeons of England, publishing his angiotome concepts in 1973. Appointments to the Royal Marsden in London and Western General and Peter MacCallum Cancer hospitals in Melbourne afforded him the opportunity of a lifetime for performing, observing and recording his cutaneous reconstructions for cancer and trauma. One of the pithy quotes that precedes each chapter of the book reads 'Insight plus hindsight equals foresight' and aptly fits Felix's evolution of the keystone concept.

The book is full of mind-boggling photographs of giant holes and flap outlines that the uninitiated could only assume are destined for failure. Photography for plastic surgeons is the department of great expectations.

The first reports of these procedures produced healthy scepticism, doubters and non-believers. To understand how to do these flaps is not simple. To mobilise half of someone's face on a few semi-mystical perforators in the bold anticipation that the tissue will move sufficiently to cover an awesome hole is not for the faint-hearted. Short of an apprenticeship with the master, this book is the next best thing.

The book commences with an introduction and a detailed discussion of the fundamental vascular anatomy of the integument, followed by the design principles of the keystone technique. From there onwards it is a photographic album of before, during and after shots of every conceivable defect involving all zones of the body; a treasure trove of ideas and delights. Each region is the subject of a chapter and each includes anatomical details of the relevant perforator system. Separate chapters are allocated to melanoma defects, radiation injury and trauma. Each illustrated case concludes with a TLC (time, life quality, complications) box. To see such spectacular results one after another without complications using design principles that, at first glance, seem counter-intuitive evokes green fingers or a lucky surgeon. But the authors have harnessed chaos using art, science and courage to develop a new concept for the transfer of tissue that is reliable and reproducible.

It is a long time since a new paradigm has appeared in reconstruction. The keystone flap allows perforator concepts to be used without the need to isolate the perforator as an axial flap, reducing operating time and technical demands. In many situations, it eliminates the need for microsurgery. It reconstructs 'like with like' and radically changes the surgeon's reconstructive mindset from distant to local options. It brings back the creativity and excitement of the art and craft movement in plastic surgery that has largely been lost with the microsurgical era. By reading this superb guidebook, you too will have the confidence and the urge to take the keystone perforator island flap principles into the trenches and the marketplace where the battle is to be won.

Professor Wayne A Morrison AM MD BS FRACS
Director, O'Brien Institute, Melbourne

Foreword by Peter C Doherty

Medical advances come about in different ways. The greatest public attention tends to be focused on the generally laboratory-based discoveries that are recognised by Nobel Prizes. Harald zur Hausen (Nobel Prize 2008), for example, established the link between human papilloma virus and cancer of the cervix, a finding that led others to develop a protective vaccine. No reasonable person could doubt that this is a great achievement of enormous human benefit. But there are so many other developments, often incremental in nature, that also make life better for millions of people and which are never celebrated in such a public way. Where, might we ask, is the Nobel Prize for the artificial hip? Is the problem that too many were involved? Nobel Prizes go to a maximum of three people. Could it be that this life-enhancing technology reflects the intelligent persistence of a spectrum of surgeons, bioengineers and even entrepreneurs who persisted in the long term?

Even if they don't win many Nobel Prizes, surgeons do sometimes enjoy great public acclaim. The drama associated with the transplantation of both cadaveric and artificial hearts made the names of Christiaan Barnard and Michael DeBakey familiar to many, at least for a time. Most of the advances in surgery that deliver enormous human benefit, though, fail to engage the attention of the media, though they do make massive contributions to the restoration of function and the alleviation of pain. These surgical pioneers proceed carefully, often by incremental steps that depend on persistence, insight, continued critical evaluation and the courage to try something new and different.

The present technical manual by plastic surgeons Felix Behan, Michael Findlay and Cheng Hean Lo describes just such an advance. Lavishly illustrated with an accompanying DVD, they detail the keystone perforator island flap principle for restoring the integrity of the outer integument following otherwise disfiguring cancer, or other surgery. Operating from the central idea that it is necessary to preserve the integrity of the dermatome with its innervation and vascularisation, the essential steps are clearly laid out and explained so that other, experienced practitioners can follow.

Rather than hunting for perforators with a Doppler audio sound prior to approximating surgical transfers, the approach detailed here has been described aptly by leading international microsurgeon Professor Fu Chan Wei: 'Felix, what we do, you do in freestyle'. In other words, there is an air of spontaneous improvisation in dragging tissue from point A to point B, with all its neural, autonomic, lymphatic and vascular support intact. In addition, these procedures that mimic nature can be completed in a half to a third of the time required by conventional microvascular repair. The resultant shorter theatre times benefit the elderly, in particular. Overall, this book makes an important and substantial contribution to the art and science of surgery.

Peter C Doherty PhD
Laureate Professor, Department of Microbiology and
Immunology, University of Melbourne, Australia
Michael F Tamer Chair of Biomedical Research,
St Jude Children's Research Hospital, Memphis, USA
1996 Nobel Laureate for Physiology or Medicine

Contents

Foreword by Wayne A Morrison v
Foreword by Peter C Doherty vi
Preface xi
Acknowledgments xii
Contributors and reviewers xiv

Section 1
The Fundamentals of Keystone Island Flaps 1

Chapter 1
Introduction to the keystone island flap 3

THE DEVELOPMENT OF THE KEYSTONE ISLAND FLAP 4

Chapter 2
Anatomy and applied physiology of fasciocutaneous flaps 10

INTRODUCTION 10

THE ANATOMY OF FASCIOCUTANEOUS TISSUES 10
Cutaneous vascularisation patterns 11
Cutaneous neurovascularisation patterns 13
Cutaneous microcirculation 16

CUTANEOUS VASCULAR PHYSIOLOGY 16

APPLIED PHYSIOLOGY: VASCULAR REGULATION WITHIN KEYSTONE ISLAND FLAPS 17
Keystone island flap elevation 18
Neural mediation of keystone island flap perfusion 20
Haemodynamic changes in the keystone flap during islanding 25

THE ROLE OF TENSION IN KEYSTONE ISLAND FLAP CLOSURE 26

SUMMARY 27

Chapter 3
Design principles and the keystone technique 28

INTRODUCTION 28

PLANNING A KEYSTONE ISLAND FLAP 28
The keystone design 28
Placement, size and orientation of keystone island flaps 28
Flap elevation 30
Flap inset and defect closure 30
Classification 31
Technical refinements 32
Design variations 34

Handling of the deep fascia/panniculus carnosus remnants 34
Shape of the skin incision 34
Type of flap movement into the defect 35
De-epithelialisation and flap subdivision 35

A NOTE ON ISLANDING 35

CLINICAL CASES 35

SUMMARY 35

Section 2
Clinical Applications of Keystone Island Flaps: Anatomical Regions 53

Chapter 4
Head and neck 55

INTRODUCTION 55

PRINCIPLES OF FLAP ELEVATION IN THE HEAD AND NECK 57
Anatomical layers of the face: preservation of the facial nerve 57
Neurovascular anatomy 58
Zones in head and neck reconstruction 60

MULTIPLE SUBUNIT RECONSTRUCTION 94

SUMMARY 97

Chapter 5
The upper limb 98

INTRODUCTION 98

PRINCIPLES OF FLAP ELEVATION IN THE UPPER LIMB 98

NEUROVASCULAR ANATOMY AND ZONES IN UPPER LIMB RECONSTRUCTION 99
Deltoid region 99
The forearm 100
Dorsum of hand and fingers 100
The palm 102

CLINICAL CASES 103

SUMMARY 113

Chapter 6
The trunk: the clavicles to the groin 114

INTRODUCTION 114

THE BACK 114
Capturing a blood supply 115
Principles of flap elevation in the back 115

THE CHEST WALL AND BREAST 116

Cutaneous blood supply of the chest wall and breast 117

Principles of flap elevation in the chest wall and breast 118

ABDOMINAL RECONSTRUCTION 120

Cutaneous vascular anatomy of the anterior abdominal wall 120

Principles of flap elevation in the abdomen 121

THE PERINEUM 127

Cutaneous vascular anatomy of the perineum 127

BUTTOCK AND PERIANAL RECONSTRUCTION 131

Cutaneous vascular anatomy of the buttock region 131

Principles of flap elevation in the buttock region 131

SUMMARY 134

Chapter 7
The lower limb 135

INTRODUCTION 135

CUTANEOUS VASCULAR ANATOMY OF THE LOWER LIMB 136

The thigh 136

The knee 137

The leg 137

The ankle and dorsum of the foot 141

The plantar surface of the foot 143

FLAP ELEVATION IN THE LOWER LIMB 143

Flap elevation in the groin and thigh 143

Flap elevation around the knee 143

Flap elevation in the leg 148

Flap elevation in the ankle and dorsum of the foot 150

Flap elevation in the plantar foot 152

SUMMARY 155

Section 3
Special Applications of Keystone Island Flaps 157

Chapter 8
Melanoma 159

INTRODUCTION 159

IMPORTANT PRINCIPLES IN KEYSTONE FLAP CLOSURE OF MELANOMA DEFECTS 160

Correct pathology and staging 160

The role of sentinel lymph node biopsy at the time of keystone reconstruction 160

Use of DRAPE in keystone closure 161

Timely commencement of adjuvant therapies in keystone flap closures 162

Quality of life and early functional recovery with low morbidity surgery 163

USE OF KEYSTONE FLAPS FOR NODAL METASTASES 163

REVISIONAL SURGERY 178

SUMMARY 178

Chapter 9

Radiotherapy 179

INTRODUCTION 179

RADIOTHERAPY EFFECTS 179
   Acute radiotherapy effects 179
   Consequential effects of radiotherapy (chronic effects of acute toxicity) 180
   Late effects of radiotherapy 180

PRESENTATIONS INVOLVING RECONSTRUCTION AND RADIOTHERAPY 180
   Reconstruction in previously irradiated tissues 181
   Reconstruction of radionecrosis 195

SUMMARY 198

Chapter 10

Trauma 199

INTRODUCTION 199

THE NATURE AND SEVERITY OF TRAUMA 199
   Isolated trauma versus multi-trauma 200
   Low-energy versus high-energy trauma 200
   Simple versus complex mechanisms 200
   Acute versus chronic trauma 200

SPECIFIC SITES 201
   Lower third of leg 201
   Hand trauma 201

MANAGEMENT OF THE PRIMARY DEFECT 201

CLINICAL CASES 205

SUMMARY 220

INDEX 221

Preface

The keystone perforator island flap represents the culmination of more than 30 years of research and operative experience by its originator, Felix C Behan. It evolved out of a clinical need for a universal locoregional flap option, solving the many problems experienced in free tissue transfer. This minimally invasive technique, providing reliable and cost-effective locally matched tissue for reconstruction of wide-ranging fasciocutaneous defects, is evolving. The benefits of this approach, especially with its low morbidity in our ageing population, are reflected in its increased acceptance within the surgical community and its adoption in numerous centres worldwide. The first publication of this technique, titled 'The keystone design perforator island flap', occurred in the *ANZ Journal of Surgery* in 2003. During this time, improved understanding of flap anatomy, physiology and vascularity has been the basis of its application in numerous body regions, with various design variants. As a result, the keystone perforator island flap concept has evolved beyond the simple geometric design inherent in its name. These keystone principles can be applied to effect reliable wound closure using geometry and designs specific to the surgical needs, whatever the site and clinical situation. The reliability of these flaps and the vascular changes observed in the clinical environment in many cases has brought into question many of the edicts we have accepted historically in our understanding of flap vascularity and physiology based on cadaveric studies. Hence, the experience gained from the use of this flap in over 3000 clinical cases over 16 years is presented here in a single text for the first time.

The aim of this book is to demonstrate the versatility and clinical applications of the keystone perforator island flap technique. As with an instruction manual, the reader may 'flick through' the book and be fascinated by the various operative series that demonstrate examples from a wider spectrum of clinical applications. Alternatively, the text can be read from front to back cover to study the finer details of perforator anatomy and applied flap physiology, including more complex case studies. It is incredible how our initial concept of using the dermatomes to assist flap design has evolved into an improved understanding of the numerous *perforator zones* throughout the body. This has been the basis of new flap developments (e.g. the omega variant keystone flap), with ongoing success of this approach.

As a teaching aid, an accompanying DVD demonstrates video footage of procedures cross-referenced in the book. In this way, the book is well suited to the inexperienced and the experienced surgeon alike. The chapters on technique (Chapter 3), upper and lower limb (Chapters 5 and 7), and melanoma reconstruction (Chapter 8) are great starting points for a broad but simple understanding of the technique. The chapters on the anatomy and applied flap physiology (Chapter 2), and head and neck reconstruction (Chapter 4) are designed to highlight the more complex features of these flaps and their variants.

The last decade has seen the emergence of improved techniques for the in-vivo assessment of vascular flow within flaps, including computed tomography angiography, laser colour Doppler ultrasound, thermal, and indocyanine green perfusion imaging modalities. Hopefully, these imaging techniques will provide unequivocal answers as to why these flaps are so reliable and heal so well. We hope that readers will see this book as the pioneering text in keystone perforator island flap surgery and use it as an inspiration to apply its principles and develop innovative techniques throughout their careers.

Felix C Behan
Michael Findlay
Cheng Hean Lo

Acknowledgments

First, I acknowledge my co-authors, Michael Findlay and Cheng Hean Lo, for their clinical, scientific and technological input in producing this tome.

Throughout my career, I acknowledge the following people and organisations: Brian Cortice, from Brisbane, who, without his input and refinement in surgical repair, the hemming suture would not have evolved; the plastic surgical training I received in Melbourne, where, thanks to a reference from the late Peter Grant, I worked with Sir Benjamin Rank at the Victorian Plastic Surgical Unit, who introduced me to plastic surgical reconstruction; Don Marshall, who taught me the refinements in surgical reconstruction; my colleague, the late Alan McLeod, who introduced me to the London surgical scene, with Ian Wilson, Charlie Westbury and Henry Shaw, all part of the St George's/Westminster/Marsden group; the Bernard Sunley Research Fellowship at the Royal College of Surgeons, without which I would not have come upon the idea of fascial-based flaps designed as angiotomes for reconstructive purposes; the Charing Cross Hospital and mortuary department, who made cadaver specimens available for educational purposes; my colleagues at the Western Hospital—Trevor Jones, Graeme Thomson, Chris Haw and the orthopaedic team—and the Peter MacCallum Cancer Centre—Michael Henderson, David Speakman, John Spillane, Simon Donohue and Mikki Pohl—without whom the referral base of cases would not have been as comprehensive; Professor Gordon Clunie, Bob Thomas, Andrew Sizeland and Steve Chan, who, without their academic input, this project may not have reached fruition; the registrars in training and junior staff for their scientific input in article and textbook preparation; and Margaret Clancy, to whom I am indebted for educational and secretarial support.

Internationally, I acknowledge Professor Bill Kuzon of Michigan, who provided editorial assistance on my first paper on the keystone flap in 2003. He saw the value of this reconstructive tool in patient care, in parallel with the microsurgical development which has been part of the Melbourne scene since Ian Taylor's first microsurgical reconstruction in the 1970s. Professor Wayne Morrison of the Bernie O'Brien Microsurgical Institute was part of the editorial process in my first keystone publication in the *ANZ Journal of Surgery*. Also, Andrew Burd of Hong Kong, former editor of the *Journal of Plastic, Reconstructive and Aesthetic Surgery*, and Jacques Baudet from Bordeaux, on the European scene, have been very supportive in the development of this idea.

I can only mention in passing the college libraries and hospital departments, who have all been most helpful. My photographic development has improved thanks to the team at the Peter MacCallum Cancer Centre.

At a personal level, my late father, when he was on the Senate of the University of Queensland, actively supported postgraduate study and was a factor in this encouragement.

In conclusion, the final acknowledgement goes to my wife, Mariette, and my children, Laurent, Amandine and Thibault, for their individual contributions, IT support and tolerance of the impositions I have placed on them throughout a surgical career. At a clinical level it was my wife, Mariette, who made the observation some years ago when doing my dressings that 'your wounds are healing better now' after I commenced using island flaps of the keystone type all over the body. It was only in retrospect that the improved vascularity was recognised as a feature of the keystone island flap concept, underlining its value as a reconstructive tool.

Felix C Behan

I owe a debt of gratitude to: Felix Behan for having the patience to put up with a trainee and now colleague who continues to ask questions and suggest that the current understanding is insufficient; Cheng Hean Lo, who has made an invaluable contribution to the text and helped us to maintain a sane collaborative environment that I hope will continue long into the future; my wife, and children Aly and Will, for putting up with all the late nights and weekends away from home during the preparation of this manuscript; and, finally, to all the patients who put their lives and well-being in our hands and agreed to allow us to catalogue their progress before, during and after their surgery so that we might teach others and improve our own technique. We hope their efforts will result in better understanding of this technique and its more widespread application as a useful option in fasciocutaneous reconstruction.

Michael Findlay

I thank my family for consistently supporting me in all my achievements: my parents, who made immense sacrifices in migrating to Australia; my wife, Elaine, who is my tower of strength; and my delightful daughter, Erica, who supports me in her own little way by surprising me with her ever-evolving curiosity of the world.

I am grateful to my co-authors, Felix Behan and Michael Findlay, for making this journey most enjoyable.

Felix Behan, Michael Leung and Heather Cleland are influential mentors in my surgical career. Their passion for their work, teaching, fortitude and willingness to lead by example are to name only a few of the attributes I have benefited from and aim to emulate.

Cheng Hean Lo

Contributors and reviewers

Authors

Felix C Behan FRCS, FRACS
Associate Professor of Surgery, University of
Melbourne
Plastic and Reconstructive Surgeon
Department of Surgical Oncology, Peter MacCallum
Cancer Centre, Melbourne, & Western Health

Michael Findlay MBBS, PhD, FRACS(Plast)
Specialist Plastic, Reconstructive and Hand Surgeon
Department of Surgical Oncology, Peter MacCallum
Cancer Centre, Melbourne, & Western Health
Adjunct Senior Lecturer, Monash University
Department of Surgery

Cheng Hean Lo MBBS
Registrar, Plastic, Hand and Faciomaxillary Surgery
Unit, The Alfred Hospital, Melbourne

Contributor

Brendon J Coventry MBBS, PhD, FRACS
Associate Professor of Surgery, University of Adelaide;
Senior Consultant Surgeon, Royal Adelaide Hospital;
Director, Adelaide Melanoma Unit, Glenelg, South
Australia

Expert reviewers

Professor Andrew Burd MB ChB, MD, FRCSEd,
FHKAM
Chief of Division of Plastic, Reconstructive and
Aesthetic Surgery, Department of Surgery,
Chinese University of Hong Kong, Prince of Wales
Hospital, Shatin, NT Hong Kong

Professor Gordon Clunie MB ChB ChM MD DSc
FRCS FRACS
Emeritus Professor of Surgery, University of
Melbourne

Michael A Henderson MD, FRACS
Associate Professor of Surgery, Department of
Surgery, University of Melbourne; Surgeon and
Head, Skin and Melanoma Service, Peter MacCallum
Cancer Centre, Melbourne

Associate Professor Trevor Jones MBBS FRACS
General Surgeon, Clinical Services Director (Surgery),
Western Health, Melbourne

Stephen Kleid MBBS, FRACS
Surgeon, Head and Neck, Skin and Melanoma
Service, Peter MacCallum Cancer Centre & Western
Hospital, Melbourne

Expert reviewers (continued)

William M Kuzon Jr MD, PhD
Reed O. Dingman Professor of Surgery; Section
Head, Plastic Surgery, University of Michigan

Andrew Sizeland MBBS, PhD, FRACS
Surgeon, Head and Neck, Skin and Melanoma
Service, Peter MacCallum Cancer Centre & Western
Hospital, Melbourne

Naveen Somia MBBS, PhD, FRACS(Plast)
Plastic Surgeon, Prince of Wales, Children's and
Westmead Hospitals, Sydney; Senior Clinical Lecturer
in Surgery, University of Sydney

David Speakman MBBS, FRACS
Surgeon and Head, Skin and Melanoma Service, Peter
MacCallum Cancer Centre, Melbourne

John Spillane MBBS, FRACS
Senior Fellow, Department of Surgery, University of
Melbourne; Surgeon, Skin and Melanoma Service,
Peter MacCallum Cancer Centre, Melbourne

Professor Robert Thomas OAM, MS, FRACS, FRCS
Former Director of Surgical Oncology, Peter
MacCallum Cancer Centre, Melbourne

External reviewers

Peter F Burke FRCS(Eng.), FRACS, FACEM,
DHMSA
Senior Consultant General Surgeon, Latrobe Regional
Hospital, Victoria; Specialty Editor, Surgical History,
ANZ Journal of Surgery

Steven T F Chan MBBS, PhD, FRACS
Professor of Surgery, Department of Surgery, The
University of Melbourne

Alan de Costa FRCS(I), FRACS
Associate Professor of Surgery, James Cook University
School of Medicine and Dentistry, Cairns

Michael Kamenjarin MBBS, FRACS, FACRRM
Visiting Surgeon, Goulburn Valley Health, Victoria

Julian Peters BMedSci, MBBS(Hons), FRACS
Senior Consultant Plastic Surgeon, The Royal
Melbourne Hospital

Christian E Sampson MD
Assistant Professor, Department of Surgery, Harvard
Medical School, Brigham & Women's Hospital,
Boston, Massachusetts

Richard Turner MBBS, BMedSci, FRACS
Professor of Surgery, School of Medicine, University
of Tasmania, Hobart

Section 1

The Fundamentals of Keystone Island Flaps

Chapter 1

Introduction to the keystone island flap

A simple solution to many reconstructive problems

Observation is the basis of scientific advancement.
Sir William Osler (1849–1919)

The keystone island flap is a unique reconstructive tool in its versatility, reliability and simplicity.

Since the development of the keystone island flap by Behan in 1995 (Behan 2003), this useful technique has become a workhorse for locoregional fasciocutaneous reconstruction in numerous body regions, both in our Victorian centre and, more recently, in centres around the globe (Pelissier et al. 2007a, 2007b). The attractiveness of locoregional reconstruction has always been offset by the need to be familiar with a very large number of named flaps in order to confidently undertake locoregional flap closure in most instances. The keystone island flap offers a solution to this dilemma by providing a single reliable flap that is easy to design, elevate and inset to effect rapid fasciocutaneous closure in most regions of the body. The technique is relatively easy to learn and forms an ideal starting point for the trainee or new surgeon undertaking their first locoregional reconstructions. In experienced hands, it permits the closure of large fasciocutaneous defects. It requires very little post-surgical care comparative to other approaches and, therefore, is not only of use in developed countries but also in developing countries where specialist postoperative nursing care is not routinely available.

Interest in this flap is increasing. The reasons stem not only from the intrinsic utility of the technique, but also from how it meets the needs of today's patients and the time-strapped surgeons who care for them. Worldwide, populations are ageing (UN Department of Economic and Social Affairs 2010). In Australia, the proportion of the population aged over 65 years is projected to almost double and those aged 85 years and over to quadruple by 2056 (Australian Bureau of Statistics 2008). These population changes place unprecedented demands on health budgets, emphasising the need for cost-effective patient management. Furthermore, multivariate analysis has revealed patient age to be a significant risk factor for medical complications following oncological surgery (Audisio et al. 2007). These two factors, in combination, place additional demands on today's surgeon to provide tissue reconstruction with minimal morbidity (and mortality) to patients and to deliver these outcomes in a cost-effective manner.

Free-tissue transfer represents a technologically advanced treatment option developed to provide reconstruction where the use of locoregional flaps alone is inadequate. The more recent developments of perforator flap and free-style free-flap surgery have further glamorised an already exciting reconstructive approach and, as a result, today's reconstructive surgical trainees are well-versed in microsurgical reconstruction at the expense of their training in locoregional flap reconstruction. Most reconstructive microsurgeons use about a dozen free flaps (with variants) as the basis for the majority of their reconstructions. This somewhat formulaic approach has simplified modern-day core microsurgery but has made training in advanced locoregional reconstruction (>500 individual flaps described to date) less appealing. Despite free-flap reconstruction being achievable in increasingly elderly and infirm patients, microsurgical reconstruction is costly for the patient's health, the surgeon's time and the health department's budget. Free-tissue transfer is associated with long operative times, prolonged in-patient stay, hyperdynamic postoperative circulatory management with concurrent risk of cardiac compromise, anticoagulation with its potential risks and poorer aesthetic outcomes when compared with locoregional fasciocutaneous reconstruction. Octogenarians with head and neck cancer suffered a higher incidence of medical complications after microvascular reconstruction, even after controlling for the level of preoperative comorbidity using the American Society of Anesthesiologists' (ASA) score (Blackwell et al. 2002). In addition, the duration of intensive care requirements was prolonged. As such, free-flap surgery is ill-suited to meeting the needs of our ageing populations except in specific instances (e.g. composite tissue or bony reconstruction).

The keystone island flap offers a single fasciocutaneous flap that is suitable for use in nearly every region of the body to achieve rapid and reliable fasciocutaneous coverage with minimal morbidity to the patient, good cosmesis and good quality of life. As such, it is well suited to meet the needs of reconstructive surgeons into the future and should appropriately limit the use of free-flap reconstruction to defects unsuitable for locoregional reconstruction and assist in the management of free-flap morbidity by assisting donor site closure.

Skin grafting is an invaluable tool, particularly where very large epithelial loss occurs, such as in burns or large pretibial ulcers. However, its use can be problematic, especially in the lower limb. For less extensive defects, the keystone island flap can provide an attractive alternative to solve the morbidity associated with skin grafting in the lower limb. Postoperative immobilisation to enhance skin graft take puts the patient at risk of venous thromboembolism, pressure ulcers and deconditioning, with loss of independent mobility (Budny et al. 1993). It ties up a valuable hospital bed with significant economic cost to the health system. Keystone island flap closure of lower limb defects can often be undertaken in the ambulatory setting, making it suitable for widespread application; it also avoids the morbidity of an additional donor site. The simple design facilitates re-excision for incompletely excised lesions, and the full-thickness fasciocutaneous closure is comfortable for most patients and has improved aesthetics compared with other reconstructive approaches. As with all islanded flaps, the design must incorporate underlying perforators or neurovascular support. Therefore, flap elevation over subcutaneous bone necessitates extension of the flap beyond the bony margin to capture perforators from the surrounding fascia and muscle. As with other flaps, the stretching of keystone flaps over sharp edges or surfaces (e.g. over the pretibial border to supply the contralateral side of the leg) should be avoided. The benefits of the keystone island flap are summarised in Box 1.1.

> **BOX 1.1 Advantages of the keystone island flap**
>
> - Simple to design
> - Robust vascular supply
> - Reliable healing
> - Short operative time
> - Minimal patient morbidity
> - Relatively pain-free surgery
> - Good aesthetic outcome
> - Cost-effective wound closure

THE DEVELOPMENT OF THE KEYSTONE ISLAND FLAP

The keystone island flap represents the culmination of nearly four decades of research and clinical reconstructive surgery. Following on from the work of Manchot (1889) and Salmon (1936), Behan undertook cadaveric injection studies (using resin and radiocontrast dye with xerography and histological examination) while undertaking a research fellowship at the Royal College of Surgeons of London in 1972. These studies demonstrated that the system of axial vessels to the integument can supply the regions of adjacent axial vessels via *linkage vessels,* as summarised in Figure 1.1 (Behan & Wilson 1973). This led to the development of the concept of the *angiotome**, which is a section of skin and underlying tissue that can be islanded on a single axial vessel so as to incorporate the integument normally supplied by that vessel and, if necessary, adjacent regions that are supplied from the central axial vessel via these linkage vessels (Behan & Wilson 1975). Thus, flap elevation within the angiotome for a given perforator permits the reliable elevation of a flap supplied to its periphery through linkage vessels from the feeding perforator to adjacent vascular territories within the flap that have lost their natural perforator supply. It is presumed that dilatation of the linkage vessels, along with an increase in their calibre and number, occurs following vascular delay, but an angiotome does not normally require vascular delay for tissue survival (although delay can maximise tissue survival/recruitment of

---

* Angiotome was coined by Behan as an extension of an existing term—the angiotome—'a segment of the vascular system of the embryo' (Dorland 1994), as a means to describe a segment of tissue (cut as a flap) that can be supplied by a single axial vessel (perforator or direct) either directly or via communications to adjacent territories (increasing the flap's size).

adjacent vascular units). In Chapter 2 we will discuss how the physiological regulation of cutaneous blood flow can be manipulated to maximise the angiotome of a given vessel and, therefore, increase the reliability of locoregional flaps.

In defining the angiotome concept, this early work permitted an improved understanding of how tissues can be either islanded or raised as free flaps while maintaining adequate blood supply to the integument. Some of the regions assessed include those that have become well-known flaps today, such as the superficial temporal artery (laterally based or total forehead flap; Fig 1.2), internal mammary perforator and thoracoacromial axis (deltopectoral flap), and deep inferior epigastric artery perforators (hypogastric flap, or more commonly known as the DIEP flap; Fig 1.3).

Unlike Manchot (1889) and Salmon (1936), who focused on the axial vessels themselves, the identification of linkage vessels and the development of the angiotome concept permitted the subsequent development of a number of direct and perforator-based fasciocutaneous flaps. Islanded flaps, such as the Bezier flap (French curvilinear V–Y island advancement) and the perforator-based keystone island flap, incorporate the principles of the angiotome to facilitate perfusion to the margins of the flap. Since then, further use of the keystone island flap in compromised tissues has allowed the development of the *immediate vascular augmentation concept (IVAC)*. These important vascular studies and their conclusions pre-date the subsequent vascular studies of others, including Cormack and Lamberty (1984a, b) and Taylor and Palmer (1987), as well as the angiosome concept. The *angiosome*, as the region of tissue autonomously supplied by a single vessel, has proven to be an invaluable concept for the description of blood supply to all the tissues of the body. However, the *angiotome* concept answers the most important clinical question for reconstructive surgeons; namely, what amount of tissue can be islanded on a single source vessel? The technique of keystone island flap elevation seeks to maximise the size of the

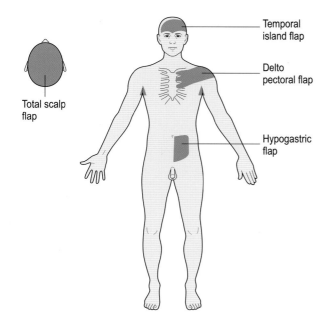

Total scalp flap

Temporal island flap

Delto pectoral flap

Hypogastric flap

◄ **FIGURE 1.1 Original diagram of the body indicating the sites of various perforator or direct vessel fasciocutaneous flaps investigated by Behan as part of his angiotome concept in 1973. The hypogastric flap has subsequently been renamed in clinical use as the deep inferior epigastric perforator (DIEP) flap, used extensively for breast reconstruction. This is the first anatomical study of the basis of this popular perforator flap. The temporal flap was used to facilitate scalp replantation clinically.**

(Reproduced with permission from Behan & Wilson 1973.)

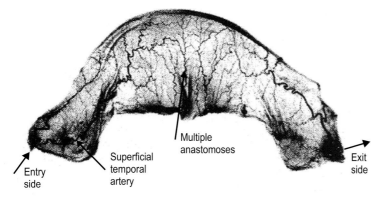

Entry side

Superficial temporal artery

Multiple anastomoses

Exit side

◄ **FIGURE 1.2 The total forehead flap— superficial temporal artery**

Injection of 50% micro-opaque dye in the anterior branch of the superficial temporal artery at various stages of filling, demonstrating the principles of angiotomes and linkage vessels.

(Reproduced with permission from Behan & Wilson 1973, Figs 3–5.)

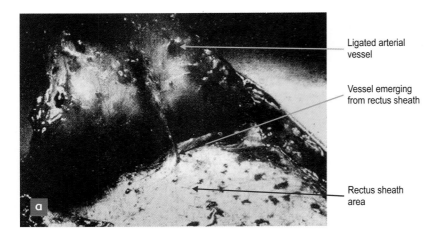

Ligated arterial
vessel

Vessel emerging
from rectus sheath

Rectus sheath
area

◄ **FIGURE 1.3 The hypogastric flap—deep inferior epigastric artery perforator**

(a) Dissection of the hypogastric flap revealing a deep inferior epigastric perforator emerging from the anterior rectus sheath. **(b)** Arterial and **(c)** venous injection studies of the hypogastric flap showing the density of vessels.

(Reproduced with permission from Behan & Wilson 1975, Figs 7–9.)

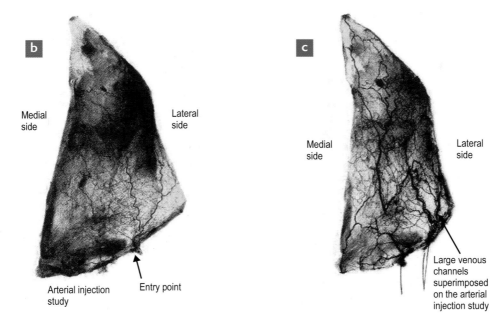

Medial
side

Lateral
side

Medial
side

Lateral
side

Arterial injection
study

Entry point

Large venous
channels
superimposed
on the arterial
injection study

angiotome from any perforator and augment this supply by providing additional (conjoint) neurovascular supply and superficial venous drainage. A comparison of the angiotome and subsequent angiosome concepts is presented in Table 1.1. The immediate vascular augmentation concept observed with islanding results in an islanded angiotome (keystone or other variants) that augments perfusion.

Cadaveric studies are useful to provide clues as to how tissues are perfused in vivo, but recent advances in computerised tomographic (CT) angiography have highlighted what almost 35 years of experience has provided clinically; namely, that cadavers are a poor substitute for the careful assessment and cataloguing of perforators, vascular patterns, skin and soft tissue viability during the raising of angiotomes (as various forms of island flaps) in live patients as part of tissue reconstruction (Rozen et al. 2009). The insight Rozen and colleagues (2009) gained through cadaveric studies has been applied in a progressive manner to raise larger

and larger direct and perforator-based island flaps in various regions of the body (often along the lines of the dermatomes of the body, as discussed in Chapter 3).

A preliminary series of locoregional flaps (approximately 200 cases) was published in 1992 and an analysis of this series provided the basis upon which the current concept of the keystone island flap is founded (Behan 1992). Fasciocutaneous island flaps were used in various anatomical regions throughout the body (Fig 1.4). Having identified a reliable method for the elevation of islanded flaps so as to incorporate sufficient perforator or direct vessel support, the focus shifted to the geometric design of the flaps in order to facilitate primary closure and to optimise aesthetics.

The Bezier or French curve flap was published in 1995 (Behan et al. 1995). It was introduced to deal with elliptical defects that are not closable by direct apposition. Developed from similar underlying principles to the keystone island flap, the Bezier flap is an elegant extension of the V–Y advancement principle

TABLE 1.1 **Angiotome versus angiosome**		
	Angiotome	**Angiosome**
Definition	An area of skin that will survive when cut as a flap supplied by an axial vessel (with its blood supply) extended by its communication with branches (or links) from an adjacent vessel.	A region of tissue supplied by a single axial (or direct) vessel without capture of linkage (or choke) vessels.
Published	Behan & Wilson1975	Taylor & Palmer 1987
Clinical utility	Defines how tissue flaps can be raised on perforating or direct vessels	Defines autonomous blood supply for tissues of body

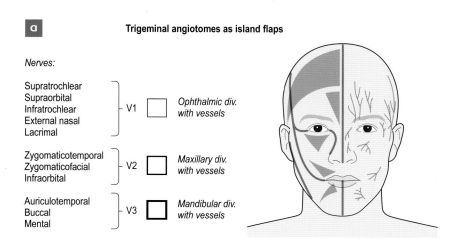

a **Trigeminal angiotomes as island flaps**

Nerves:

Supratrochlear
Supraorbital
Infratrochlear   V1   *Ophthalmic div.*
External nasal   *with vessels*
Lacrimal

Zygomaticotemporal
Zygomaticofacial   V2   *Maxillary div.*
Infraorbital   *with vessels*

Auriculotemporal
Buccal   V3   *Mandibular div.*
Mental   *with vessels*

Major island flaps

Forehead	11
Eyebrow	1
Eyelid	6
Temple	3
Ear A	4
Ear C.F.	4
Nose	12
Lip	7
Chin	1
Neck ant.	2
Cheek	1
Total	**53**

Total to the 1st April 1992. Excluding small or minor flaps with subcutaneous pedicles

Fasciocutaneous angiotomes as island flaps

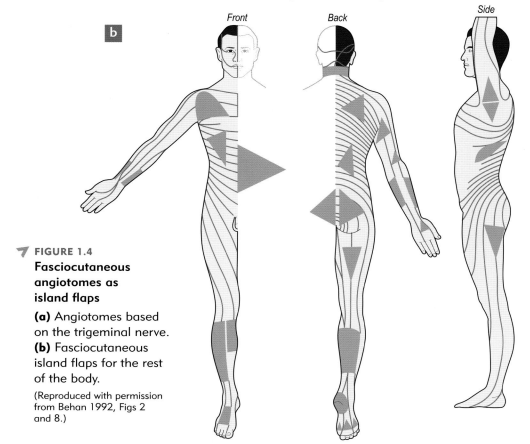

Front   *Back*   *Side*

b

Major island flaps

Neck	2
Scalp	13
Axilla	5
Chest wall	3
Abdomen	1
Upper limb:	
– upper arm	9
– forearm	6
Back	5
Hand	40
Sacral area	16 + 16
Lower limb:	
– thigh	3
– leg	24
Foot	10
Total	**137 + 16**

Total to the 1st April 1992. Excluding small or minor flaps with subcutaneous pedicles

◥ **FIGURE 1.4**

Fasciocutaneous angiotomes as island flaps

(a) Angiotomes based on the trigeminal nerve.
(b) Fasciocutaneous island flaps for the rest of the body.

(Reproduced with permission from Behan 1992, Figs 2 and 8.)

(i.e. limited in terms of advancement). The gentle curve of the Bezier flap uses Langer's lines to minimise the visibility of scars and maximise the aesthetic result.

In subsequent years, the design of the Bezier flap evolved. The gentle curve of this design was retained at the wound margin, but it was identified that having two regions for V–Y advancement and moving these areas further away from the long axis of the wound would provide improved tissue laxity and greatly aid the primary closure of larger defects. This resulted in an arc of tissue being raised on underlying perforators; hence, it was initially coined the 'arc' flap.

It was renamed a keystone flap** due to its resemblance to the keystone of archways. A keystone is the central, apical, wedge-shaped stone of Roman (and other) arches that lies in such a manner as to provide arch support through the action of gravity and friction. This architectural development facilitated the building of multistorey structures, including the Colosseum (Fig 1.5). In an analogous manner, the shape of the keystone island flap seems to lock into the defect and provide structural advantages for wound closure, employing double V–Y advancement (Dieffenbach).

In 2003, the keystone island flap concept—as the keystone design perforator island flap—was first published (Behan 2003). Described as a curvilinear-shaped trapezoidal design flap, it fits well into body contours. Since that time, it has been used extensively to effect wound closure in various regions of the body. The ease of use, short operative time, minimal morbidity, reliable healing and avoidance of costly and morbid free-flap reconstruction in our ageing population has led to an explosion in the use of this technique in recent years, both in Australasia and overseas.

** The term 'keystone' was suggested as a more appropriate descriptive term for Behan's arc flap by Mr Alan Breidahl, a Melbourne plastic surgeon.

It is also gaining popularity in the management of defects following radiotherapy. Tissue reconstruction in irradiated fields remains a complex and challenging problem, marred by poor wound healing, flap necrosis and eventual wound breakdown. Local flap reconstruction is usually to be avoided following radiotherapy; however, the reliable healing and robust vascular supply seen with keystone island flaps resulted in the keystone island flap being used extensively for the closure of irradiated defects (Chapter 9). The experience with keystone island flaps in irradiated defects was published in 2006 (Behan et al. 2006) and demonstrated the utility of these flaps for reliable wound closure in irradiated fields. Since then, the excellent wound healing demonstrated with these flaps in irradiated fields has made their use commonplace for this purpose.

The purpose of this text is to assemble, in one book, an easy-to-understand guide to the development, design and surgical application of the keystone island flap. The extensive use of clinical defects, followed by intraoperative series of photographs and videos, is deliberate so as to maximise transfer of the relevant concepts. Additional information, such as the history, neurovascular anatomy, reconstructive alternatives and technical refinements, are presented in boxes for the interest of the reader.

In the following chapters we will discuss in detail the design elements and flap physiology upon which the keystone island flap is based. Following a general discussion of the flap and the basis of how it works, we will look at specific defects in various regions of the body and examine how keystone island flaps have been used to close these defects successfully. Following this, the use of the keystone island flap for specific surgical entities, such as melanoma and trauma, is addressed. A summary can be found at the end of each chapter, which may be of use where the reader wishes to gain a

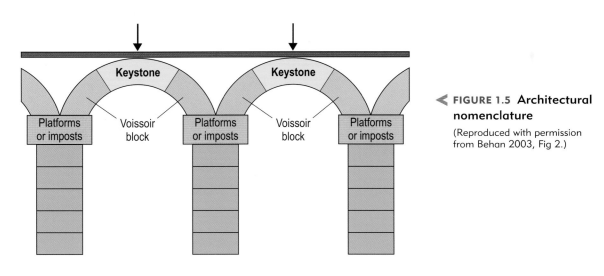

◄ **FIGURE 1.5 Architectural nomenclature**

(Reproduced with permission from Behan 2003, Fig 2.)

rapid understanding of each of the chapter's contents. Surgeons new to locoregional flaps will find Chapter 3 on the design and technique of keystone flap elevation to be invaluable and should then consider reading Chapters 5 and 7 on the lower and upper limbs as starting points for the incorporation of this technique into their own practice.

In the current era of microsurgical free-tissue transfers, free perforator flaps and free-style free flaps, the aim of reconstruction should be more than soft tissue coverage. The reconstructive surgeon must not lose the art of functional aesthetic reconstruction, focusing on aesthetics and quality of life. We are firmly of the belief that free-tissue transfer has revolutionised reconstructive surgery and will maintain an invaluable role in patient care for many years to come. However, we challenge today's reconstructive surgeon to have equal familiarity with locoregional reconstruction, such as the keystone island flap, as a less invasive, simpler and more time-efficient means to achieve similar results in many instances. We see the keystone island flap and microsurgical free-tissue transfer as complementary reconstructive techniques, which should be part of any reconstructive arsenal in the 21st century.

BIBLIOGRAPHY

Audisio R A, Zbar A P, Jaklitsch M T 2007 Surgical management of oncogeriatric patients. J Clin Oncol 25(14):1924–9.

Australian Bureau of Statistics 2008 Population projections Australia 2006 to 2101. Australian Bureau of Statistics, Canberra: pp 46–9.

Behan F C 1992 The fasciocutaneous island flap: an extension of the angiotome concept. Aust N Z J Surg 62(11):874–86.

Behan F C 2003 The keystone design perforator island flap in reconstructive surgery. Aust N Z J Surg 73(3):112–20.

Behan F, Sizeland A, Porcedu S, Somia N, Wilson J 2006 Keystone island flap: an alternative reconstructive option to free flaps in irradiated tissue. Aust N Z J Surg 76(5):407–13.

Behan F C, Terrill P J, Breidahl A, Cavallo A, Ashton M, Bennett T, Moss C, Archer B 1995 Island flaps including the Bezier type in the treatment of malignant melanoma. Aust N Z J Surg 65(12):870–80.

Behan F C, Wilson J 1973 The vascular basis of laterally based forehead island flaps, and their clinical applications. Plast Reconstr Surg (European Section), Madrid.

Behan F C, Wilson J 1975 The principle of the angiotome, a system of linked axial pattern flaps. Sixth International Congress of Plastic and Reconstructive Surgery, Paris.

Blackwell K E, Azizzadeh B, Ayala C, Rawnsley J D 2002 Octogenarian free flap reconstruction: complications and cost of therapy. Otolaryngol Head Neck Surg 126(3):301–6.

Budny P G, Lavelle J, Regan P J, Roberts A H 1993 Pretibial injuries in the elderly: a prospective trial of early mobilisation versus bed rest following surgical treatment. Br J Plast Surg 46(7):594–8.

Cormack G C, Lamberty B G H 1984a Fasciocutaneous flap nomenclature. Plast Reconstr Surg 73(6):996.

Cormack G C, Lamberty B G H 1984b Fasciocutaneous vessels in the upper arm: application to the design of new fasciocutaneous flaps. Plast Reconstr Surg 74(2): 244–50.

Dorland W A N 1994 Dorland's illustrated medical dictionary, 28th edn. Saunders, Philadelphia.

Manchot C 1889 *Die Hautarterien des Menschlichen Korpers.* FC Vogel, Leipzig.

Pelissier P, Gardet H, Pinsolle V, Santoul M, Behan F 2007a The keystone design perforator island flap. Part II: clinical applications. J Plast Reconstr Aesthet Surg 60(8):888–91.

Pelissier P, Santoul M, Pinsolle V, Casoli V, Behan F 2007b The keystone design perforator island flap. Part I: anatomic study. J Plast Reconstr Aesthet Surg 60(8):883–7.

Rozen W M, Chubb D, Stella D L, Taylor G I, Ashton M W 2009 Evaluating anatomical research in surgery: a prospective comparison of cadaveric and living anatomical studies of the abdominal wall. Aust N Z J Surg 79(12):913–17.

Salmon M 1936 *Arteres de la peau.* Masson, Paris.

Taylor G I, Palmer J H 1987 The vascular territories (angiosomes) of the body: experimental study and clinical applications. Br J Plast Surg 40(2):113–41.

United Nations Department of Economic and Social Affairs, Population Division 2010 Population ageing and development 2009. United Nations, New York.

Chapter 2

Anatomy and applied physiology of fasciocutaneous flaps

with Brendon Coventry

To study the phenomena of disease without books is to sail an uncharted sea. To study books without patients is not to go to sea at all.

Sir William Osler (1849–1919)

Safe fasciocutaneous flap elevation is facilitated by a thorough understanding of the anatomy and applied vascular physiology of skin and subcutaneous tissues.

INTRODUCTION

The body of knowledge amassed regarding skin anatomy and physiology is immense. The function of the skin is manyfold (Box 2.1), but of particular importance to the reconstructive surgeon are its roles as a protective barrier (following oncological surgery +/− chemoradiotherapy) and in social interaction (aesthetics). This chapter serves to provide or refresh a basic overview of fasciocutaneous anatomy and physiology of relevance to the everyday practice of fasciocutaneous flap surgery.

BOX 2.1 Functions of skin

- Protective barrier (physical, chemical, radiation)
- Immune function/antigen presentation
- Sensation (largest sense organ)
- Thermoregulation
- Metabolic—vitamin D, adipose tissue stores

THE ANATOMY OF FASCIOCUTANEOUS TISSUES

The anatomical layers of the integument include the epidermis, dermis, subcutaneous fat and fascia. Skin may be classified into glabrous (non-hair bearing) and non-glabrous (hair-bearing) types. Structural characteristics and features, such as colour, texture, thickness, size and density of hair follicles, nature and density of sweat glands and sensory receptors, vary considerably in different body regions and between people.

The epidermis has a number of layers (Box 2.2). The outer layer of the epidermis is shed continuously and replaced by progressive movement and maturation of keratinocytes from the germinal basal layer, a process taking 25–50 days (Young & Heath 2002). Other cells present include melanocytes for pigment production, Langerhans cells for antigen presentation, and Merkel cells, a form of specialised touch receptor, among others. Epidermal appendages, such as hair follicles and sweat glands, appear as down-growths into the dermis and are enmeshed in the rich dermal plexus of vessels. They are

- Stratum corneum: cornified layer of dead or dying cell remnants primarily composed of keratin
- Stratum lucidum: found only in the thicker skin of the palms of hands and soles of feet
- Stratum granulosum: characterised by intracellular granules
- Stratum spinosum: this prickle cell layer has a 'prickly' appearance at high magnification
- Stratum basale: germinal layer

sympathetically innervated to regulate their functions in thermoregulation and fight–flight responses.

The basement membrane separates the epidermis from the dermis, which is anchored to the underlying subcutaneous tissue and muscle by fibrous insertions. The dermis forms the main structural support for the skin, with prominent connective tissue elements, such as collagen and elastin admixed with fibroblasts and smaller numbers of other cell types, such as mast cells, lymphocytes and macrophages. This highly vascularised layer plays a pivotal role in wound healing and skin graft take. It is supported by numerous underlying vascular plexuses and also plays an important role in thermoregulation. The dermis is further separated into two distinct layers: papillary dermis (superficial, thin, loose with fine, interlacing collagen fibres) and reticular dermis (more extensive, deeper, with coarse, irregularly placed bundles of collagen).

The subcutaneous tissue lying between the skin and the deeper fascia or bone plays an important role in energy storage, thermal insulation and cushioning against mechanical shock. The subcutaneous tissue is composed of delicate lobules separated by fibrous septa that are connected to both dermis and deep fascia. Each lobule, containing hundreds of adipocytes, is vascularised through a single pedicle entering the centre

of the lobule and is drained to a vein on the periphery. Within the panniculus adiposus layer of subcutaneous tissue lies a layer referred to in furred mammals as the panniculus carnosus. In humans, muscles such as the occipitofrontalis, platysma, palmaris brevis, corrugator cutis ani, dartos muscle of scrotum and subareolar muscle of nipple are remnants of this layer and their close association with the skin (e.g. platysma) makes them useful for inclusion within island flaps to maximise flap perfusion. Radiographic injection studies demonstrate that this layer in the forehead (originally labelled as fascia) richly perfuses the overlying skin (Behan & Wilson 1973), leading to the origin of the angiotome concept (Behan & Wilson 1973, 1975). Island flaps formed in this way are, therefore, musculocutaneous flaps rather than fasciocutaneous flaps.

Where structures from the panniculus carnosus are poorly developed in humans (such as in the limbs and trunk), the deep fascia replaces these structures in being a point of transit for perforating vessels to ramify to the overlying skin. The deep fascia is a membrane of fibrous tissue varying in thickness. For example, it is well-developed in the iliotibial tract and absent in the face (McMinn 1994). Over bone, it is anchored firmly to periosteum. The cutaneous nerve supplying the overlying skin usually innervates it. According to Cormack and Lamberty (1994), there are two distinct types of deep fascia. In the trunk, the deep fascia forms an elastic and well-developed epimysial covering on the muscles, permitting expansion of the chest and abdominal wall. In the limbs, the deep fascia forms a more rigid structure in continuity with intercompartmental fascial septa. It acts as a point of origin for muscle fibres and contributes to retinacula around joints (Cormack & Lamberty 1994).

Cutaneous vascularisation patterns

The circulatory network of skin, fat and fascia consists of multiple interconnecting horizontal plexuses (Fig 2.1). The density of these plexuses varies by body region; for

Skin circulation

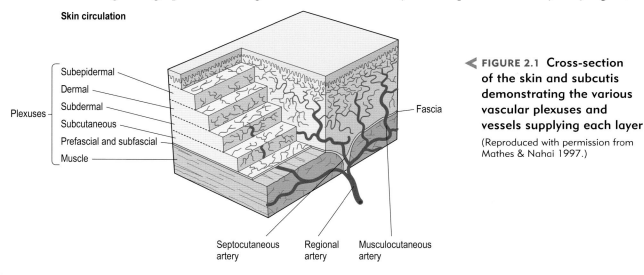

Plexuses
- Subepidermal
- Dermal
- Subdermal
- Subcutaneous
- Prefascial and subfascial
- Muscle

Fascia

Septocutaneous artery   Regional artery   Musculocutaneous artery

◀ FIGURE 2.1 **Cross-section of the skin and subcutis demonstrating the various vascular plexuses and vessels supplying each layer**

(Reproduced with permission from Mathes & Nahai 1997.)

example, the density of vessels in the reticular dermis in the face is five times greater than in the sole of the foot (Cormack & Lamberty 1994). This has clinical implications in raising flaps. These cutaneous plexuses are fed by either direct cutaneous vessels (as seen in the scalp) or cutaneous perforators. The cutaneous perforators can reach the skin by numerous different courses involving fascial septae, fascia, muscle or bone, as summarised in Figure 2.2. These arteries are usually accompanied by two smaller venae comitantes.

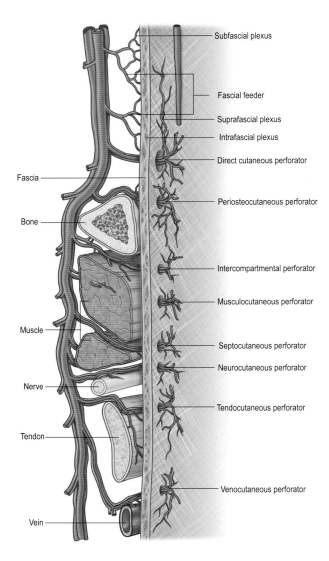

Subfascial plexus

Fascial feeder

Suprafascial plexus

Intrafascial plexus

Direct cutaneous perforator

Periosteocutaneous perforator

Intercompartmental perforator

Musculocutaneous perforator

Septocutaneous perforator

Neurocutaneous perforator

Tendocutaneous perforator

Venocutaneous perforator

Fascia

Bone

Muscle

Nerve

Tendon

Vein

▲ **FIGURE 2.2 Overview of the types of arterial perforators to the skin. One or more types of these perforators must be included within island flaps for their survival and healing. Knowledge of the perforators supplying a flap improves safety and permits modification of the flap design and movement to maximise the aesthetic outcome.**

(Reproduced with permission from Gray H, Standring S 2005 Gray's anatomy: the anatomical basis of clinical practice, 39th edn. Churchill Livingstone, New York, Fig 79.6.)

The density of these vessels varies; for example, the density of vessels in the reticular dermis in the face is five times greater compared to those in the sole of the foot (Cormack & Lamberty 1994). This has clinical implications in raising flaps.

On the basis of patterns of vascularisation, two classification schemes have been developed to describe the patterns of vascularisation in these flaps; these schemes are complementary (see below). An understanding of these patterns aids in the assessment of the available vasculature upon which to base locoregional fasciocutaneous flaps, even in the setting of complex defects. Cormack and Lamberty (1994) divided fasciocutaneous flaps into three different types (Fig 2.3):

Type A flap: This flap depends on multiple fasciocutaneous vessels entering its base orientated with the long axis of the arterial plexus within the deep fascia of the flap (including Ponten's (1981) lower leg superflaps).

Type B flap: This flap is based on a single fasciocutaneous perforator of moderate size, which is consistent both in its presence and its location. Examples include scapular, parascapular and saphenous artery flaps. The flap may be modified such that the perforator is removed in continuity with the more major vessel from which it arises (initially classified as a fifth type).

Type C flap: This flap is supported by multiple small fasciocutaneous perforators. An example would be the radial forearm flap, which may also be harvested with a portion of radius (subsequently classified as a type D flap).

Cormack and Lamberty type A flaps are usually the most common pattern for keystone flaps, particularly in the lower limb and where Doppler ultrasound or surgical isolation of perforators has not been undertaken. This is a safe approach as long as there is sufficient attachment of the flap to capture some good perforators.

Mathes and Nahai (1997) also described three vascular patterns in relation to fasciocutaneous flaps:

Type A flap: This flap has a direct cutaneous pedicle (e.g. groin, digital artery, temporoparietal fascia).

Type B flap: This flap relies on a septocutaneous pedicle. It includes all fasciocutaneous flaps with a pedicle coursing either between a recognised intermuscular septum or in the space between adjacent muscles (e.g. radial forearm, lateral arm, anterolateral thigh).

Type C flap: This flap is based on a musculocutaneous pedicle. The pedicle length may be increased by dissecting out the pedicle proximally through the muscle to its regional source (e.g. deep inferior epigastric, anterolateral thigh).

Direct cutaneous pedicles (Mathes and Nahai type A) generally allow the most movement, followed by those that are musculocutaneous (type C) because

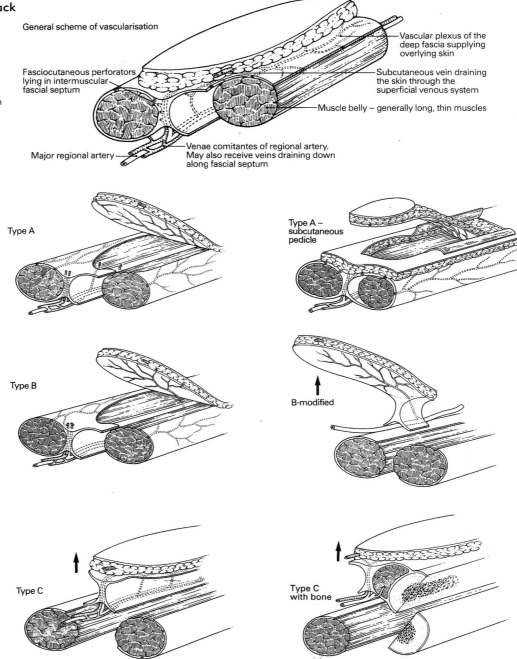

FIGURE 2.3 The Cormack and Lamberty (1994) classification of the vascular patterns for fasciocutaneous flaps (types A, B and C).

(Reproduced with permission from Cormack & Lamberty 1994, Fig 5.24.)

General scheme of vascularisation

Vascular plexus of the deep fascia supplying overlying skin

Fasciocutaneous perforators lying in intermuscular fascial septum

Subcutaneous vein draining the skin through the superficial venous system

Muscle belly – generally long, thin muscles

Major regional artery

Venae comitantes of regional artery. May also receive veins draining down along fascial septum

Type A

Type A – subcutaneous pedicle

Type B

B-modified

Type C

Type C with bone

the fascia can be divided circumferentially to allow the most movement. The movement of type B flaps is limited in the axis of the septum through which it perforates, so where a septocutaneous perforator is expected, flaps should be planned to move perpendicular to this axis. An arterial network courses through the fasciocutaneous tissue planes to accompany and supply peripheral nerves and veins separately. Via cadaveric and histological studies, one or more small arteries have been demonstrated within the perivenous areolar tissue of the long saphenous, short saphenous and cephalic veins (Shalaby & Saad 1993). An intrinsic venocutaneous vascular system (intimate vascular network on the vascular wall accompanying all veins) coexists with an extrinsic venocutaneous vascular system (accompanying arteries which run within 10 mm of the venous wall with obvious branches to the skin) (Nakajima et al. 1998). This latter plexus communicates with septocutaneous and musculocutaneous perforators of the deep arteries.

Cutaneous neurovascularisation patterns

Lundborg (1977) defined the blood supply of nerves as either extrinsic or intrinsic. Sunderland (1945) coined the term 'vasa nervorum' to refer to vessels that originate externally to the nerve and terminate intraneurally. Nakajima and colleagues (1998) demonstrated an intrinsic neurocutaneous vascular system (arteries exist on the epineurium of every nerve along its entire length, giving off branches to the skin at 2–5 cm intervals) and an extrinsic neurocutaneous vascular system (nearby accompanying arteries located within 5 mm of the nerve, with branches to the skin and communications with septocutaneous and musculocutaneous perforators). Breidenbach and Terzis (1986) carried out cadaveric and injection studies to classify the vascular pattern of peripheral nerves into three types:

Type I: This type has no dominant pedicle. The nerve receives its blood supply through either the intrinsic system or extrinsic vessels originating from musculocutaneous or septocutaneous perforators, which directly enter the nerve and do not run along its length (e.g. lateral cutaneous nerve of thigh, lateral antebrachial cutaneous nerve of forearm).

Type II: This type has one dominant vessel that runs with the nerve for at least a significant majority of its length (e.g. superficial radial nerve, superficial peroneal nerve, posterior cutaneous nerve of thigh, lateral antebrachial cutaneous nerve of forearm).

Type III: This type has multiple dominant pedicles (e.g. saphenous nerve).

Based on these accompanying arteries of superficial veins and nerves, flaps have been previously investigated and reported (Nakajima et al. 1998, Masquelet et al. 1992, Bertelli & Khoury 1992). Behan has used this neurovascular supply to augment the neurovascular supply of keystone island flaps (conjoint arterial and neuro-arterial supply) and, therefore, has found that the dermatomal precincts are of use in the planning of keystone flaps (Fig 2.4). This principle can be extrapolated to the use of named cutaneous nerve territories as the basis for neurovascular-based keystone island flaps, as shown schematically in Figure 2.5 and demonstrated clinically in Figure 2.6.

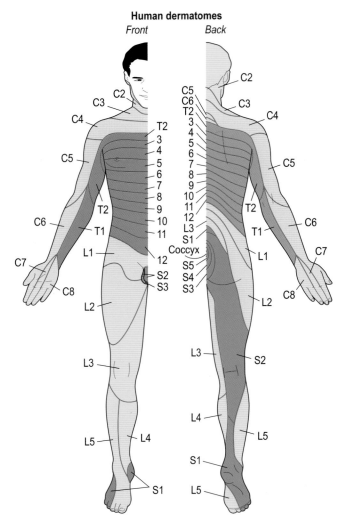

Human dermatomes

▲ FIGURE 2.4 **Dermatomal roadmap used as an aide-mémoire to the planning and axis of keystone island flaps, which have a remarkable similarity to the designated perforator zones in various regions of the body**

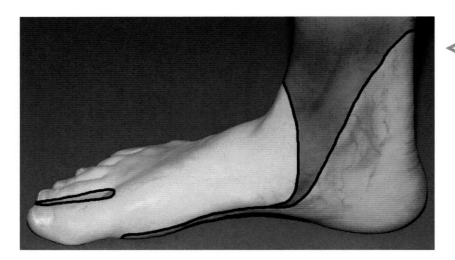

◄ FIGURE 2.5 **Named cutaneous nerve territories may be used to elevate keystone island flaps based on specific cutaneous nerves (with their accompanying vessels)**

Here the cutaneous nerve territories are: saphenous nerve— grey; posterior tibial nerve—pink; superficial peroneal nerve—yellow; deep peroneal nerve—green.

FIGURE 2.6

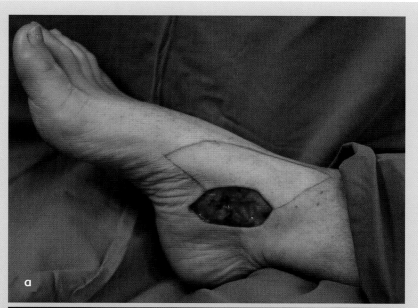

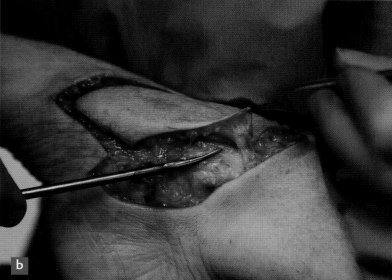

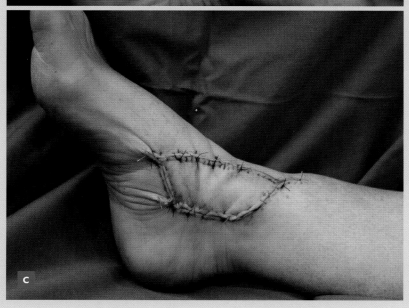

FIGURE 2.6 Clinical demonstration of neurovascular-based keystone island flap

(**a**) Fasciocutaneous defect from wide local excision of primary melanoma. Saphenous neurovascular-based keystone island flap marked out.

(**b**) Islanding and elevation of the flap, demonstrating the saphenous nerve entering and the great saphenous vein exiting the undersurface of the flap.

(**c**) Final inset of the flap with subsequent uncomplicated wound healing and function.

TLC

Time (operation/cost)
60 minutes
Life quality (and aesthetics)
Early mobilisation and acceptable aesthetics
Complications
Nil

Cutaneous microcirculation

Arterioles and venules of cutaneous microcirculation form two main plexuses in the dermis: an upper horizontal network in the papillary dermis (from which nutritive capillary loops of the dermal papillae arise) and a lower horizontal plexus at the dermal–subcutaneous interface (Braverman 1997, 2000). As previously discussed, interconnecting vessels of various patterns exist between deep vessels from the underlying muscles and subcutaneous fat and the two horizontal cutaneous plexuses. Ascending arterioles from the lower horizontal plexus, accompanied by a post-capillary venule, communicate with the upper horizontal plexus at randomly spaced intervals of 1.5–7 mm (Braverman 2000). Most of the microvasculature is contained in the papillary dermis 1–2 mm below the epidermal surface.

Vessels in the papillary dermis consist of arterioles, arterial and venous capillaries, and post-capillary venules. Arterioles are characterised by an internal elastic lamina (Braverman 2000). The vessel wall of arterioles consists of endothelial cells, elastic lamina, two layers of smooth muscle cells (innervated by vasoconstrictive noradrenergic nerve fibres) and the basement membrane. With a diameter of 17–26 μm, they are the major site of resistance to blood flow (Braverman 2000). Terminal arterioles are also called metarterioles. When vessel diameter decreases below 15 μm, smooth muscle cells are completely replaced by a single cell that functions as a pre-capillary sphincter and as the pacemaker for vasomotor activity. It appears that the pre-capillary sphincters are not innervated but that they respond to local or circulating vasoconstrictor substances instead.

Capillaries are characterised by a thin vascular wall made up of: pericytes, which have contractile properties and which can release a variety of vasoactive agents and regulate flow through the junctions between endothelial cells; and veil cells (exact nature and function undetermined) (Braverman 2000). Arterial capillaries have an outside diameter of 10–12 μm. Venous capillaries, with a diameter that increases from 12 to 35 μm, connect with post-capillary venules. These venules have thicker walls without elastic fibres, representing the most physiologically reactive segment of the microcirculation—intercellular gap formation, increased vascular permeability and cell migration in response to acute inflammation (Ganong 1999).

In the fingers, palms, toes, nose and ears, shunts or arteriovenous anastomoses (AVAs) connect arterioles to venules directly, bypassing the capillaries (Ganong 1999). These AVAs, or shunts, have thick, muscular walls and are abundantly innervated (densely innervated in comparison to vessels either side of them) by post-ganglionic sympathetic vasoconstrictor fibres. Changes in the levels of firing of these sympathetic neurons can lead to dramatic thermoregulatory changes in regional blood flow within the skin. Through variations in the amount of blood being shunted through these AVAs, blood flow can vary from 1 to 150 mL/100 g of skin/min (Ganong 1999).

CUTANEOUS VASCULAR PHYSIOLOGY

Attempts to interpret the literature on cutaneous circulation are complicated by terminology, differences in experimental techniques and whether these different techniques result in comparable data (Bell & Robbins 1997). The control of cutaneous blood flow is multifactorial, complex and not fully understood. The mechanisms affecting it may be distant or local, neurological or hormonal, providing acute or basal long-term control (Fig 2.7).

The autonomic nervous system innervates the cutaneous vasculature via sympathetic and parasympathetic pathways. Most autonomic post-ganglionic fibres reach the cutaneous vasculature in a segmental fashion, travelling with the sensory fibres in cutaneous branches of the spinal nerves and also by following the main arteries supplying the skin. As a result, their territories loosely correspond with the cutaneous sensory dermatomes (Gibbins 1997).

The bulk of the sympathetic innervation is noradrenergic (mediating vasoconstriction). Tonic activation of these sympathetic vasoconstrictor neurons results in significant vasomotor tone or a submaximal level of cutaneous blood flow (Morris 1997). If the normal tonic activity of these sympathetic vasoconstrictors is down-regulated or turned off, it causes a passive increase in cutaneous blood flow (Gibbins 1997, Holzer 1997, Low & Kennedy 1997). In addition, a non-adrenergic sympathetic vasodilator pathway exists, innervating selected regions of the cutaneous vasculature (e.g. sympathetic vasodilatation seen with emotional blushing) (Gibbins 1997). The distribution of parasympathetic neurons to the skin is limited; they are associated with arteries in the facial region (in particular, lips and forehead), where they mediate vasodilatation (Gibbins 1997). They may also be involved in the flushing of the face—the afferent pathway is the trigeminal nerve and the efferent pathway is via parasympathetic fibres in the facial nerve, then via the greater superficial petrosal nerve to innervate the face (Holzer 1997, Low & Kennedy 1997).

A group of primary afferent sensory neurons mediates non-adrenergic, non-cholinergic vasodilatation and increases vascular permeability in the skin. During the inflammatory response, nociceptive C and A-δ axons are activated with antidromic conduction of nerve impulses in these afferent nerve fibres. This results in the release of peptides (substance P and calcitonin gene-related peptide, CGRP) from sensory terminals

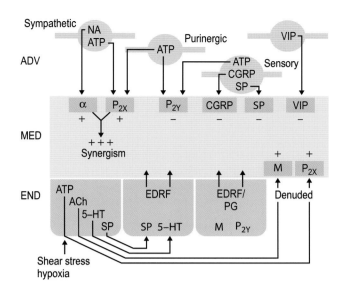

▲ **FIGURE 2.7** Schematic representation of potential modes of regulation of vascular tone by endothelial cell-related mechanisms. In addition to the effects of temperature, a number of mediators act locally to influence vessel tone. Noradrenaline (NA), adenosine triphosphate (ATP), calcitonin gene-related peptide (CGRP), substance P (SP) and vasoactive intestinal polypeptide (VIP) can be released from nerves in the adventitia (ADV) to act on their respective receptors in the media (MED) and cause vasoconstriction or vasodilation. ATP, acetylcholine (ACh), 5-hydroxytryptamine (5-HT) and SP released from endothelial cells (END) by shear stress or hypoxia act on their receptors on endothelial cells to cause release of endothelium-derived relaxing factors (EDRF) or prostaglandins (PG), which act on smooth muscle to cause relaxation. In areas denuded of endothelial cells, opposite effects may be produced by receptors on smooth muscle. α: noradrenaline receptor; M: muscarinic receptor; P_{2X}: purinoceptor; P_{2Y}: purinoceptor.

(Reproduced with permission from Lincoln J, Burnstock G 1990 Neural-endothelial interactions in control of local blood flow. In Warren J, ed. The endothelium: an introduction to current research. Wiley-Liss, New York, p 21.)

and histamine and kinins from mast cells. These afferent neurons have been implicated in the triple response (local reddening, weal and hyperaemic flare) resulting from focal irritation of human skin. Several theories have been proposed to explain the spread of flare: the axon reflex hypothesis—one axon branch is activated by an irritant stimulus, nerve impulses travel centrally but at the branching point also pass antidromically down other branches, which may come close to arterioles, releasing vasodilator transmitters and causing arteriolar dilatation; chemical coupling—the release of mast cell–derived histamine and other factors that are able to activate adjacent nerve fibres; and electrical coupling—between two afferent nerve fibres leading to the flare response spreading beyond the collateral network of a single afferent nerve fibre (Holzer 1997).

The metabolic theory of autoregulation states that vasoactive substances or metabolites accumulate in active tissues, contributing to autoregulation. With low blood flow these metabolites accumulate and vessels dilate, while an increase in blood flow washes them away. The metabolic changes and substances influencing cutaneous vasculature include oxygen tension, carbon dioxide tension, potassium, lactate, osmolality and pH. In response to various stimuli, endothelial cells play an important role by secreting vasoactive substances, including prostaglandins and thromboxanes, nitric oxide and endothelins (Ganong 1999).

According to the myogenic theory of autoregulation, vascular beds have an intrinsic capacity to maintain relatively constant blood flow by changing vascular resistance to compensate for changes in perfusion pressure (Ganong 1999). As the pressure rises, the blood vessels distend and the vascular smooth muscle fibres respond by contracting. A decrease in distending pressure results in relaxation and lowering of vascular resistance. This process occurs independently of innervation and bloodborne vasoactive agents (Cormack & Lamberty 1994). It is probably due to the intrinsic contractile response of smooth muscle to stretch (Ganong 1999).

APPLIED PHYSIOLOGY: VASCULAR REGULATION WITHIN KEYSTONE ISLAND FLAPS

Keystone island flap designs are useful because of their mobility and capacity to be rotated, stretched and manoeuvred to span often large defects to create skin (and soft-tissue) cover. The success of these flaps derives from the blood supply arising from the base of the flaps via fascial perforators and/or direct vessels, but there appears to be some quite special vascular dynamics that permit excellent flap survival, which we hypothesise is due, at least in part, to sympathetic autoregulatory responses.

This hypothesis derives from information already known concerning sympathetic nerve supplies to vascular beds, as well as from correlations with multiple observations made during keystone island flap reconstructions over the years.

Some of the theoretical and practical considerations surrounding the blood supply and the apparent paradox of demonstrable excellent perfusion, despite much of the natural blood supply being removed during the act of forming the flap, are described below.

Keystone island flap elevation

Raising a keystone island flap involves circumferential division of skin, some subcutaneous tissue and, to a varying extent, division of the deep fascia. When small cutaneous blood vessels are transected, the injury initiates a series of events leading to clot formation and haemostasis. The initial event is constriction of the vessel and formation of a temporary haemostatic platelet plug, which is triggered when platelets bind to collagen and aggregate. The constriction or spasm of an injured arteriole may be significant, sufficient to occlude the vessel lumen at least temporarily and cause blanching of skin in the perioperative field. The mechanism for this arterial vasoconstriction is attributable to sympathetic vasoconstrictor nerves, a direct response of the vascular smooth muscle cell to injury and vasoconstrictor agents (thromboxane A_2, serotonin, noradrenaline, adrenaline) released from platelets that adhere to the wall of damaged vessels (Cormack & Lamberty 1994). This is followed by conversion of the platelet plug into the definitive fibrin clot, involving a cascade of enzymatic reactions and a series of numbered clotting factors.

Despite this vasoconstriction, which occurs initially during surgery, within minutes of islanding, keystone island flaps appear more erythematous than the surrounding skin. This clinical finding is just one of a group of observations regularly made during keystone island flap elevation and is called the *quaternary response* (Box 2.3). In order of occurrence, this response includes a hyperaemic flare within the flap, the development of *red dot signs* during flap inset and an associated relatively pain-free postoperative period for the patient consistent with temporary local neurapraxia of cutaneous nerves and subsequent return of sensation. The hyperaemia has been noted to persist for more than 2 years in some

---

BOX 2.3 Quaternary response

Immediate phase
1. Red dot sign
2. Vascular flare

Delayed phase
3. Pain-free postoperatively (PFP)
4. Rapid and reliable healing

FIGURE 2.8

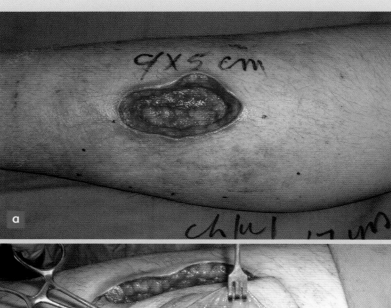
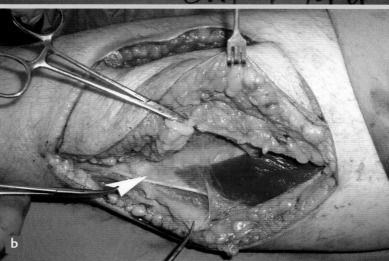

FIGURE 2.8 Keystone island flap procedure in a 22-year-old male with a chronic calf ulcer, 9 × 5 cm, following a motor vehicle accident 18 months earlier, demonstrating the quaternary response and the immediate vascular augmentation concept (IVAC)

(a) Wound debridement followed by keystone island flap mark-out on the posterior margins of the defect. (If the diagonal of the distant points of the keystone are joined, we have two V–Y flaps at an angle to each other and directed into the defect. By incorporating this into a single flap, the larger surface area of this flap increases the likelihood of perforator capture.)

(b) Dividing fascia along the base with preservation of the superficial peroneal nerve (arrow).

patients. The *red dot sign* was coined because more bleeding is often observed from suture needle holes through the flap than from those in the surrounding skin, producing a red dot of blood at these sites on the flap side (Fig 2.8). Postoperatively, patients with keystone island flaps often do not report much pain, require minimal opioid analgesia and remain in their near normal functional level.

The pathophysiology and significance of these observations remain uncertain. However, it may be

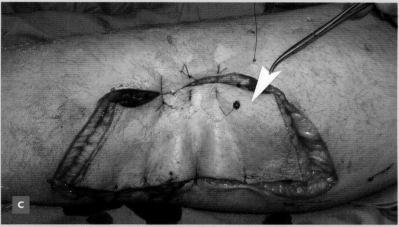

(c) Direct closure at key points with strategic vertical mattress sutures, showing lines of tension and variations in vascular flow in the subdermal plexus. The *red dot sign* on the flap (the suture site) indicates the increase in vascular perfusion compared with the surrounding tissue. These white lines are indicators of the effect of linear tension on perfusion within the subdermal plexus. If this pattern remains, flap reliability will suffer.

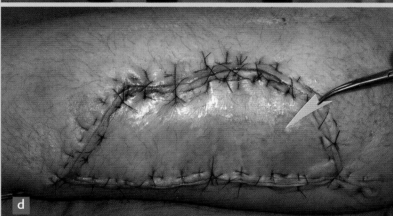

(d) The white lines of tension have disappeared following circumferential suturing and flap inset under even physiological tension throughout the flap. A hyperaemic flare (arrow) is the result of this combination of islanding and even tension throughout the flap. Reactive hyperaemia is more intense than the surrounding tissue.

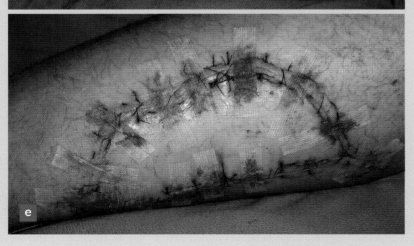

(e) Appearance at 7 days when the wound feels tight but is pain-free for the patient (third component of the quaternary response).

TLC

Time (operation/cost)		
60 minutes		
Life quality (and aesthetics)		
Early mobility and acceptable aesthetics		
Complications		
Nil		

(Reproduced with permission from Behan FC, Rozen WM, Kapila S Ng SK 2001 Two for the price of one: a keystone design equals two conjoined V–Y flaps. ANZ J Surg 81(6):405–6.)

explained by the complex interplay resulting from the denervation of autonomic and somatic afferent nervous systems and local haemodynamic changes. Normal skin maintains significant vasomotor tone, and denervation results in major alterations of skin blood flow. Noxious stimuli produce cutaneous constriction (thought primarily to be due to the activation of sympathetic noradrenergic neurons) followed by dilatation (Ganong 1999). Sympathetic vasoconstriction overrides antidromic vasodilatation during active simultaneous stimulation of both afferent and sympathetic fibres (Ochoa et al. 1993). However, in contrast to sympathetic vasoconstriction, which is short-lasting, the resulting antidromic vasodilatation and hyperaemia outlasts the period of nerve stimulation. After terminating stimulation, vasodilatation and warming (statistically significant increase in temperature) has been recorded via thermography (Ochoa et al. 1993).

Neural mediation of keystone island flap perfusion

We believe that circumferential division and flap islanding results in at least partial sympathectomy of the flap and, hence, down-regulation of sympathetic vasoconstrictor tone. This may explain the similarities in clinical observations made in keystone island flaps (Figs 2.9 and 2.10) and those following lumbar sympathectomy, a procedure used to alleviate rest pain in patients with lower limb peripheral vascular disease. After division of the lumbar sympathetic chain, cutaneous blood flow is increased in ischaemic lower limbs (vascular flare and *red dot sign* in keystone island flaps) and rest pain is improved (relatively pain-free postoperative period observed in our patients). It has been shown via immunohistochemical methods that lumbar sympathectomy severs both vasomotor and sensory fibres (nociceptive sensory denervation), which contributes to the relief of rest pain (Coventry & Walsh 2003). Sympathetic blockade may increase skin blood flow up to five times and raise skin temperature by more than 2°C. The temperature returns to near normal over the next 2–5 weeks and sympathetic regeneration occurs after 1 year.

FIGURE 2.9

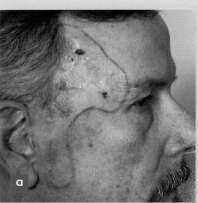
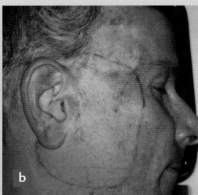
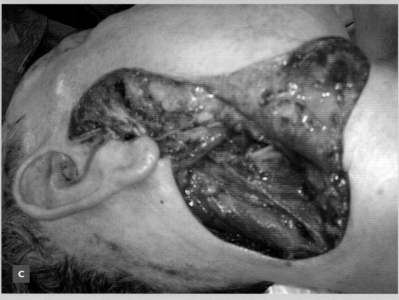

FIGURE 2.9 Keystone island flap procedure in a 45-year-old yachtsman with multiple skin cancers of the face

(a) The patient prior to surgery.

(b) Following excision and skin grafting for multifocal basal cell carcinoma (4 × 4 cm). On subsequent surveillance, he was noted to have a lump in the right parotid consistent with lymphatic spread (the Australian disease*). Fine needle aspiration cytology and computerised tomographic (CT) scanning confirmed a likely metastatic squamous cell carcinoma with involvement of the overlying skin.

(c) Following superficial parotidectomy and selective neck dissection (levels II–V), an undermined defect is produced with the neck flap tip demonstrating signs of potential vascular compromise (undersurface shown).

* The late Arnold Levine, Professor of Pathology at the Marsden Hospital to the mid 1980s, coined the phrase the 'Australian disease' for nodal dissemination involving the parotid gland from cutaneous malignancies of the head region.

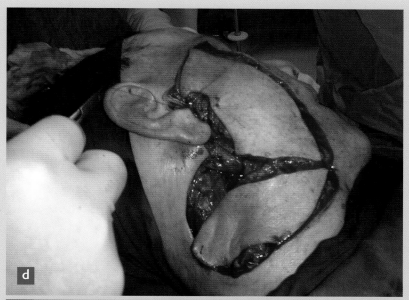

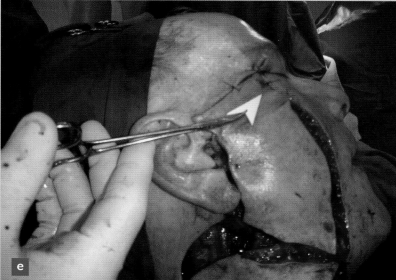

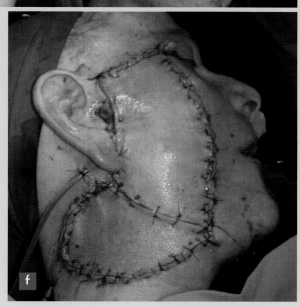

(d) The upper defect (4 × 6 cm) was closed by elevation of a keystone island flap (approximately 1:1 ratio of defect to flap width), based on facial artery branches (not visualised), by sharp dissection through the skin followed by blunt dissection of the subcutaneous tissues, particularly the anterior limit, using a claw retractor for counter-traction. The dissection can usually be safely teased down to the plane of the facial nerve. This is the first case where islanding was used to improve circulation to the apex of a vascularly compromised flap using the immediate vascular augmentation concept (IVAC, see Chapter 3 and Fig 2.11). It is also the first case where double flaps were used—one to revascularise the compromised neck flap and the second to close the defect. A 1:1 ratio of undermined flap to non-undermined flap within the island helps ensure perforator/direct vessels capture for revascularisation. The success of this early case has led to the utilisation of this technique where necessary to facilitate preservation of existing tissue as much as possible.

(e) A *red dot sign* (arrow), one of the cardinal signs of the quaternary response of keystone flap islanding.

(f) Vascular flare of the flaps following completion of suturing—another of the signs of the quaternary response.

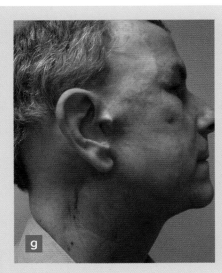

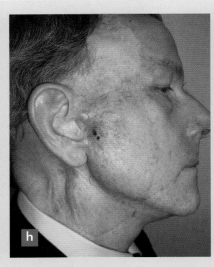

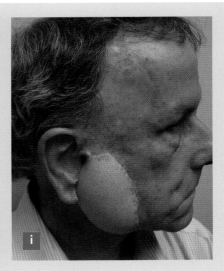

(g) The appearance after 5 years before the onset of local recurrence needing the free flap reconstruction. Trimming of the posterior border of the neck flap should have been undertaken during surgery to minimise the contour irregularity evident here in this early case.

(h) Local recurrence after 5 years warranting the use of a free-flap reconstruction following additional oncological clearance at this early stage of the development of the keystone island flap for reconstruction of head and neck defects.

(i) Appearance following free-tissue transfer, demonstrating adequate closure of the defect, but poor colour match, contour and developing flap ptosis.

See video for Figure 2.9

TLC

Time (operation/cost)
120 minutes
Life quality (and aesthetics)
Good with acceptable aesthetics prior to free flap
Complications
Recurrence of disease after 5 years disease-free

FIGURE 2.10

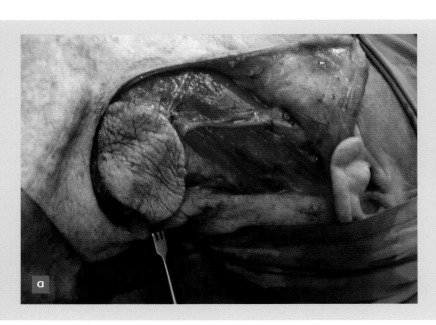

FIGURE 2.10 Keystone island flap procedure in a 65-year-old male with a supraclavicular mass (4 × 4 cm) confirmed as metastatic melanoma by fine-needle aspiration cytology preoperatively (unknown primary)

(a) Clearance of nodal levels 2–4 and extended into the clavicular region. Oncological clearance was achieved.

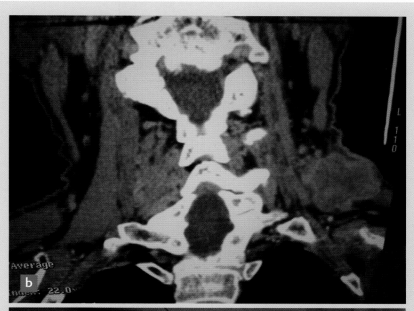

(b) Preoperative CT scan, demonstrating the size and position of the tumour deposit (4 cm diameter) with cutaneous attachment.

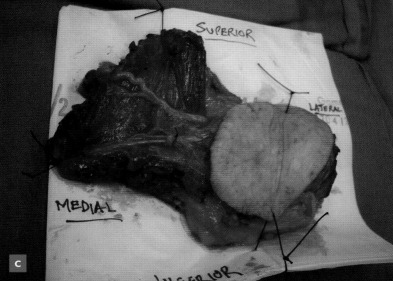

(c) The resected specimen, demonstrating the skin excision with underlying structures of the neck dissection—attached with orientation.

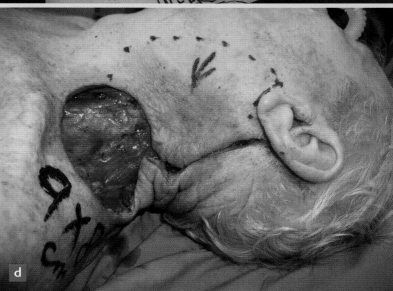

(d) The resective defect showing an undermined (to black arrow) upper neck skin flap with early vascular compromise. The undermining of the neck dissection is at the arrow, and the dotted line over the attached masseter complex is the design for the keystone island mark-out to increase perfusional dynamics and overcome the compromised state of the flap apex.

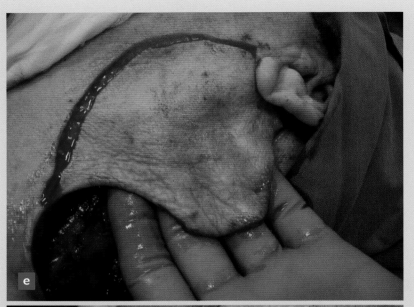

(e) Islanding of the compromised tissue to ensure capture of facial artery perforators and utilisation of the IVAC principle to improve vascularity to the undermined flap.

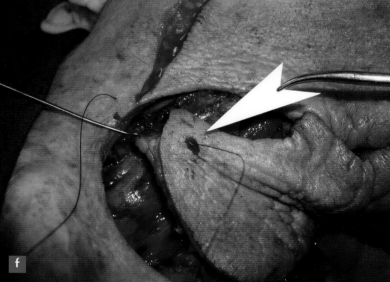

(f) A *red dot sign* in the posterior keystone flap—a sign of the quaternary response to islanding as an indicator of reliable perfusion and optimisation of healing. This posterior keystone flap, based on trapezius perforators, was used to facilitate defect closure, while preserving the accessory nerve during flap elevation.

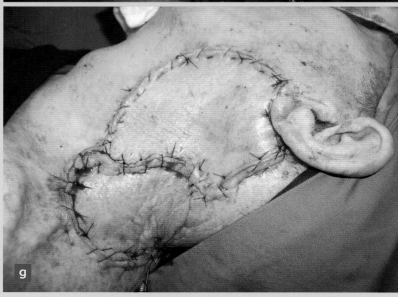

(g) Closure is complete, demonstrating vascular flare and good blood supply to the previously compromised neck flap.

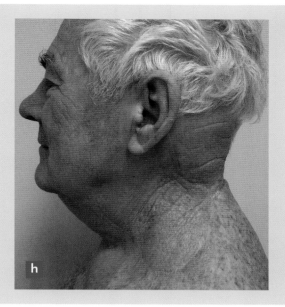

(h) Postoperative appearance following irradiation.

TLC

Time (operation/cost)		
Approximately 90 minutes		
Life quality (and aesthetics)		
Good, with acceptable aesthetics		
Complications		
Nil		

Haemodynamic changes in the keystone flap during islanding

Haemodynamic changes are also important in islanding. Rubino and colleagues (2006) examined haemodynamic enhancement in perforator flaps using echo colour Doppler ultrasound measurement of vessel diameters, velocity and flow before and after flap islanding. Normal systemic skin circulation has its points of resistance in parallel (like a tree), whereas Rubino and colleagues (2006) describe the inversion phenomenon in perforator flaps where the flap skin is perfused through long vessels whose calibre decreases from origin to skin surface, creating a flap with a resistance in series. This leads to an inversion of the gradient of blood velocity between pedicle artery and perforator artery, with the velocity of blood and the rate of flow reaching the skin being higher in such perforator flaps. This may explain the vascular dynamics that we have recorded in the series of keystone island flaps we have conducted since 2003.

Keystone island flaps are not exactly the same as the perforator flaps used in Rubino and colleagues' clinical series. Keystone island flaps have a conjoined vascular supply, including perforators, direct vessels (where present) and blood vessels, travelling with nerves that enter these flaps. They have both somatic and autonomic innervation that can be influenced by surgical manipulation and, in view of the clinical findings of no apparent surrounding oedema (Cormack & Lamberty 1994), one may conclude that lymphatic drainage is also likely enhanced, or at least not impeded, presenting another potential difference for keystone island flaps. These differences increase their reliability but can make interpretation of their haemodynamics somewhat challenging. However, their islanded nature is likely to lead to similar vessel diameter, velocity and flow changes as observed with free perforator flaps.

The success of the keystone island flap over 15 years is based on the following clinical observations. These are a sequential development based on the original angiotome principle. Neurocutaneous perforator zones throughout the body are the basis of the design of the keystone island flap and facilitate its movement. Islanding of the flaps creates evidence of increased vascular perfusion within the flap—the *immediate vascular augmentation concept* (IVAC; Fig 2.11). This is characterised by four clinical signs (the quaternary response, see Box 2.3), namely the:

1. *red dot sign*
2. vascular flare, which slowly eliminates any lines of surgical tension
3. rapid sequential healing
4. frequently observed relatively pain-free postoperative phase.

> **FIGURE 2.11 Factors affecting perfusion of keystone island flaps during islanding**

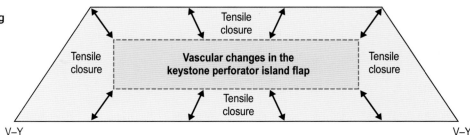

This phenomenon is still poorly understood, but we attribute the putative mechanism to the following features of keystone island flap elevation:

- Blunt dissection of axial flap vessels produces an initial transient vasoconstriction, likely by sympathetic discharge, followed by either sympathectomy where prolonged vasodilatation occurs and/or additional nociceptor input from the conjoint supply aiding this dilatation (Coventry & Walsh 2003). This effect creates vasodilatation within the flap.
- The keystone island flap design eliminates the subdermal plexus input from the flap periphery, minimising zones of stasis and maximising unidirectional flow.
- The white lines of tensile closure at the sites of the mattress sutures are a temporary phenomenon and are eventually eliminated by the increase in vascular flow and even distribution of tension following complete closure (similar to the crease-free tension of an open umbrella).
- Thus, an end effect produces an increase in vascular perfusion to help explain the colour changes from the initial white ischaemic, through the blue cyanotic stage to a pink perfused phase (the hyperaemic flare). Randomly, at the strategic points where mattress sutures are inserted, the *red dot sign* (increased bleeding from flap suture holes than from non-flap suture holes) is apparent.
- Inversion of the velocity gradient and the increase of blood flow to the skin are forms of a haemodynamic enhancement that has been found in perforator flaps (Rubino et al. 2006). In the keystone island flap, we hypothesise that the conjoined axis with an intact neurovascular support increases the blood supply.
- Historically, this is a similar effect to the use of the 'delay procedure' but here it is done in an immediate setting (i.e. IVAC).

THE ROLE OF TENSION IN KEYSTONE ISLAND FLAP CLOSURE

It is traditional plastic surgery teaching that closing a defect under excessive tension results in decreased blood flow and wound breakdown. The keystone island flap facilitates wound closure by decreasing the maximal defect closing tension across the widest point of the elliptical defect and redistributing the tension over a larger area (Fig 2.12). Despite the defect closing tension remaining relatively high in some cases (wounds closed with types I–III keystone island flaps), flap necrosis remains an uncommon problem. Larrabee and colleagues (1984) carried out porcine biomechanical flap studies to conclude that flap survival is ensured despite high closing tension if the flap length remains short. As a result of their perforator-based nature without undermining, types I–III keystone island

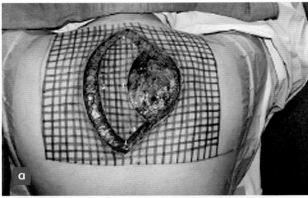

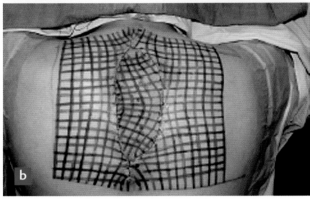

▲ **FIGURE 2.12 Demonstrating the application of a grid pattern at the time of excision of a lesion**

(a) From the back. **(b)** The changes in the distribution of tension following keystone island flap closure of the defect.

(Reproduced with permission from Pelissier P, Santoul M, Pinsolle V, Casoli V, Behan F 2007 The keystone design perforator island flap. Part 1: anatomic study. J Plast Reconstr Aesthet Surg 60:883–7.)

flaps are relatively short in comparison to other dermal pedicled designs, including rotation and transposition flaps. Hence, the robust vascular network of the keystone island flap appears to withstand the tension.

Numerous observations have been documented when skin is stretched, expanded or placed under tension. Soft tissue expansion led to epidermal thickening and an increase in total collagen content but dermal thinning (Johnson et al. 1988). Tissue expansion in humans induced a rise in mitotic activity and a significant increase in the number of basal and suprabasal keratinocytes (Olenius et al. 1993). Angiographic evidence of vasodilatation and an increase in vascularity were demonstrated in expanded porcine skin (Cherry et al. 1983, Marks et al. 1986). In addition, the surviving length of random flaps raised in previously expanded skin were greater in comparison to delayed flaps (not statistically significant), further contributing to the notion that the vascularity of expanded skin may be augmented, comparable to that seen in delay procedures (Cherry et al. 1983). The influence of mechanical tension on the formation of new cutaneous tissue and angiogenesis has been previously investigated for decades (Nugent & O'Connor 1983).

SUMMARY

The survival and function of skin and its appendages as a unit relies upon the maintenance of its blood supply. Flap elevation and inset to effect fasciocutaneous wound closure mandates the maintenance of this blood supply. The keystone flap (and its islanded variants) demonstrates robust vascular perfusion that appears to be better than the surrounding skin clinically. The quaternary response is a quartet of clinical findings that represents evidence of this phenomenon, along with a potential neural basis among other putative mechanisms. This improved vascularity of islanding enhances the reliability of these flaps and improves their wound healing, with benefits for patients.

BIBLIOGRAPHY

Behan F C, Wilson J (eds) 1975 The principle of the angiotome, a system of linked axial pattern flaps. Sixth International Congress of Plastic and Reconstructive Surgery, Paris.

Behan F C, Wilson J 1973 The vascular basis of laterally based forehead island flaps, and their clinical applications. Plast Reconstr Surg (European Section), Madrid.

Bell C, Robbins S 1997 Autonomic vasodilatation in the skin. In: Gibbins I L, Morris J L (eds) Autonomic innervation of the skin. Harwood Academic Publishers, Amsterdam, pp 87–110.

Bertelli J A, Khoury Z 1992 Neurocutaneous island flaps in the hand: anatomical basis and preliminary results. Br J Plast Surg 45(8):586–90.

Braverman I M 1997 The cutaneous microcirculation: ultrastructure and microanatomical organization. Microcirculation 4(3):329–40.

Braverman I M 2000 The cutaneous microcirculation. J Invest Dermatol Symp Proc 5(1):3–9.

Breidenbach W C, Terzis J K 1986 The blood supply of vascularized nerve grafts. J Reconstr Microsurg 3(1):43–58.

Cherry G W, Austad E, Pasyk K, McClatchey K, Rohrich R J 1983 Increased survival and vascularity of random-pattern skin flaps elevated in controlled, expanded skin. Plast Reconstr Surg 72(5):680–7.

Cormack G C, Lamberty B G H 1994 The arterial anatomy of skin flaps, 2nd edn. Churchill Livingstone, Edinburgh.

Coventry B J, Walsh J A 2003 Cutaneous innervation in man before and after lumbar sympathectomy: evidence for interruption of both sensory and vasomotor nerve fibres. Aust N Z J Surg 73(1–2):14–18.

Ganong W G 1999 Review of medical physiology. McGraw-Hill, New York.

Gibbins I L 1997 Autonomic pathways to cutaneous effectors. In: Gibbins I L, Morris J L (eds) Autonomic innervation of the skin. Harwood Academic Publishers, Amsterdam, pp 1–56.

Holzer P 1997 Control of the cutaneous vascular system by afferent neurons. In: Gibbins I L, Morris J L (eds) Autonomic innervation of the skin. Harwood Academic Publishers, Amsterdam, p 213–67.

Johnson P E, Kernahan D A, Bauer B S 1988 Dermal and epidermal response to soft-tissue expansion in the pig. Plast Reconstr Surg 81(3):390–7.

Larrabee W F Jr, Holloway G A Jr, Sutton D 1984 Wound tension and blood flow in skin flaps. Ann Otol Rhinol Laryngol 93(2 Pt 1):112–15.

Low P A, Kennedy W R 1997 Cutaneous effectors as indicators of abnormal sympathetic function. In: Gibbins I L, Morris J L (eds) Autonomic innervation of the skin. Harwood Academic Publishers, Amsterdam, pp 165–212.

Lundborg G 1977 Intraneural microvascular pathophysiology as related to ischaemia and nerve injury. In: Daniel R K, Terzis J K (eds) Reconstructive microsurgery. Little, Brown & Co., Boston.

Marks M W, Burney R E, Mackenzie J R, Knight P R 1986 Enhanced capillary blood flow in rapidly expanded random pattern flaps. J Trauma 26(10):913–15.

Masquelet A C, Romana M C, Wolf G 1992 Skin island flaps supplied by the vascular axis of the sensitive superficial nerves: anatomic study and clinical experience in the leg. Plast Reconstr Surg 89(6):1115–21.

Mathes S J, Nahai F 1997 Reconstructive surgery, principles, anatomy and technique. Churchill Livingstone, Edinburgh.

McMinn R M H 1994 Last's anatomy, 9th edn. Churchill Livingstone, Edinburgh.

Morris J L 1997 Autonomic vasoconstriction in the skin. In: Gibbins I L, Morris J L (eds) Autonomic innervation of the skin. Harwood Academic Publishers, Amsterdam, pp 57–85.

Nakajima H, Imanishi N, Fukuzumi S, Minabe T, Aiso S, Fujino T 1998 Accompanying arteries of the cutaneous veins and cutaneous nerves in the extremities: anatomical study and a concept of the venoadipofascial and/or neuroadipofascial pedicled fasciocutaneous flap. Plast Reconstr Surg 102(3):779–91.

Nugent J, O'Connor M 1983 Physical factors and angiogenesis. In: Ryan T J, Barnhill R L (eds) Ciba Foundation Symposium 100 – Development of the vascular system. Pitman Books, London, pp 80–94.

Ochoa J L, Yarnitsky D, Marchettini P, Dotson R, Cline M 1993 Interactions between sympathetic vasoconstrictor outflow and C nociceptor-induced antidromic vasodilatation. Pain 54(2):191–6.

Olenius M, Dalsgaard C J, Wickman M 1993 Mitotic activity in expanded human skin. Plast Reconstr Surg 91(2):213–16.

Ponten B 1981 The fasciocutaneous flap: its use in soft tissue defects of the lower leg. Br J Plast Surg 34(2):215–20.

Rubino C, Coscia V, Cavazzuti A M, Canu V 2006 Haemodynamic enhancement in perforator flaps: the inversion phenomenon and its clinical significance. A study of the relation of blood velocity and flow between pedicle and perforator vessels in perforator flaps. J Plast Reconstr Aesthet Surg 59(6):636–43.

Shalaby H A, Saad M A 1993 The venous island flap: is it purely venous? Br J Plast Surg 46(4):285–7.

Sunderland S 1945 Blood supply of peripheral nerves: practical considerations. Arch Neurol Psychiatry 54:280–2.

Young B, Heath J W 2002 Wheater's functional histology, 4th edn. Churchill Livingstone, Edinburgh.

Chapter 3

Design principles and the keystone technique

Logic will get you from A to B, imagination will get you everywhere.

Albert Einstein (1879–1955)

INTRODUCTION

The keystone island flap is an easy reconstructive tool to master. As a single flap, it offers the greatest versatility of any locoregional flap design. It has a simple design that can be applied as a direct extension of elliptical defects, and its diameter can be increased readily to improve the chances of perforator/vessel incorporation when the local neurovascular anatomy is uncertain. Unlike various random pattern flaps that rely on ratios of length to breadth of dermal attachment with significant variation for different body regions, the keystone perforator island flap can be used in any region where perforator or neurovascular support exists. Having examined the vascular basis of these flaps in Chapter 2, the purpose of this chapter is to look at the design of a standard keystone island flap and demonstrate some of the variations that can be undertaken in specific circumstances to optimise its functional and aesthetic results. Numerous variations in design are possible, including skin island shape, basis of vascular support, and presence or absence of incorporated named nerves. The islanded nature of the flap permits various flap manipulations to facilitate closure, such as advancement, rotation, folding and flap-on-flap techniques with inset of these islanded flaps, producing even physiological tension for good wound healing. The eventual scars are difficult to see due to the combination of non-parallel straight lines and parallel arcs of different lengths, with good aesthetics as a result.

PLANNING A KEYSTONE ISLAND FLAP

The keystone design

The classic design of all keystone flaps bears a resemblance to the keystone of archways (see Fig 1.4). This consists of a trapezoid bent into the shape of an arc, with the longest side on the convex surface

of the arc. Variations in the angles and relative lengths of each of the sides of the keystone can be used but, most commonly, the shape consists of a short arc formed by the margin of the defect (with or without lateral extensions to form an ellipse), followed by incisions formed at right angles to the tangent of the ends of this short arc (Fig 3.1). These incisions are made the same or a greater length than the transverse width of the defect. A long, curving arc-shaped incision then joins the tips of these two incisions, staying parallel to the short arc to complete the keystone shape (Behan 2003).

With certain characteristics of a bipedicled flap, the keystone flap is actually two V–Y flaps side by side but at an angle to each other so that their advancements are directed towards the centre of the defect (Fig 3.2). In a conventional bipedicled flap design, the secondary defect is usually larger than the primary defect and may require skin grafting. By converting this bipedicled flap into an island with V–Y advancement at each end, the longitudinal tension in the flap is released, thus maximising elasticity in the transverse direction and aiding defect and donor site closure. V–Y closure at the periphery narrows the whole defect complex so that the flap does not have to move as far transversely. Similarly, the secondary defect on the opposite side of the flap is reduced by this manoeuvre (see Fig 2.11) (Behan 2003).

Placement, size and orientation of keystone island flaps

Beyond the basic flap geometry, there are further considerations when planning keystone flaps so as to facilitate replacement of like tissues with like, ease wound and donor site closure, and incorporate appropriate neurovascular support. While many flap types necessitate the use of preoperative imaging (e.g. computed tomographic or magnetic resonance angiography, Doppler ultrasonography), this has not been our practice for the vast majority of defects

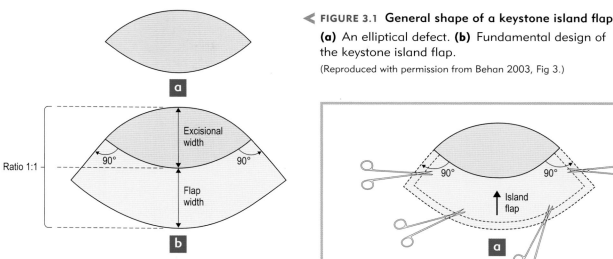

◀ **FIGURE 3.1 General shape of a keystone island flap**

(a) An elliptical defect. **(b)** Fundamental design of the keystone island flap.

(Reproduced with permission from Behan 2003, Fig 3.)

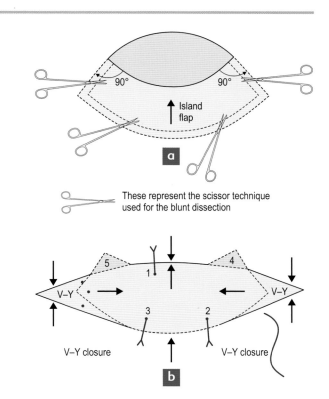

These represent the scissor technique used for the blunt dissection

▶ **FIGURE 3.2 Advancement and closure of V–Y flaps into an island**

(a) Blunt dissection mobilisation around the limits of the flap. **(b)** Vertical mattress sutures (numbered 1–3) bring the flap into alignment, creating lines of tension. Closure of the double V–Y apposition points at the limits of the flap creates a relative redundancy in the central portion of the flap. The redundant shaded areas (numbered 4 and 5) are excised. The wound closure is completed with the hemming suture.

(Reproduced with permission from Behan 2003, Fig 4.)

because of the reliability of perforator supply where a minimum of a 1:1 ratio of defect width to flap width is maintained (Behan 2003). One simple method to assist flap placement is to design the flaps so that their longitudinal axis runs in the lines of the dermatomes. A pinch test is then used to assess whether sufficient tissue elasticity and laxity are present to permit elevation and closure (elasticity is better than laxity). The keystone island flaps are commonly raised parallel to the long axis of dermatomes similar to the elongation of tissue during intrauterine development, often within a single dermatome and placed over muscle bellies wherever possible to improve perforator incorporation and flap movement during closure. Where the underlying neurovascular anatomy is uncertain, this approach increases the chance that the flaps will run parallel to longitudinal neurovascular structures, which can then be incorporated into the flap as their lateral mobility facilitates ready advancement of the flap into the defect (Behan 1992, 2003).

While flap planning should be included as part of the planning for the excision of lesions so that the orientation of the excision occurs in an axis that permits easy flap formation and advancement, the robust nature of the vascular supply to these flaps and their numerous variations for wound closure does not make this mandatory. The simplest approach is to excise lesions in an elliptical manner with their long axis parallel to the line of cutaneous nerves, veins and/or known vascular perforators (Fig 3.3)—in the extremities, the defect is generally longitudinally or obliquely placed (Behan 2003). To facilitate closure of the secondary defect, the flap should be sited along the side of the excision margin that has the greater tissue laxity and may include division of the deep fascia to facilitate movement. It is the tissue beyond the flap itself that must, ultimately, move to close the secondary defect. It is this recruitment of peripheral tissue that enables direct closure of the secondary defect (see Fig 2.11). In the lower leg, the flap is best located posterior to the defect so that the skin laxity over the posterior compartment can be exploited to close the secondary defect. Mobilisation of keystone island flaps directly over the sharp pretibial border should be avoided due to the linear pressure this puts on the flaps, combined with the paucity of perforators in the region and the relative immobility of the pretibial skin. Every effort is made to place incisions along lines of election or natural junction lines to hide the scar among wrinkles and render the scar less conspicuous.

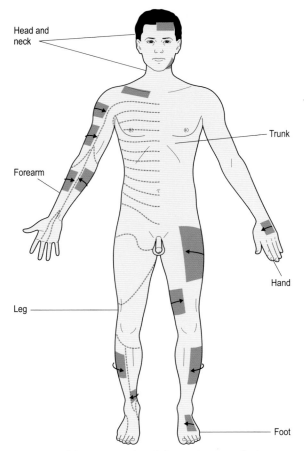

⋀ **FIGURE 3.3 Keystone island flaps designed along dermatomal axes—perforator zones**

The longitudinal axis of flaps superimposed over septocutaneous, musculocutaneous, fasciocutaneous and direct vessels permits maximal transverse movement for defect closure (longitudinal movement will be poor due to tethering from the underlying tissues). This pattern may be altered to site the elliptical defect in the line of the relaxed skin tension lines; therefore, the keystone island flap will also be slightly oblique.

(Reproduced with permission from Behan 2003, Fig 1.)

Flap elevation

Skin, fat and fascia/panniculus carnosus remnants (e.g. platysma) are incorporated as a trilaminate unit in the flap, and associated subcutaneous venous or neural supports are preserved wherever possible (Behan 1992). After incision of the skin, blunt dissection through the subcutaneous plane allows retention of these superficial veins and cutaneous nerves—to preserve long-term sensory function, the arterial network accompanying cutaneous nerves and veins, and the venous outflow (see Fig 3.2) (Behan 1992, Nakajima et al. 1998). Cadaveric injection studies have confirmed the preservation of the dual (conjoint) blood supply of the keystone island flap (superficial vascular network and deep musculocutaneous and septocutaneous

perforators) with this dissection technique (Pelissier et al. 2007). Careful teasing of the circumferential tissues is performed without the need for flap undermining so as to preserve the integrity of perforators. The next step in keystone island flap elevation is division of the deep fascia (where appropriate) along the convex surface of the flap. Division here allows the island flap, pedicled on perforators, to sway as a single unit between the primary and secondary defects (similar to the historical bridge/bipedicled flap principle).

Flap inset and defect closure

Keystone island flaps are mobilised by advancement, rotation or transposition to close the primary defect. Vertical mattress (or figure-of-eight) sutures are placed at strategic points, initially across the midpoint of the defect, followed by two sutures bisecting the donor defect on the contralateral side of the defect (see Fig 3.2). Early placement of these sutures maximises the use of biological and mechanical creep to minimise tension during wound closure (Wilhelmi et al. 1998). Additional sutures, including occasional deep dermal absorbable sutures, are added as required to approximate the dermal edges, facilitate two-layer apposition and obliterate dead space, with the inset being completed by the use of a running mattress (Hemming) suture around the periphery of the flap in order to produce good wound eversion and even physiological tension, and maximise wound healing (Behan 2003). White lines of tension, suggestive of poor subdermal plexus perfusion, may be a temporary feature during flap insertion. However, these disappear after the flap is fully inserted and tension is equally distributed circumferentially. Elements of tension at the V–Y points and the limits of flap insertion are assessed to determine whether non-physiological wound tension is present (tension beyond the normal tension on skin by movement and contact with surrounding skin). Sometimes it is appropriate to insert a small full-thickness skin graft on the side of the donor defect to ease this tension, while maintaining appropriate fasciocutaneous coverage of the defect site (type IIB keystone flap, see over). Flap inset can be undertaken over a drain if it is thought necessary by positioning the drain in a U-shape under the flap to permit the use of a single drain for both sites.

Postoperatively, continuous suture loops are cut at 5–10 days depending on the location (5 days on the face and 10 days elsewhere). The tension sutures stay in for 2–4 weeks, depending on the amount of tension. Even for large reconstructions, postoperative intensive flap and patient monitoring are often not necessary. Postoperative pain is usually negligible and opioid analgesia is rarely needed. In our experience, the use of a keystone island flap with its relatively low complication rate without the need for intensive care unit admissions and surgical re-explorations has a marked bearing on the patient's clinical well-being.

Classification

Depending on the extent of flap mobilisation required to achieve defect closure, keystone island flaps have been classified into four types (Behan 2003):

Type I: In this type, the deep fascia on the convex border of the keystone island flap is left intact. This flap is suitable for smaller defects up to 2 cm in width over most areas of the body.

Type II (Fig 3.4): In this type, the deep fascia along the convex border of the keystone island flap is divided to permit further mobilisation. These flaps are further subdivided into type IIA, when the secondary defect is closed primarily, and type IIB, when the secondary defect is skin-grafted. Skin grafting is useful where excess tension exists, allowing the flap to cover vital structures while the graft allows wound healing (e.g. distal third of the lower leg and distal third of the forearm). These flaps are particularly useful for the upper and lower limbs.

Type III (Fig 3.5): In this type, a double keystone may be designed to exploit maximum laxity of the surrounding tissues for considerably larger defects (5–10 cm). It is suitable for large defects in the calf, trunk or sacral regions and can either be performed as a direct symmetrical circumferential advancement or in a Yin Yang manner, where there is asymmetrical movement of the opposing flap ends, giving a twisting or serpiginous appearance (similar to the Yin Yang symbol, see Fig 6.13).

Type IV (including cervicosubmental, omega (Ω) and goblet variants) (Fig 3.6): In this type, a portion of the keystone island flap, based either proximally or distally, is undermined, raised in the subfascial plane and mobilised to facilitate closure. With the extent of undermining approaching up to

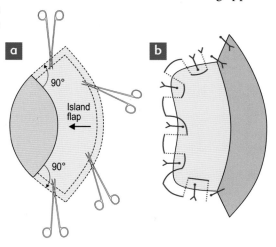

> **FIGURE 3.4 Type II keystone island flaps**
>
> **(a)** Type IIA closure of the defect is facilitated by division of the fascia along the outer curvilinear incision. **(b)** In type IIB closure, where non-physiological wound tension is present, a skin graft is placed in the secondary defect.
>
> (Reproduced with permission from Behan 2003, Fig 9.)

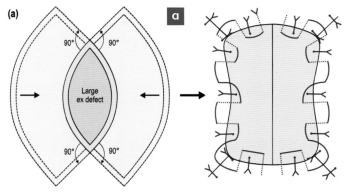

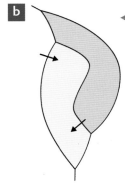

> **FIGURE 3.5 Two identical opposing type II keystone island flaps are (a)** advanced perpendicularly to the long axis of the flaps or **(b)** opposing ends are advanced with an element of rotation to produce the Yin Yang variant
>
> (**(a)** Reproduced with permission from Behan 2003, Fig 11.)

> **FIGURE 3.6 A type IV keystone island flap**
>
> Part of the flap is elevated and undermined deep to fascia (or platysma) and transposed into the defect with or without skin grafting of the secondary defect. In the omega (Ω) variant, one end of the flap is undermined, then turned 180 degrees to be sutured to the other end of the flap (creating a shape similar to an omega symbol).
>
> (Reproduced with permission from Behan 2003, Fig 13.)

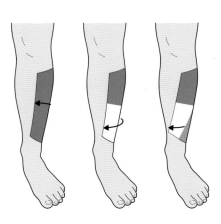

two-thirds of the flap surface area, the secondary defect often requires complementary grafting. In areas of bony protrusion, this type of flap is not suitable because V–Y closure advances poorly over the prominence. It is useful around joints (neck, wrist, ankle and knee) to cover vital structures, such as neurovascular bundles, bone, joint and tendon. The observed hypervascularity of the flaps allows development of the omega (Ω) variant (horseshoe or 180-degree fold on itself) and one of the arms of the keystone can be divided longitudinally to create a goblet appearance for closure.

If undermining is necessary (e.g. type IV cervicosubmental and omega (Ω) variant flaps), it is performed with a sequential method of sharp and blunt dissection; sharp dissection to get through the planes of dermis and deep fascia, and blunt dissection (scissor technique or using a finger/blunt) to get through subcutaneous fat and develop the subfascial/subplatysmal plane back to the pivot point of rotation or transposition. We do not routinely isolate and skeletonise perforators. This adds operating time, unnecessary complexity and postoperative scarring. The risk of perforator damage is increased, and the absence of soft tissue support may contribute towards vessel kinking or occlusion.

Technical refinements

Flap siting/position is based on principles associated with anatomical regions, which include the following:

1 For flap types I–III, design flaps along the long axis of nerves/underlying muscles so that advancement into the defect is perpendicular to the long axis of these structures (see Fig 3.3).

2 Flap type IV needs a definable vascular base within the attached region of the flap, even though these neurovascular structures (e.g. branches of external carotid artery in the region of the middle third of the sternocleidomastoid/C2–C3 cervical plexus to assist with neurovascular support) do not necessarily need to be identified specifically pre- or intraoperatively (Fig 3.7).

3 Be cautious closing over convex structures (e.g. scalp) and over the pretibial border. Omega (Ω) and goblet variants, which naturally try to take on a convex structure, will be best suited to such closure; otherwise, straight advancements can lead to necrosis or delayed healing of part of the flap. In the operative case shown in Figure 3.7, the site of the transposition was planned so that the 'dog ear'—small remnant evident at the margin of the flap—would lie near the angle of the mandible (a natural convexity).

4 Maintain a fascial/muscular base so as to maximise the integrity of vascular plexuses. This also permits immediate excision of dog ears as long as the underlying fascia or muscle layer is preserved.

5 Knowledge of the dermatomes is useful. Maintaining the long axis of keystone island flaps to match the axis of dermatomes is very helpful in their planning with positioning around neurovascular axes (e.g. L1–L2 dermatome for planning a quadriceps keystone island flap in groin reconstruction and C2–C3 for the cervicosubmental island flap in the head and neck; see Chapter 4).

6 Maintain named nerves (e.g. accessory, sural, saphenous, superficial peroneal, superficial radial nerve) as conduits through flaps (minor nerves can be sacrificed) and plan to incorporate these into flaps so as to utilise their neurovascular input (conjoint supply).

7 Perioperative Doppler ultrasound studies are not routinely used. They can be useful in specific circumstances where the positioning of orthopaedic pins or wires limit the normal safe dimensions of flaps. Here, the identification of feeding vessels by Doppler ultrasound in these regions can ensure appropriate safety of non-ideal flap geometry.

FIGURE 3.7

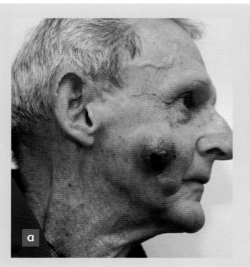

FIGURE 3.7 A clinical case illustrating the use of a cervicosubmental (CSM) keystone island flap and demonstrating a number of the principles of keystone island flap elevation

(a) A 73-year-old man with radio-recurrent Merkel cell tumour of the right cheek.

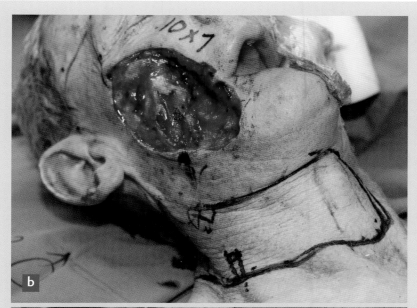

(b) A 10 × 7 cm defect is formed following tumour resection. A cervicosubmental keystone island flap is marked out and a perforator identified (X mark in top left of flap) by Doppler ultrasound.

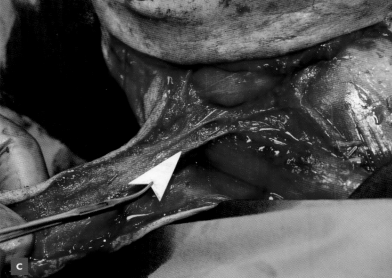

(c) Following elevation of the flap from medial to lateral by blunt dissection in the subplatysmal plane, a perforating vessel is visualised (not necessary for flap elevation but obvious in this case).

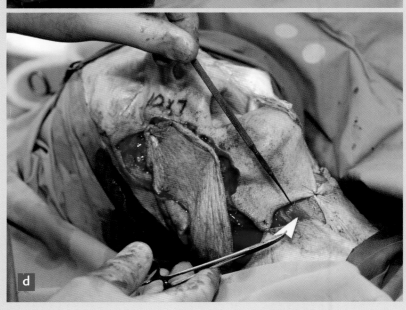

(d) Transposition of the flap with a few strategic mattress sutures to encourage skin creep and commencement of direct closure of the secondary defect.

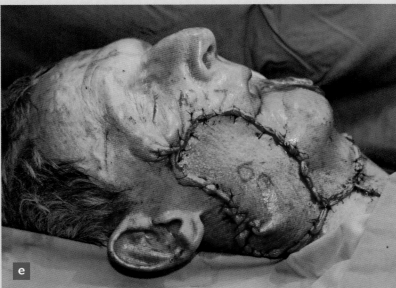

(e) Intraoperative appearance immediately following completion of wound closure over a suction drain, including immediate supraplatysma resection of the dog ear of the flap (small remnant evident at posterior margin of flap) without any effect on flap vascularisation.

(f) Appearance at 9 months showing disease-free survival following appropriate oncological management. Focus now shifts to improving aesthetics relating to his unilateral facial nerve palsy.

TLC

Time (operation/cost)
60 minutes

Life quality (and aesthetics)
Acceptable after radiotherapy, acceptable aesthetics

Complications
Nil

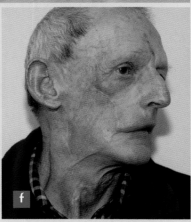

Design variations

Multiple facets of the keystone island flap can be altered to suit the requirements of the defect and the available donor tissue. The four types of keystone island flap that have been described above can have numerous design variations. These variations can be categorised into the following, which are outlined below:

1 Handling of deep fascia/panniculus remnants
2 Shape of skin incision
3 Type of movement of flap into defect
4 Degree of islanding
5 De-epithelialisation and removal of dog ears

Handling of the deep fascia/panniculus carnosus remnants

The site at which vessels perforate the deep fascia forms a fixed point around which the flap is advanced, rotated or transposed. Where insufficient flap movement occurs by islanding and blunt dissection alone, division of the fascia at the flap periphery can be used to gain extra flap mobilisation. This can be done on the far convex edge alone or around the entire circumference of the flap. Where thin flaps are required (e.g. periorbital reconstruction), the deep fascia/panniculus remnants of the leading edge may be excluded from the flap (see Fig 4.15).

Shape of the skin incision

The geometry of the basic keystone design can be modified to suit the defect shape and donor site limitations. The most common variation is forming asymmetrical limbs, where there is either greater laxity at one end of the flap than the other or to fit the flap into creases (e.g. cervicosubmental flap in neck skin creases, Fig 3.7), resulting in a wider flap at one end than the other. The angles at which the V–Y points come off can also be varied to fit better into natural skin creases, and some surgeons have even included an additional V–Y point in the middle of the long convex arc (crown flap variant) to limit tension across the closure, even though this has never been necessary in our experience. A number of related flaps have been developed, some as a natural progression from the keystone flap for specific defects, and include the Bezier flap (see Fig 3.8),* the bridge flap (Fig 3.15) and the goblet flap, all of which share common principles of keystone islanding (see Fig 4.17).

Type of flap movement into the defect

The islanded nature of the keystone flap and the degree to which undermining and flap elevation can be undertaken, while maintaining its vascular supply, allows multiple different forms of flap movement into the defect. The most common is advancement by V–Y closure at the two flap corners away from the defect. Elevation of one end of the flap permits either rotation or transposition into the defect. This can be undertaken to the point where one limb of the flap is transposed to meet the other as an omega (Ω) variant (see Fig 4.12).

De-epithelialisation and flap subdivision

The conjoint supply into the subdermal plexuses of the flap permits surgical manipulations that would risk partial flap loss in non-islanded local flaps. These include de-epithelialising central regions of the flap and trimming dog ears in the primary surgery. De-epithelialisation is particularly useful in central defects of the ear where a rim of pinna is maintained. Keystone flap reconstruction of these defects can be undertaken with a strip of skin removed from the flap to allow inset of the detached edge of the pinna to improve aesthetics. This can be undertaken safely without risk to the tip of the flap. Dog-ear removal can similarly be undertaken in a judicious fashion to minimise revisional surgery without significant risk to the flaps. Where dog ears are present over convex surfaces, a variable degree of settling will occur depending on the degree of convexity and the elasticity of the patient's skin. If insufficient softening occurs at any residual dog-ear sites, simple revision can be undertaken after a delay of 6–12 months. This is very rare due to frequent settling and immediate dog-ear revision in most cases.

A NOTE ON ISLANDING

Incompletely islanded keystone flaps via the maintenance of a skin bridge have been described (Moncrieff et al., 2008). Proponents of this approach argue that this improves vascularity to the flap by retention of a dermal blood supply. In our experience, the keystone island flap is characterised by hypervascularity, including the hyperaemic flare, *red dot sign*, reliable flap survival and prompt wound healing (components of the quaternary response). Therefore, we have not sought to alter the island design concept. The clinical success of the islanded keystone flap in irradiated fields (Behan 2003) in patients with vascular disease and poor wound healing supports our approach.

CLINICAL CASES

Variations in the design of keystone island flaps and the circumstances in which these can be undertaken to optimise their functional and aesthetic results are shown in Figures 3.8 to 3.15.

SUMMARY

Following these design principles of the keystone flap leads to safe and timely flap elevation, closure and healing. The principles include creation of a skin island by sharp incision of skin, blunt dissection of subcutaneous tissues while maintaining neurovascular structures where possible, incorporation of a platysma or fascial base, and closure under even physiological tension. Using this method, numerous variants can be devised depending on the geometry of the defect, donor tissue availability and experience of the surgeon. Application of these principles enables fasciocutaneous reconstruction in an expeditious and safe manner, with good functional and aesthetic outcomes. Surgical dissection is less extensive and the operating time is shorter. The learning curve is not as steep as with free-tissue transfer and microsurgical skills are not required. Disease control with best functional outcome is prioritised and multi-staged surgery with a lengthy hospital stay is avoided.

BIBLIOGRAPHY

Behan F C 1992 The fasciocutaneous island flap: an extension of the angiotome concept. Aust N Z J Surg 62(11):874–86.

Behan F C 2003 The keystone design perforator island flap in reconstructive surgery. Aust N Z J Surg 73(3):112–20.

Moncrieff M D, Bowen F, Thompson J F, Saw R P, Shannon K F, Spillane A J, Quinn M J, Stretch J R 2008 Keystone flap reconstruction of primary melanoma excision defects of the leg: the end of the skin graft? Ann Surg Oncol 15(10):2867–73.

Nakajima H, Imanishi N, Fukuzumi S, Minabe T, Aiso S, Fujino T 1998 Accompanying arteries of the cutaneous veins and cutaneous nerves in the extremities: anatomical study and a concept of the venoadipofascial and/or neuroadipofascial pedicled fasciocutaneous flap. Plast Reconstr Surg 102(3):779–91.

Pelissier P, Santoul M, Pinsolle V, Casoli V, Behan F 2007 The keystone design perforator island flap. Part I: anatomic study. J Plast Reconstr Aesthet Surg 60(8):883–7.

Wilhelmi B J, Blackwell S J, Mancoll J S, Phillips L G 1998 Creep vs. stretch: a review of the viscoelastic properties of skin. Ann Plast Surg 41(2):215–19.

---

* Development of the Bezier flap pre-dated the keystone flap, but both share similar principles, as discussed in Chapter 1.

FIGURE 3.8

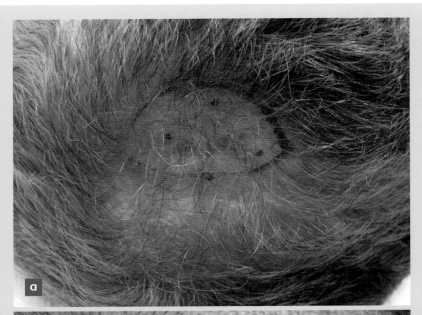

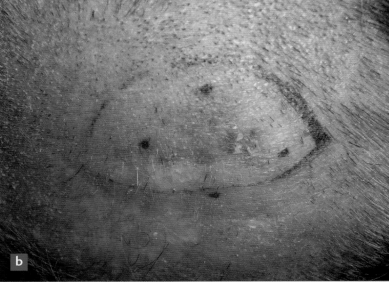

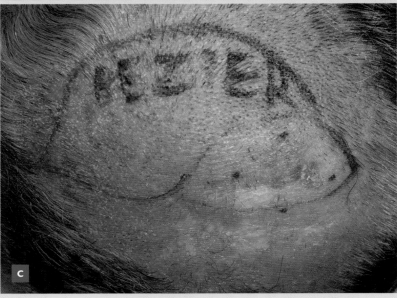

FIGURE 3.8 A 55-year-old male sports car enthusiast with recurrent Hutchinson's freckle (lentigo maligna)

(a) Mark-out of the Hutchinson's melanotic freckle (HMF) on the scalp. (*Note*: Six years earlier a transverse keystone island flap was performed for an HMF of the scalp behind the present lesion.)

(b) Close-up of the pigmented lesion with 1-cm clearance.

(c) Bezier (sinusoidal ellipse) with V–Y flaps at either end to close the defect in anteroposterior direction.

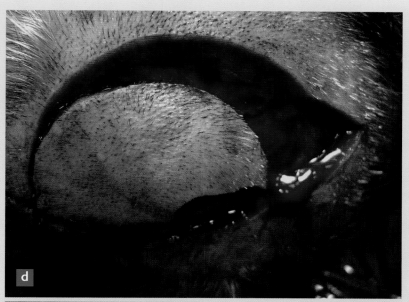

(d) A flap raised. (*Note*: The flap is designed to be much larger than normal on the basis that it must cover a convex surface and, therefore, a smaller flap would not be sufficient to permit closure. Also, instead of the tip of the flap being drawn from the midpoint of the defect, it is drawn closer to the tip of the defect to assist in closure due to limited advancement present within the scalp.)

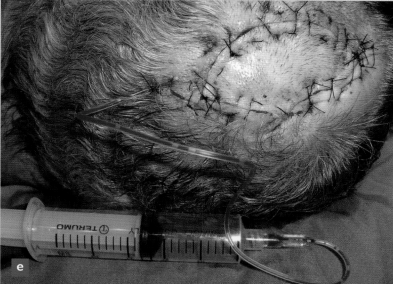

(e) On insertion under physiological tension, showing sufficient vascularisation despite the presence of the previous keystone scar across the flap (a relative contraindication to the use of non-islanded flaps).

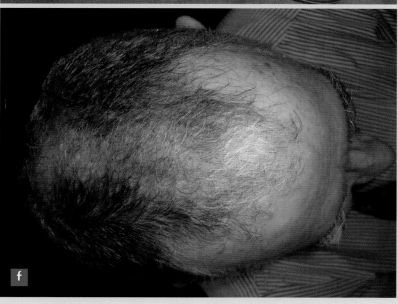

(f) Appearance 12 months postoperatively, with the patient reporting increased hair growth from the region of the island flap. This is a common reported finding by patients with these flaps in the scalp. This may indicate persistent improved local cutaneous vascularity.

TLC

Time (operation/cost)
40 minutes
Life quality (and aesthetics)
Improved hair quality in flap and good aesthetics
Complications
Crusting of wound anteriorly, healed without further problems

FIGURE 3.9

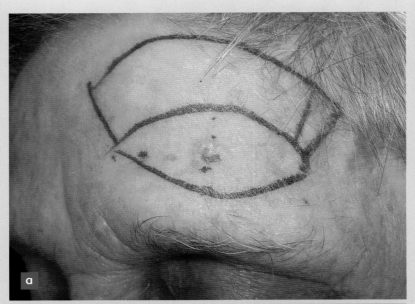

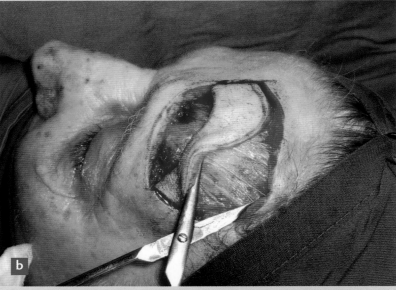

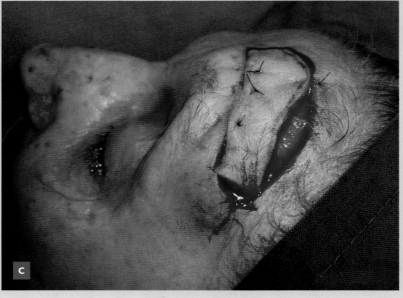

FIGURE 3.9 Case of a 65-year-old female demonstrating the use of an early type I keystone flap

(a) Basal cell carcinoma of the left supraorbital ridge with a transverse mark-out planned, along with the keystone flap for closure. (Usually, excisions in the supraorbital region are planned vertically to avoid unilateral eyebrow elevation but the patient had a planned supraorbital keystone flap from the opposite forehead for nasal reconstruction.)

(b) A 4 × 2 cm defect is formed and, following islanding of the keystone flap, blunt dissection is used to mobilise the flap while preserving neurovascular structures.

(c) Strategic mattress sutures are used to align the structures prior to definitive closure.

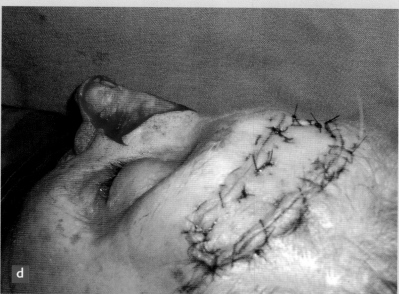

(d) Defect on nose to be reconstructed with similar transversely oriented keystone flap from contralateral side to maintain symmetry.

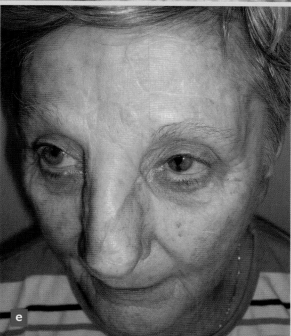

(e) Appearance at 6 months showing good aesthetics and symmetry of the eyebrow position following contralateral use of a keystone flap for nasal reconstruction.

TLC

Time (operation/cost)
40 minutes
Life quality (and aesthetics)
Intact supraorbital nerve and acceptable aesthetics
Complications
Nil

FIGURE 3.10

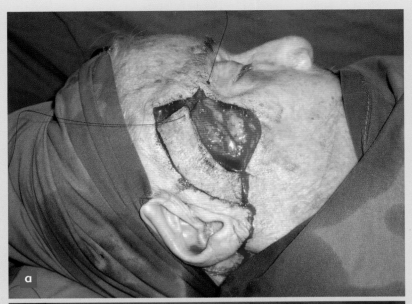

FIGURE 3.10 An 82-year-old female with a basal cell carcinoma (BCC) of the right malar eminence, demonstrating the use of a neurovascular axis as the basis for flap orientation

(a) Excision of BCC producing a defect and islanding of the keystone flap along the axis of the superficial temporal artery branches.

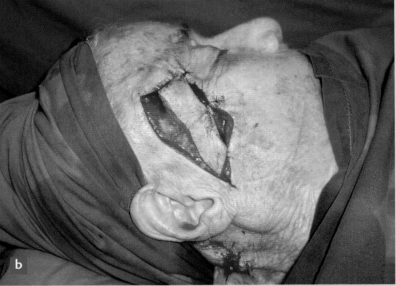

(b) Strategic mattress sutures used to facilitate closure.

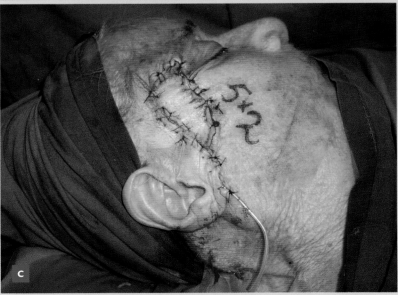

(c) Final closure with a hemming suture, demonstrating physiological wound tension and elevation of the cheek in an aesthetically acceptable manner.

TLC

Time (operation/cost)		
30 minutes		
Life quality (and aesthetics)		
Good, with acceptable aesthetics		
Complications		
Nil		

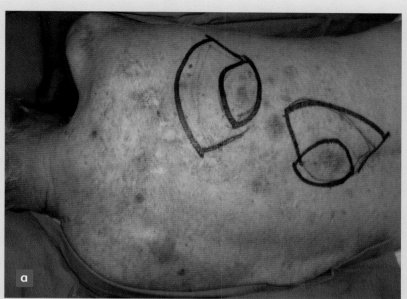

FIGURE 3.11 Elderly patient with two superficial multifocal basal cell carcinomas of the back

(a) Lesion 1 along the inferior pole of the right scapula shows an orientation that is different from that for lesion 2, which is paraspinal at the T11–T12 level and, therefore, longitudinal in its axis. Keystone flaps in parallel would be very difficult to close. Hence, the medial flap straddles two intercostal zones.

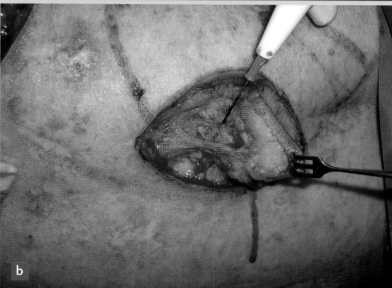

(b) Diathermy of the defect base during excision, often showing prominent vessels consistent with angiogenesis of tumour growth.

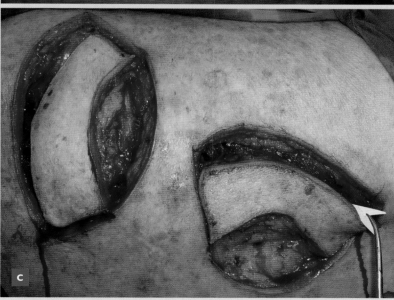

(c) The two keystone flaps islanded on intercostal and paraspinous muscle perforators, respectively, including blunt dissection of the subcutaneous structures to facilitate flap advancement without undermining.

FIGURE 3.11

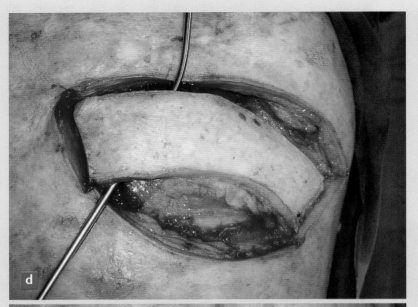

(d) Insertion of the drain tube under the attached region of the flap permits use of a single flap for both the primary and secondary defect sites.

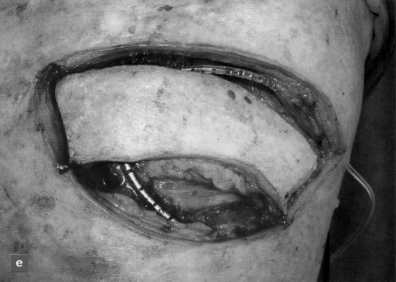

(e) The drain is in place ready for wound closure.

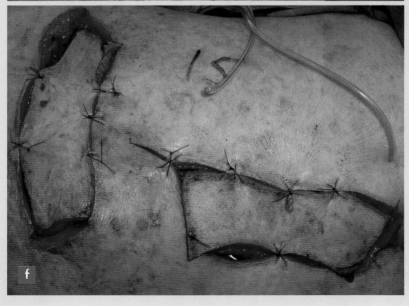

(f) Initial wound closure with strategic mattress sutures.

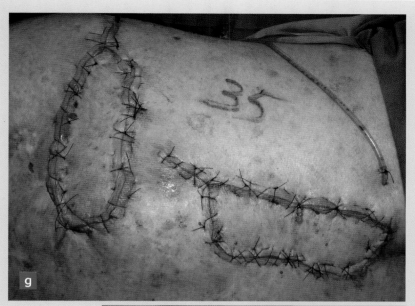

(g) A continuous horizontal everting mattress suture is added to produce accurate wound apposition.

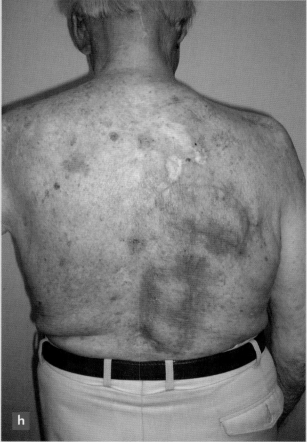

(h) Appearance 6 weeks following surgery, with good movement and healing evident.

See **video** for Figure 3.11

TLC

Time (operation/cost)
45 minutes (for both with two operators)
Life quality (and aesthetics)
Good, with acceptable aesthetics
Complications
Haematoma on anticoagulants—resolved without intervention

FIGURE 3.12

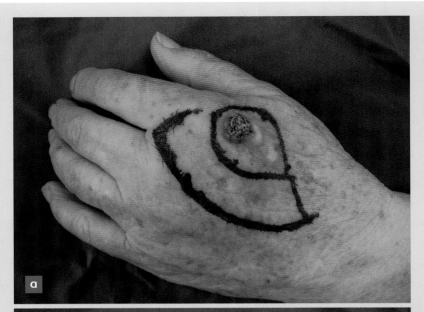

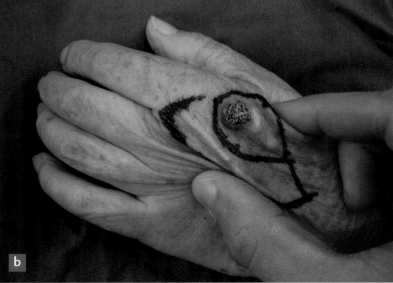

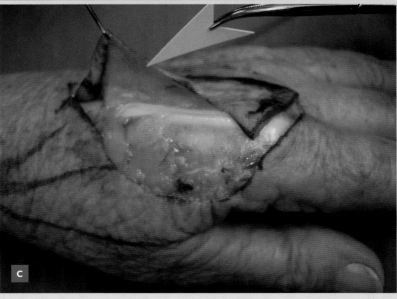

FIGURE 3.12 Squamous cell carcinoma over the metacarpophalangeal joint of the index finger of the left hand

(a) A keystone island flap was designed longitudinally to permit incorporation of the longitudinally oriented neurovascular structures, while maximising movement.

(b) The pinch test is performed to assess the laxity of tissue for designing the medial or lateral orientation of the keystone.

(c) The excisional defect is approximately 4 × 2 cm. The leading edge of the flap (arrow) is mobilised on small perforators, leaving paratenon on the underlying extensor tendons.

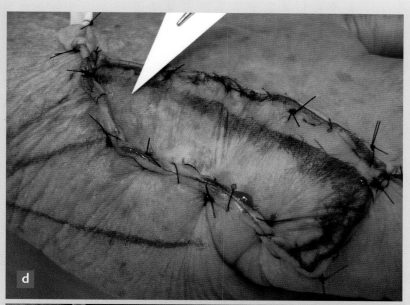

(d) Following mattress suturing, the tourniquet is released. A hyperaemic vascular flare is more noticeable in the flap than the surrounding tissues.

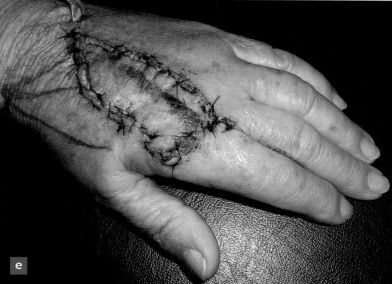

(e) Appearance at 5 days for removal of the drain tube. The continuous sutures are cut to reduce tension and removed later (2 weeks). The strategic mattress sutures stay in for 3 weeks.

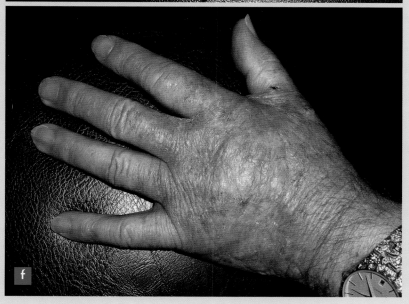

(f) Appearance at 6 months.

TLC

Time (operation/cost)	
45 minutes	
Life quality (and aesthetics)	
Early mobilisation and acceptable aesthetics	
Complications	
Nil	

FIGURE 3.13

FIGURE 3.13 Melanoma of the right arm in a young woman

(a) This melanoma was classified as Breslow thickness 0.6 mm, Clark's level II, requiring wide local excision. A 1-cm re-excisional margin was used, creating a 5 × 3 cm defect. A keystone flap was outlined along the lateral arc to avoid damage to the biceps, along the longitudinal axis of the limb (can be placed obliquely if this assists closure).

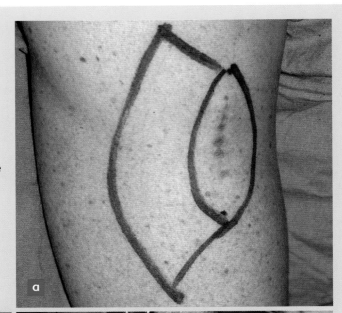

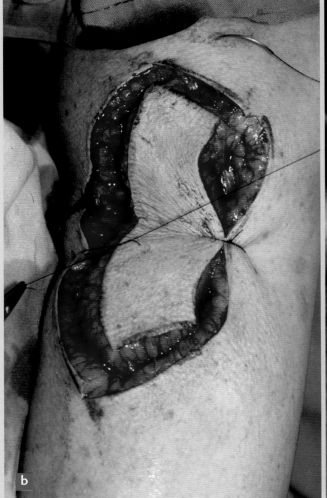

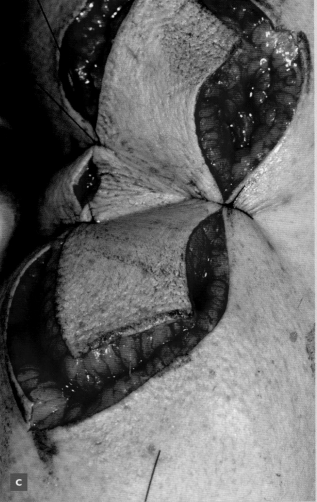

(b) Initial suturing closes the defect.

(c) The white lines of tension are created to close the surgical site. This appearance should not cause anxiety as the subdermal plexus has been bypassed and the perforator supply is the dominant circulation.

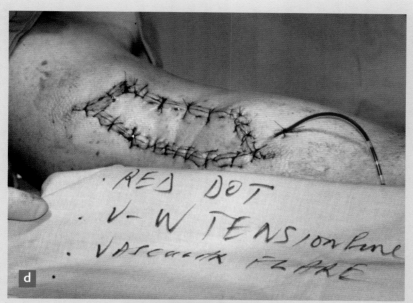

(d) On completion of suturing, with the lines of tension in the subdermal plexus now fully perfused and the pink flare developing (part of the initial phase of the quaternary response in these flaps; see Chapter 2). The drainage is complete, with the tubing bent in a U-shape to service both sides.

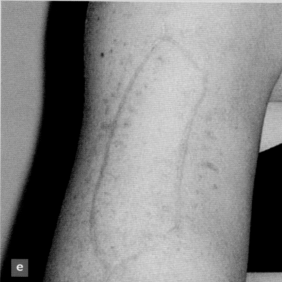

(e) Early postoperative appearance at 4 months.

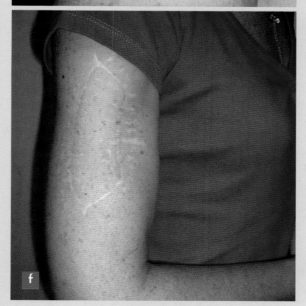

(f) Appearance at 4 years showing appropriate summer clothing, reflecting patient comfort with aesthetics.

TLC

Time (operation/cost)
50 minutes
Life quality (and aesthetics)
Good—can wear short-sleeved blouses, acceptable aesthetics
Complications
Nil

FIGURE 3.14

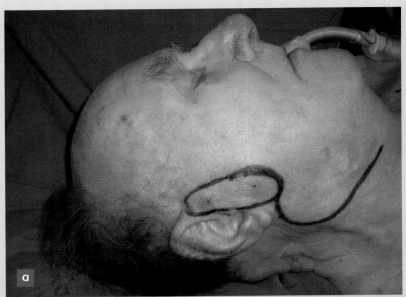

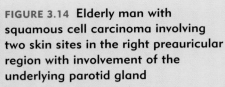

FIGURE 3.14 **Elderly man with squamous cell carcinoma involving two skin sites in the right preauricular region with involvement of the underlying parotid gland**

(a) Preoperative view demonstrating the skin mark-out for surgical excision and elective neck dissection.

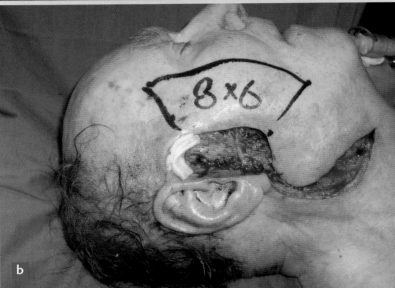

(b) Following excision, a cheek-based keystone flap (facial and zygomaticofacial vessels) is planned anterior to the defect, with the anterior border made relatively convex in the periorbital region to minimise distortion of the eyelids.

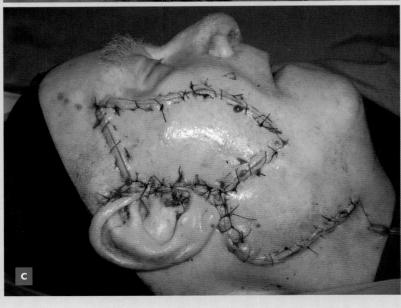

(c) Inset and closure demonstrating even tension and good flap perfusion (multiple red dots are evident, including in the anterior border of the flap in this picture).

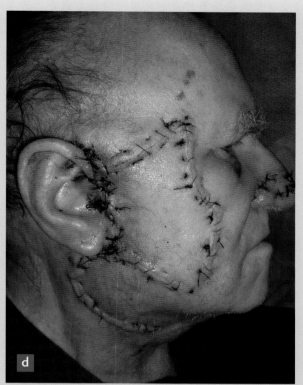

(d) Ten days postoperatively the wound shows good healing.

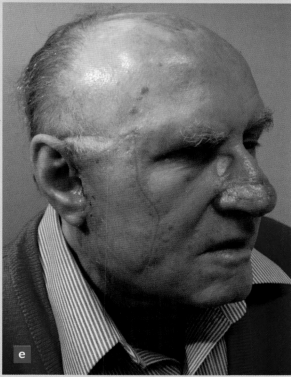

(e) Appearance at 6 weeks postoperatively, with good early contour, colour match and minimal facial distortion.

See [video] for Figure 3.14

TLC

Time (operation/cost)
50 minutes
Life quality (and aesthetics)
Good, with acceptable aesthetics
Complications
Nil

FIGURE 3.15

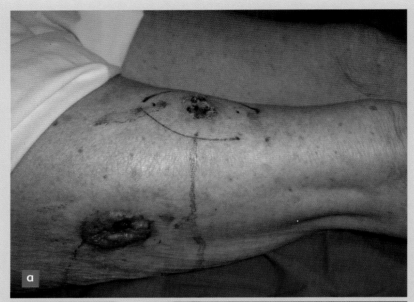

FIGURE 3.15 **The bridge flap variant of the keystone island flap used in an 84-year-old woman with two ulcerative lesions of her right thigh**

(a) Appearance of the thigh preoperatively, demonstrating the two lesions following injection with local anaesthetic (in combination with general anaesthetic).

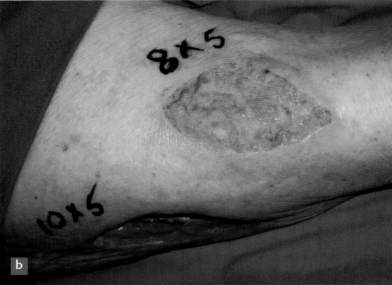

(b) Defect sizes following excision of the lesions are 8 × 5 cm and 10 × 5 cm, respectively.

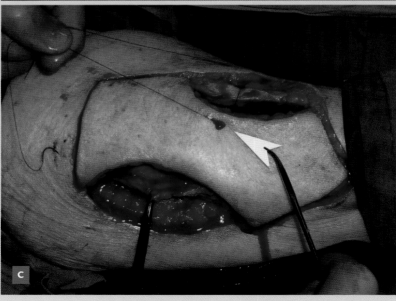

(c) The bridge of skin, fat and fascia between the two lesions is islanded as a bridge flap using slight extensions at either end. The fascia is divided to aid mobilisation (arrow showing free fascial edge), but the flap is not otherwise undermined and, where possible, neurovascular structures are kept intact. A *red dot sign* is evident on wound closure, with bright red blood oozing from the flap side of the suture and not the surrounding skin.

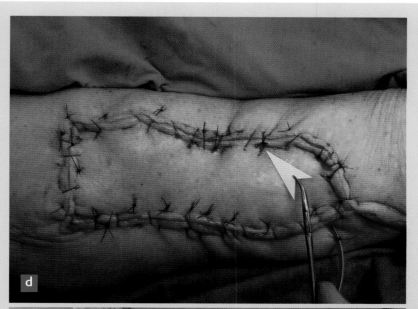

(d) Approximation is complete and a number of the suture sites on the flap are still bleeding (red dots).

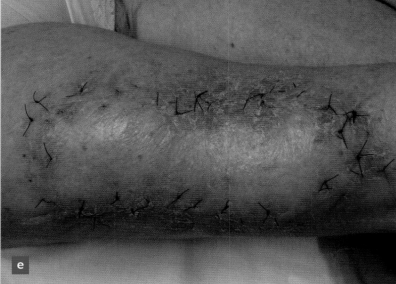

(e) Three weeks postoperatively: the hemming sutures are removed by the second week and the remaining mattress sutures by the third week.

TLC

Time (operation/cost)
55 minutes
Life quality (and aesthetics)
Good, with acceptable aesthetics
Complications
Nil

Clinical Applications of Keystone Island Flaps: Anatomical Regions

Chapter 4
Head and neck

Progress is impossible without change, and those who cannot change their minds cannot change anything.

George Bernard Shaw (1856–1950)

The usefulness of the keystone and other island flaps is almost unparalleled for the reconstruction of small and large oncological defects of the head and neck where bony reconstruction is not necessary. It adheres to the Gillies' principle of replacing 'like with like' and the next best tissue is the next best tissue.

INTRODUCTION

The head and neck region is a very specialised area of the body. Despite constituting less than one-tenth of the total body surface area, it houses most of the special senses (e.g. vision, hearing, taste and smell) and forms the portal through which we eat, drink and socially interact with our world. Lifestyle factors, such as sun exposure, tobacco smoking, alcohol consumption and poor dental hygiene, contribute to the head and neck region being the most densely affected site for cutaneous and mucosal malignancies (Raasch et al. 2006). Lymphatic spread of these tumours adds to the burden of disease by involving the parotid (the Australian disease) and cervical lymph nodes. As a group, patients affected by head and neck malignancy are often elderly with multiple comorbidities relating to their age, lifestyle factors, nutrition and low socioeconomic status. The combination of these factors makes patient selection, preoperative optimisation and perioperative planning paramount.

The majority of head and neck defects are amenable to fasciocutaneous (skin and soft tissue without bone) reconstruction alone. The management of patients with invasive disease is characterised by multimodal therapy combining surgical extirpation with radio- and/or chemotherapy. This biases reconstructive approaches away from skin grafts to those approaches that provide robust vasculature and rapid healing so as not to delay the commencement of adjuvant therapies. Developments in microsurgery have made free-flap reconstruction achievable in elderly well patients where the demands of the defect mandate the use of free tissue (e.g. bony reconstruction). However, its poor colour match with the surrounding skin and frequent ptosis of the transplanted tissue lead to suboptimal aesthetics/quality of life, with frequent social isolation despite otherwise successful surgery. The donor defects can also be problematic. For example, closure of the radial free forearm flap donor site can necessitate the use of skin grafting with the potential for tendon exposure. As a result, postoperative quality of life has become an important issue.

The relative frequency of new primary lesions and the recurrence of previous disease and metachronous (second) tumours, often in irradiated fields, makes the use of reliable local reconstructive approaches ideal, with their lower morbidity, shorter operative times and fewer complications. An excellent blood supply and numerous natural skin creases provide a rich canvas for the planning of locoregional flaps in this area. Our experience of robust vascularity, despite previous radiotherapy within these flaps, leads to timely healing through the use of local tissues. The reliable vascularity with such fasciocutaneous island flaps even allows scars to be incorporated into the flap design, a previous contraindication to the use of these flaps in non-irradiated beds (Fig 4.1). Local flap reconstruction preserves important regional 'lifeboats', such as the pectoralis major flap, and permits future salvage procedures should recurrence of disease occur. Therefore, locoregional flap reconstruction offers the best opportunity to meet the specific reconstructive needs of patients with head and neck defects by combining good functional and aesthetic results through the rapid transfer of vascularised, locally sourced tissue. It can also be of use for optimising functional and aesthetic

FIGURE 4.1

FIGURE 4.1 A 79-year-old woman with recurrent melanoma involving the parotid following previous wide local excision and cervicosubmental (CSM) keystone island flap reconstruction to her right cheek 7 years previously

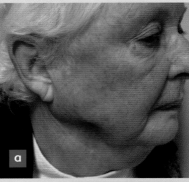

(a) Careful examination demonstrates a fine line scar of a previous keystone island flap oriented vertically on the cheek up to the zygomatic arch.

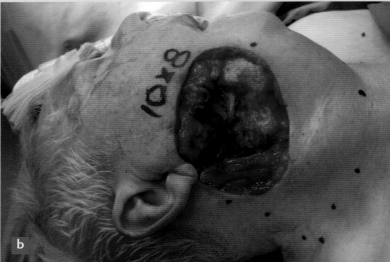

(b) Following parotidectomy and removal of the affected overlying skin, a 10 × 8 cm fasciocutaneous defect is created. The dots demonstrate the planned mark-out of a CSM keystone island flap.

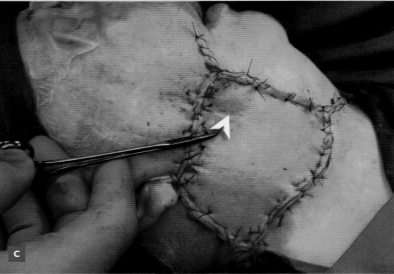

(c) Following flap inset and defect closure, the tip of the flap beyond the previous surgical scar is slightly different in colour (arrow). The presence of a previous surgical scar does not complicate the vascular dynamics.

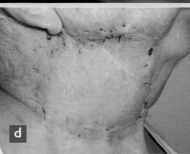

(d) Appearance at 3 weeks following surgery, with good healing despite the obvious existing scar within the newly devised flap.

TLC

Time (operation/cost)
60 minutes
Life quality (and aesthetics)
Good, with acceptable aesthetics
Complications
Nil, despite previous scar traversing flap

outcomes by facilitating free-flap donor sites where these are thought unavoidable (e.g. radial forearm flap).

One of the potential barriers to more widespread use of locoregional flaps in head and neck surgery is the vast array of flaps described during the extensive history of head and neck reconstruction (Strauch et al. 2009).* Few of the described flaps have the versatility necessary to permit reconstruction of different subunits of the head and neck. Many flaps are site-specific in their application, necessitating a significant breadth of experience for confident locoregional reconstruction in the head and neck. The keystone island flap, with its capacity to reconstruct defects in many regions and in defects of various sizes, demonstrates this versatility. This has created a whole new perspective.

The keystone flap and its geometric variants are well-suited to close head and neck defects. It has a reliable blood supply, demonstrates good healing even in irradiated tissues, is quick to perform and can be used in small or large defects in various subregions of the head and neck. Its geometry renders it difficult to see once the scar outline has matured, and the technique of islanding keystone flaps benefits patients by minimising postoperative pain. It is often the closest match to the missing tissue (like for like, the next best skin is the next best skin) in terms of skin colour, tissue quality and its response to age and gravity, resulting in improved aesthetics compared to other approaches. Other specific flaps can be utilised for the

---

* The earliest published local flaps for head and neck reconstruction are recorded in the *Sushruta* papyrus, which is over 2000 years old.

reconstruction of specific defects with excellent results, but few will be able to be applied in so many different areas and defects.

The purpose of this chapter is to illustrate, through the knowledge of neurovascular anatomy, potential donor sites and the principles of island flap elevation, as well as how keystone island flaps can be planned (with variants), raised and transferred in a reliable manner so as to solve numerous reconstructive challenges in this region. These principles will provide a sound basis upon which readers may develop their own surgical variations to suit the nature of each defect, the available donor tissues and the surrounding structures so as to maximise the functional and aesthetic outcomes.

PRINCIPLES OF FLAP ELEVATION IN THE HEAD AND NECK

The principles of raising keystone flaps in the head and neck are similar to those in other regions but with particular emphasis on the preservation of important neurovascular structures and closure of defects without distorting the surrounding features.

Anatomical layers of the face: preservation of the facial nerve

The facial nerve and its branches are essential to the resting tone and appearance of the face during facial expression. Facial nerve injury can result in functional issues, such as exposure keratitis of the eye with blindness, external nasal valving and drooling from the corner of the mouth. Asymmetrical appearance, worsened upon spontaneous facial movements, leads to significant social dysfunction, affecting numerous aspects of the patient's life.

When knowledge of the surface landmarks of these nerve branches (Fig 4.2) is combined with an understanding of the layers of the face and neck (Fig 4.3), it becomes possible to minimise the risk of facial nerve injury during flap dissection. The facial nerve is most at

◄ **FIGURE 4.2 Relevant landmarks for the facial nerve branches**

Of the five main branches, the frontal and marginal mandibular branches are most at risk due to their relatively superficial course. Pitanguy's line marks the frontal branch passage from the lower border of the tragus to a point 1.5 cm above the lateral brow.

(Reproduced with permission from Putz R, Pabtz R 2009 Sobotta – Atlas of human anatomy, English/Latin single volume edition, 14th edn, Elsevier, Munich.)

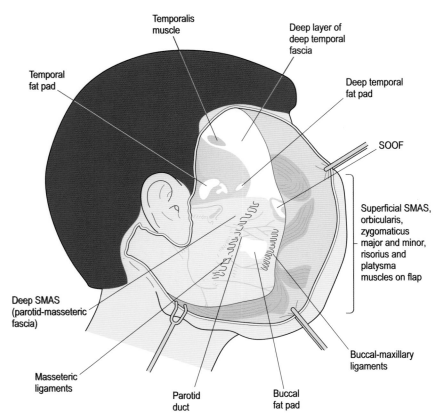

Temporalis
muscle

Deep layer of
deep temporal
fascia

Temporal
fat pad

Deep temporal
fat pad

SOOF

Superficial SMAS,
orbicularis,
zygomaticus
major and minor,
risorius and
platysma
muscles on flap

Deep SMAS
(parotid-masseteric
fascia)

Masseteric
ligaments

Parotid
duct

Buccal
fat pad

Buccal-maxillary
ligaments

◀ **FIGURE 4.3** **Dissection**
deep to the subcutaneous
musculo-aponeurotic system
(SMAS), demonstrating the
anatomical layer in which the
nerve branches lie following
their exit from within the
parotid gland

Any dissection down to or
deep to this plane should be
undertaken bluntly to avoid
nerve injury.

(Reproduced with permission from
Rees T, La Trenta G S 1994 Aesthetic
plastic surgery, 2nd edn, WB
Saunders, Philadelphia.)

risk during reconstruction of periauricular, temple, cheek or neck defects due to inadvertent nerve injury during flap elevation. The frontal branch can be damaged due to its relatively superficial course. The marginal mandibular branch may have variable anatomy around the angle of the mandible, leading to increased risk of injury. Staying above the muscular layer of the face and superficial to the investing layer of deep cervical fascia in the neck is the best way to avoid entering the plane of these nerves. Preoperative identification of the nerve branches potentially in the operative field, restriction of the depth of surgery where nerve branches could be at risk and use of blunt dissection in deep tissue planes all contribute to maintaining the functional integrity of the facial nerve branches.

Where facial nerve injury is expected due to tumour involvement, the geometry of the keystone flap closure can be modified to produce facial elevation on the affected side and, hence, help with static appearance. This can be combined with a tarsorrhaphy (immediate or delayed, temporary or permanent) to protect the eye.

Distortion of surrounding structures upon wound closure can also be an issue in the use of locoregional flaps in the head and neck. This is particularly important in cheek, periorbital and perioral reconstruction, where lower lid ectropion may result from a poorly planned and executed flap. Distortion from locoregional flaps can be minimised by: greater mobilisation of the keystone flaps than in other regions; suture inset either into deep tissues, such as periosteum, for greater support; or being designed so that lines of tension

bypass at-risk areas (i.e. sutured medially and laterally in the periorbital region). Increased flap mobilisation necessitates a thorough understanding of the neurovascular anatomy, with inclusion of fascia/muscle within the deepest layer of the flap where possible.

Neurovascular anatomy

All tissue flaps need a reliable arteriovenous supply. The head and neck offer a rich network of cutaneous vessels upon which flaps can be based (Figs 4.4 and 4.5). Previous surgery (particularly neck dissection) and/or radiotherapy and previous surgery can make locoregional flap elevation a challenge—such surgical sites in the elderly in Australia are rarely pristine. Part of the appropriate analysis of head and neck defects is the identification of arteriovenous or neurovascular structures as the basis for flap reconstruction (Table 4.1). Where possible, flaps should be planned to incorporate known, intact vessels and/or cutaneous nerves, improving their reliability, even following undermining, rotation or transposition. The vessels need not be formally explored unless it is likely that they have been ligated or damaged by previous surgery. Orienting keystone flaps along dermatomal axes is a useful guide to surgeons in their early use of the keystone flap, but it is no replacement for experience or careful assessment of the local neurovascular anatomy.**

** The first series of keystone island flaps by Behan were the size of thumbnails but now, after having performed more than 3000 keystone island flaps, the defect sizes may be over 22 × 20 cm for coverage of a scapula.

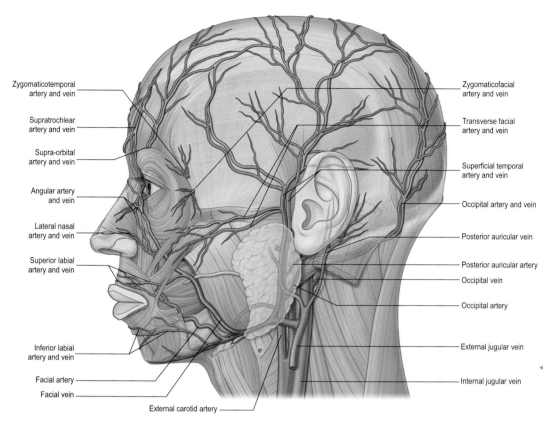

Zygomaticotemporal artery and vein
Supratrochlear artery and vein
Supra-orbital artery and vein
Angular artery and vein
Lateral nasal artery and vein
Superior labial artery and vein
Inferior labial artery and vein
Facial artery
Facial vein
External carotid artery

Zygomaticofacial artery and vein
Transverse facial artery and vein
Superficial temporal artery and vein
Occipital artery and vein
Posterior auricular vein
Posterior auricular artery
Occipital vein
Occipital artery
External jugular vein
Internal jugular vein

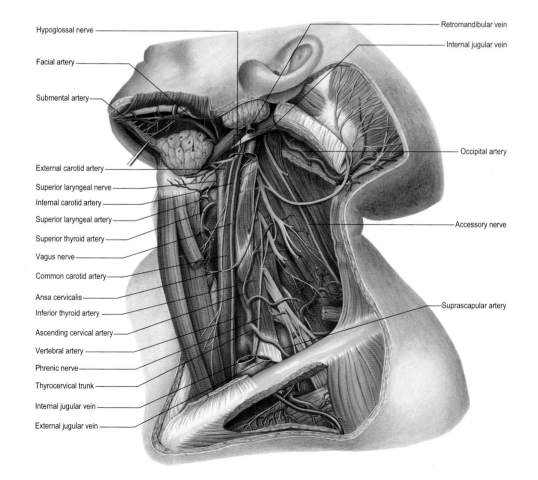

Hypoglossal nerve
Facial artery
Submental artery
External carotid artery
Superior laryngeal nerve
Internal carotid artery
Superior laryngeal artery
Superior thyroid artery
Vagus nerve
Common carotid artery
Ansa cervicalis
Inferior thyroid artery
Ascending cervical artery
Vertebral artery
Phrenic nerve
Thyrocervical trunk
Internal jugular vein
External jugular vein

Retromandibular vein
Internal jugular vein
Occipital artery
Accessory nerve
Suprascapular artery

◀ FIGURE 4.4 Diagrams demonstrating the major vessels and nerves supplying the skin of the head and neck

Note the predominance of supply from the external carotid artery and its branches. This parent vessel forms the basis for the majority of keystone flaps used in the neck and face, including the cervicosubmental island flap.

(Reproduced with permission from Gray H, Standring S 2005 Gray's anatomy: the anatomical basis of clinical practice, 39th edn. Churchill Livingstone, New York, Figs 28.7A, 29.13.)

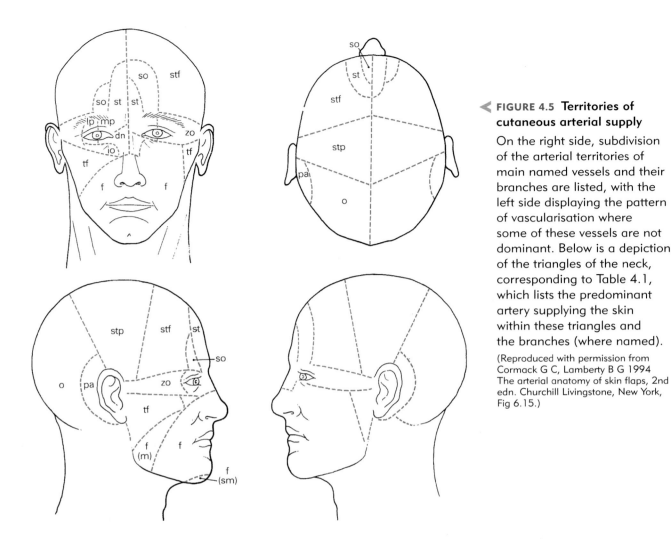

◀ **FIGURE 4.5 Territories of cutaneous arterial supply**

On the right side, subdivision of the arterial territories of main named vessels and their branches are listed, with the left side displaying the pattern of vascularisation where some of these vessels are not dominant. Below is a depiction of the triangles of the neck, corresponding to Table 4.1, which lists the predominant artery supplying the skin within these triangles and the branches (where named).

(Reproduced with permission from Cormack G C, Lamberty B G 1994 The arterial anatomy of skin flaps, 2nd edn. Churchill Livingstone, New York, Fig 6.15.)

Islanding is the key to our vascular success and acts as a buffer to partial flap necrosis by enhancing the vascular reliability of the perforator or direct supply to the periphery of the flap. This mandates sufficient perforator or direct supply. As a single flap, this makes the keystone island flap an invaluable tool for head and neck reconstruction.

Zones in head and neck reconstruction

To aid discussion of the neurovascular anatomy and of the ways that keystone island flaps can be applied to close various defects, we have subclassified the head and neck region into seven zones to aid this process. These zones are as follows:

1 periauricular
2 cheek
3 periorbital
4 perioral
5 scalp
6 nose
7 neck

The vascular basis of keystone island flaps in each of these zones can be either on remaining intact vessels within the zone or via vessels in adjacent zones to the defect, depending upon how the skin incision is planned. To understand the planning of these flaps, we will examine the specific requirements of each reconstructive zone with illustrative cases.

PERIAURICULAR

The periauricular region is a common and problematic area for reconstruction due to the prevalence of both primary and secondary cancer in this region. Defects may be in fields that have already undergone radiotherapy, making the use of local flaps problematic in some instances, and bone exposure is common following extirpation of disease or as a consequence of osteoradionecrosis in the mastoid. We have subclassified the periauricular region into the following defects:

1 central (Fig 4.6)
2 preauricular (Fig 4.7)
3 infra-auricular (Fig 4.8)
4 postauricular (Fig 4.9)
5 supra-auricular (Fig 4.10)

TABLE 4.1 Summary of cutaneous blood supply by regions

Skin over	Supplied by
NECK	
Submental triangle	Facial artery via submental branch
Digastrics triangle	Facial artery via direct branches
Carotid triangle	Superior thyroid artery via infrahyoid and sternomastoid branches
Muscular triangle	Superior thyroid artery Inferior thyroid artery via very small musculocutaneous perforators
Sternomastoid muscle	
Upper part	Posterior auricular artery via direct branches Occipital artery via descending branches Occipital artery via musculocutaneous perforators
Middle part	Superior thyroid artery
Lower part	Subclavian artery via direct branch
Occipital triangle	Occipital artery via descending branches
Omoclavicular triangle	Transverse cervical artery via direct branch Supraclavicular artery
Trapezius	
Upper part	Occipital artery and ascending ramus of superficial branch of transverse cervical artery
Lateral part	Supraclavicular artery and superficial branch of transverse cervical artery via musculocutaneous perforators
HEAD	
Scalp	
Forehead	Supratrochlear artery } of ophthalmic artery Supraorbital artery Frontal branch of superficial temporal artery
Temporoparietal region	Frontal branch of superficial temporal artery Parietal branch of superficial temporal artery
Occipital region	Occipital artery Posterior auricular artery
Periorbital region	Supraorbital artery Supratrochlear artery Lacrimal branch Zygomatico-orbital branch of superficial temporal artery Infraorbital branch of maxillary artery Angular artery—continuation of facial artery
Nose	External nasal branch of ophthalmic artery and its dorsal nasal branch Lateral nasal branch of facial artery Collumellar and alar branches of superior labial artery
Cheek	Infraorbital branch of maxillary artery Branches of facial artery/angular artery Premasseteric artery if present Transverse facial branch of superficial temporal artery
Lips	Superior labial artery Inferior labial artery Mental branch of inferior alveolar artery
Chin	Mental branch of inferior alveolar artery Submental branch of facial artery
Ear	
External surface	Anterior auricular branches of superficial temporal artery Perforating branches of posterior auricular artery
Cranial surface	Unnamed branch of superficial temporal artery Posterior auricular artery
Nasolabial fold	Direct branches of facial artery Terminal branches of infraorbital artery and transverse facial artery

(Reproduced with permission from Cormack G C, Lamberty B G H 1994 The arterial anatomy of skin flaps, 2nd edn. Churchill Livingstone, New York, Table 6.1.)

FIGURE 4.6

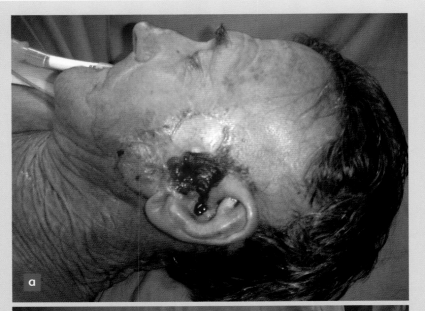

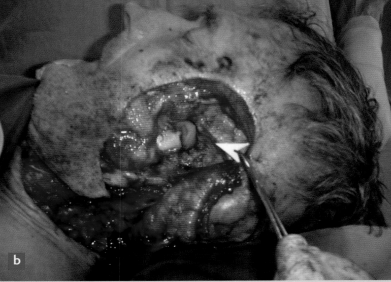

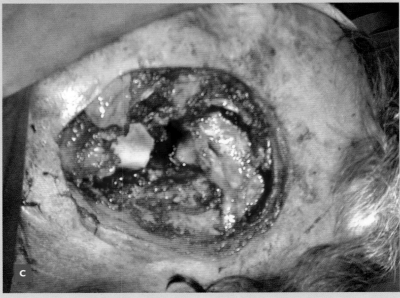

FIGURE 4.6 Management of a central periauricular defect by the use of the keystone island flap

(a) Preoperative appearance, demonstrating a fungating preauricular lesion. A secondary deposit of squamous cell carcinoma involving the parotid, conchal fossa of the ear.

(b) Part of the mastoid bone is removed during excision of the tumour.

(c) Following excision of the parotid disease, including the temporomandibular joint, a 10 × 8 cm defect is produced.

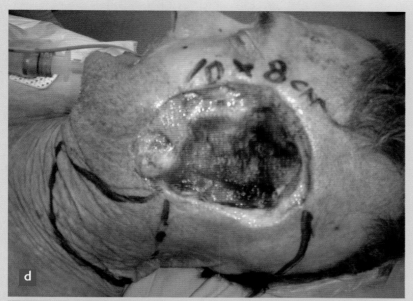

(d) A cervicosubmental (CSM) keystone island flap is designed across the midline in the submental area to permit sufficient reach to cover the defect to above the level of the zygomatic arch.

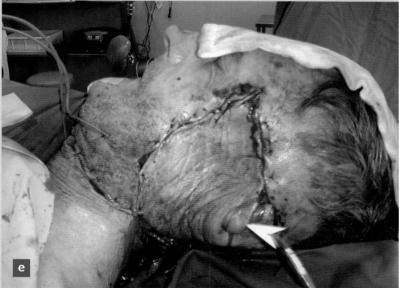

(e) The flap is inset and, due to the degree of transposition of the flap as an omega (Ω) variant, a significant dog ear is produced (arrow). This is excised in the primary operation (skin with minimal fat only) and the neck defect closed directly over a suction drain.

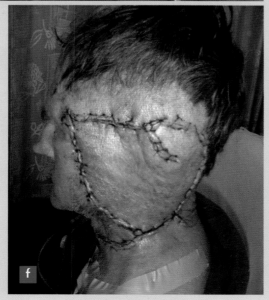

(f) Postoperative appearance demonstrating the vascular changes in the flap and good appearance with trimming of the dog ear. Good initial contour restoration.

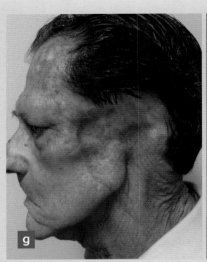

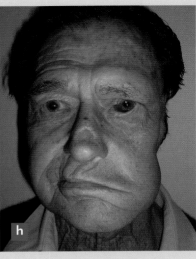

(Reproduced with permission from Behan F, Sizeland A 2006. Reiteration of the core principles of the Keystone island flap. ANZ J Surg 76(12):1127–9.)

(g) Appearance 3 years following surgery and radiotherapy, showing good skin colour match but loss of flap volume with time and radiotherapy. A late tarsorrhaphy has been performed.

(h) The stigmata of facial nerve paralysis are the most significant aesthetic issue for the patient, and his recurrent lower lid ectropion needed subsequent correction.

TLC

Time (operation/cost)
120 minutes

Life quality (and aesthetics)
Good, with ability to socialise in his town without embarrassment

Complications
Physiological tension provided static facial nerve reconstruction; after 3 years, his ectropion needed a tarsorrhaphy

FIGURE 4.7

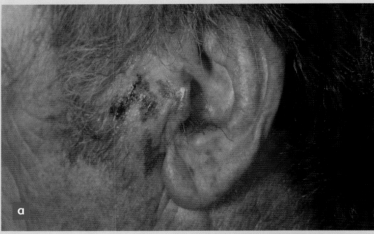

FIGURE 4.7 Anterior periauricular defect for reconstruction

A 63-year-old male with superficial spreading melanoma of the root of the helix: **(a)** with subsequent development of nodal disease within the preauricular and parotid nodes (4 × 4 cm)

(b) clinically and

(c) by computerised tomographic (CT) scanning.

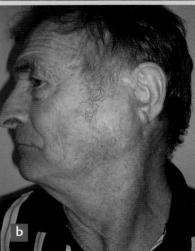

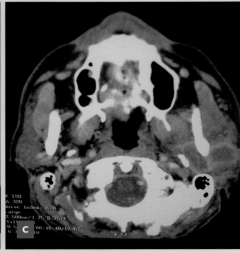

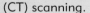

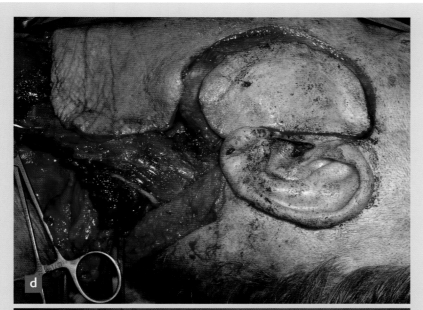

(d) Following neck dissection, the parotid and overlying involved skin are about to be removed to produce a 10 × 6 cm defect in the preauricular region with

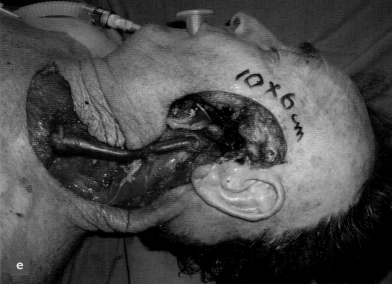

(e) sacrifice of the facial nerve.

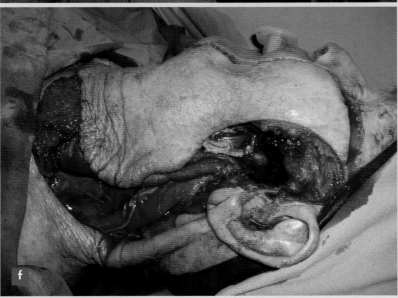

(f) A large anterior cheek and neck keystone island flap, based on facial artery perforators (retrograde) and the infraorbital neurovascular bundle, is raised (a composite SMAS and CSM flap). The undermined neck skin shows poor colour consistent with compromised vascularity. The immediate vascular augmentation concept (IVAC) principle is applied by incorporating this skin as part of the island flap to improve its functional perfusion. Note the improved colour relative to its appearance in **(e)**—pre-islanding.

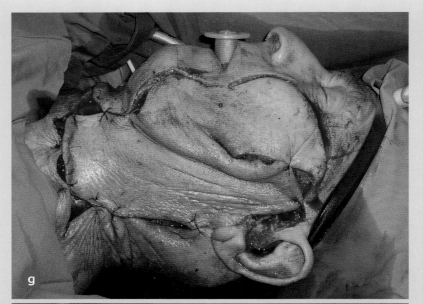

(g) The omega (Ω) variant closure allows the inferior limit of the flap to be transposed into the defect. The physiological tension produced aids in static reconstruction of the facial nerve.

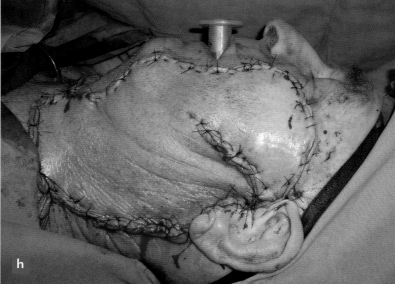

(h) Good vascular perfusion on completion of flap inset, with immediate revision of the dog ear.

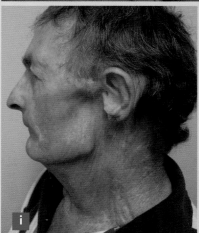

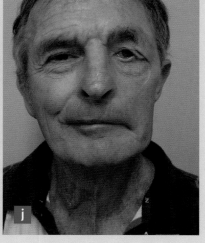

See video for Figure 4.7

TLC

Time (operation/cost)		
90 minutes		
Life quality (and aesthetics)		
Good, acceptable—continued work as an auctioneer		
Complications		
Vascular embarrassment of the undermined neck flap was eliminated by IVAC, no complications		

(i) Lateral view 18 months post operation.

(j) Frontal view showing acceptable appearance despite facial nerve palsy with delayed tarsorrhaphy.

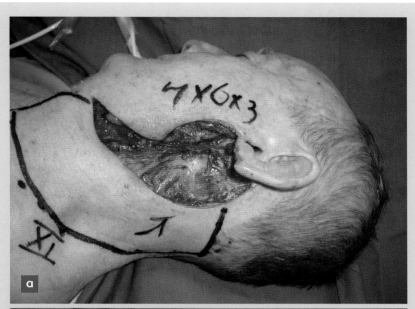

FIGURE 4.8 Infra-auricular defect for closure

(a) Squamous cell carcinoma involving the parotid gland and requiring a mastoidectomy that resulted in a 4 × 6 cm defect that was 3 cm deep. An inferiorly designed keystone based on sternocleidomastoid branches is designed for defect closure.

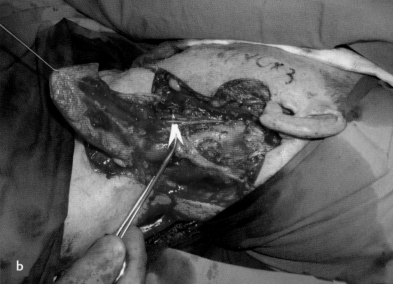

(b) Flap elevation deep to the platysma demonstrates the intact vascular perforator entering the base of the flap. (It is not necessary to visualise these, only to preserve them.)

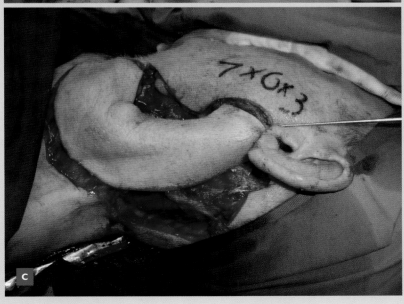

(c) Initial transposition of the flap under minimal tension to effect wound closure.

FIGURE 4.8

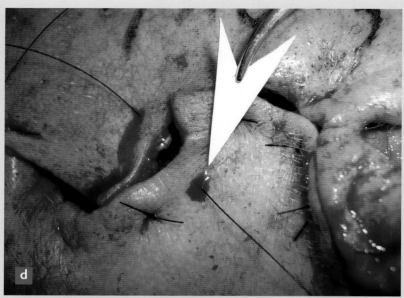

(d) A *red dot sign* on the flap demonstrating increased bright red bleeding from the flap side relative to the non-flap side.

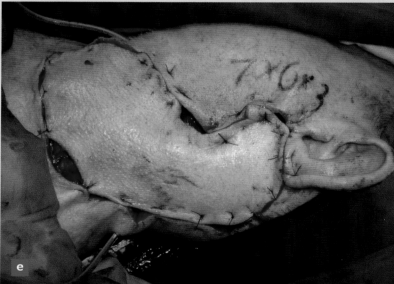

(e) Strategic mattress suturing used to effect flap positioning prior to definitive continuous everting mattress suturing to even out tension across the flap. Note the mild pallor of the tip of the flap prior to evening out tension.

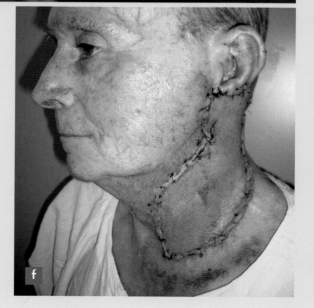

(f) Postoperative view demonstrating good flap survival and healing.

See video for Figure 4.8

TLC

Time (operation/cost)
50 minutes
Life quality (and aesthetics)
Good, observe sequential change in appearance after radiotherapy (with the patient smiling on completion of treatment)
Complications
Nil

FIGURE 4.9

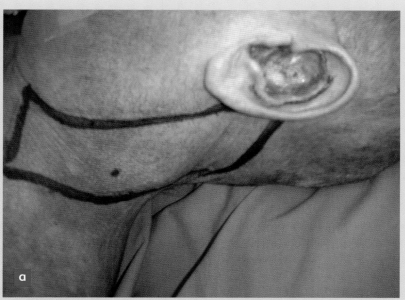

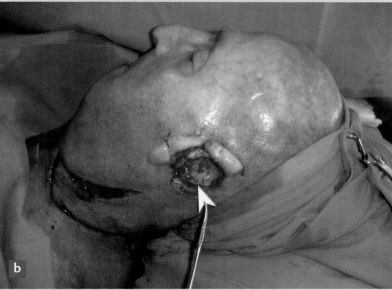

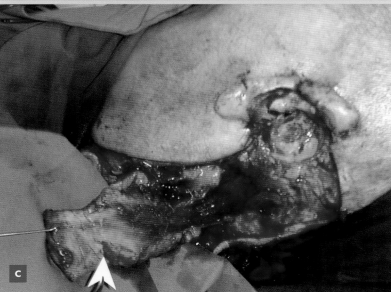

FIGURE 4.9 Postauricular defect reconstruction with keystone island flap

(a) An 84-year-old male with a basal cell carcinoma of the left conchal bowl extending to the external auditory canal and measuring approximately 4 × 3 cm. The mark-out of the posterior keystone island flap sits along the line of the C3 dermatome and is planned to include the great auricular nerve and branches of the cervical plexus, along with perforators from the sternocleidomastoid muscle.

(b) Surgical defect 4 × 3 cm down to the mastoid process. The helix is displaced anteriorly to facilitate the reconstruction of the external auditory canal by the keystone island flap.

(c) The keystone island flap is raised in its upper half and the arrow indicates the flap during the hyperaemic phase of increased vascular perfusion associated with islanding.

(Reproduced with permission from Behan F, Sizeland A, Gilmour F, Hui A, Seel M, Lo CH 2010 Use of the keystone island flap for advanced head and neck cancer in the elderly—a principle of amelioriation. J Plast Reconstr Aesthet Surg 63(5):739–45.)

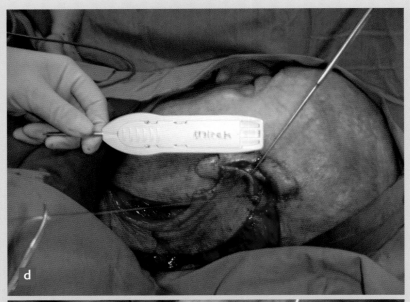

(d) A bone anchoring suture is used to stabilise the attachment at the external auditory canal.

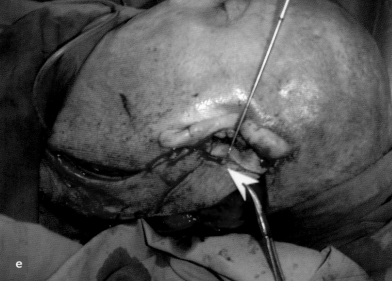

(e) Sufficient vascularity is gained by islanding a bridge of skin across the distal third of the flap, which can be de-epithelialised to allow inset of the retracted pinna of the ear in order to optimise aesthetics.

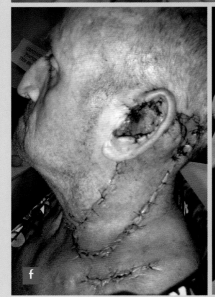

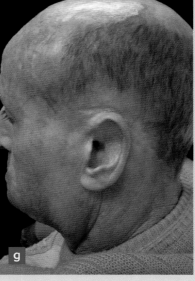

(f) Appearance at 1 week following surgery, demonstrating robust survival of the flap despite de-epithelialisation below the level of the tip.

(g) Good aesthetic result obvious on longer follow-up following an uneventful 6-week course of radiotherapy.

TLC

Time (operation/cost)
100 minutes
Life quality (and aesthetics)
Good, aesthetic preservation of the helix by immediate inset into the keystone island flap
Complications
Nil

FIGURE 4.10

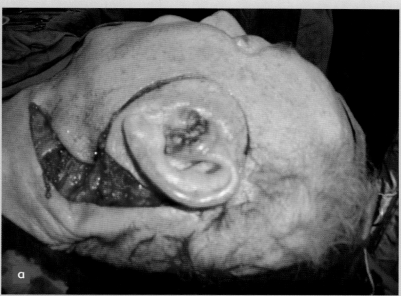

FIGURE 4.10 **Supra-auricular defect reconstruction in a 78-year-old male with squamous cell carcinoma of the conchal fossa extending down the left external auditory canal**

(a) Surgical specimen, including auriculectomy and dissection of level II, III and IV nodes.

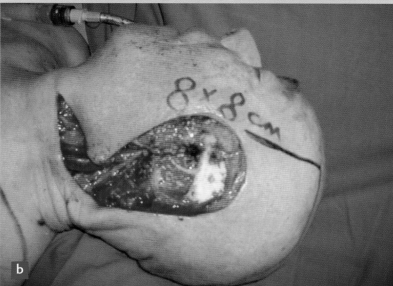

(b) An 8 × 8 cm defect is produced, including exposed cranium (without pericranium/periosteum).

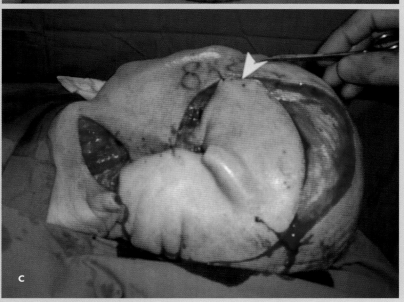

(c) A keystone island flap is designed superior to the defect with its base extending down posterior to the defect to incorporate the posterior auricular artery.

(Reproduced with permission from Behan F, Sizeland A, Gilmour F, Hui A, Seel M, Lo CH 2010 Use of the keystone island flap for advanced head and neck cancer in the elderly—a principle of amelioriation. J Plast Reconstr Aesthet Surg 63(5):739–45.)

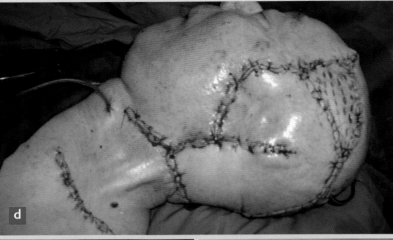

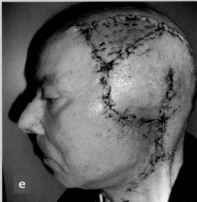

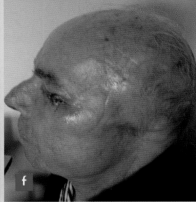

(d) Insertion over the external auditory canal site (for delayed reconstruction of the canal if the patient desires). Note the increase in vascularity in this omega (Ω) flap variant of the keystone. The secondary defect in the scalp will not close directly, therefore, a fenestrated full-thickness skin graft is applied from the supraclavicular area.

(e) Appearance at 10 days.

(f) Appearance at 2 years with delayed tarsorrhaphy to assist with eye closure following facial nerve palsy.

TLC

Time (operation/cost)
120 minutes
Life quality (and aesthetics)
Good, reasonable aesthetics—full-thickness graft provided good contour match
Complications
Static facial nerve support with tarsorrhaphy after 3 years and radiotherapy

The keystone island flaps most commonly used to close these defects can be classified as follows (Fig 4.11):

1 anterior (SMAS) keystone island flap
2 posterior (nuchal) keystone island flap
3 inferior (cervicosubmental) keystone island flap
4 superior (scalp) keystone island flap.

The flaps are named by the principle fascial components and location from which they are derived. The SMAS refers to the superficial musculoaponeurotic system of the face, and the natural elasticity or laxity of the cheek skin can be raised, based upon this system, with its associated neurovascular support, and mobilised posteriorly for periauricular closure. The postauricular region is characterised by well-developed deep fascia that requires circumferential division for full mobilisation during flap inset. This fascia (prior to division) is in continuity with the ligamentum nuchae of the occipital region and has, therefore, been termed a nuchal keystone island flap. The cervicosubmental (CSM) island flap (see Fig 4.1) is raised to include the platysma and its overlying fat, fascia and skin within the C2–C3 dermatome, and is based upon perforators from the external carotid artery branches. The scalp keystone island flaps are specific subtypes on the basis of their vascular supply. There are very few (if any) perforators in this region, but numerous direct vessels

permitting easy flap elevation, as long as these feeding vessels are retained at the margin of the flap.

Existing techniques for reconstruction of this region are encompassed in only a few types of flap. The pectoralis major flap (Ariyan 1979) is a major flap for the reconstruction of defects in this region as long as they do not extend above the level of the zygomatic arch. Our practice is to try to preserve this flap as a lifeboat for salvage surgery. The pectoralis major flap clearly provides significant benefit over other approaches in instances where there is a significant volume defect and with exposure of major vessels, such as the internal jugular vein. Keystone island flaps can be used effectively for robust fasciocutaneous coverage in these cases but they lack the bulk of the pectoralis major flap in such instances. Keystone island flaps can be used in conjunction with the pectoralis major flap to minimise skin paddle size and permit direct closure of the chest donor site (Fig 4.12). Other flaps used locoregionally include the cervicofacial flap, temporalis fascia flaps combined with skin grafting (or in combination with keystone island flaps in our practice) and the deltopectoral flap (Bakamjian et al. 1971) and its variants. A number of additional approaches have been published in relatively small series within the literature, but are not in widespread practice (Strauch 2009).

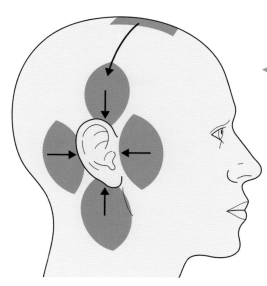

◀ **FIGURE 4.11 Diagrammatic representation of the types of keystone island flaps used for periauricular reconstruction, including the anterior (SMAS), posterior (nuchal), inferior (cervicosubmental) keystone and superior (scalp) keystone island flaps**

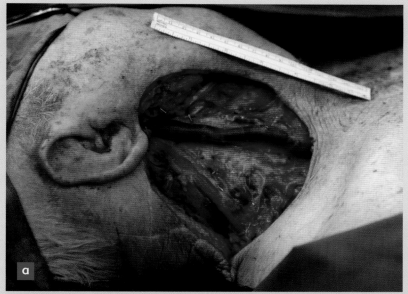

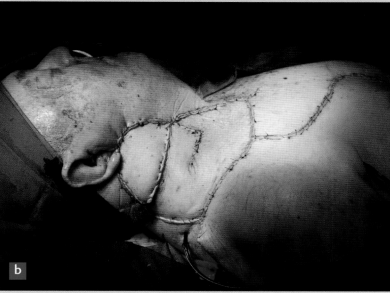

FIGURE 4.12 Demonstration of the capacity to undermine keystone island flaps while preserving their neurovascular supply

(a) An 8 × 12 cm defect with exposed internal jugular vein following excision of fungating secondary squamous cell carcinoma involving the jugular chain of cervical nodes in a patient with chronic lymphocytic leukaemia (CLL). A pectoralis major flap was selected as the reconstruction of choice given the patient's comorbidities and need to cover the internal jugular vein, where postoperative radiotherapy was planned; however, the size of the skin defect would result in a sizeable skin graft to the chest wall. Therefore, a keystone island flap, based on the transverse cervical artery, was raised to minimise the skin defect.

(b) The keystone is closed against itself (omega (Ω) variant) and the pectoralis major flap tunnelled under the flap to be delivered into the residual skin defect. In this way the entire distal muscle was used to cover the internal jugular vein, with the keystone flap covering its lower half.

FIGURE 4.12

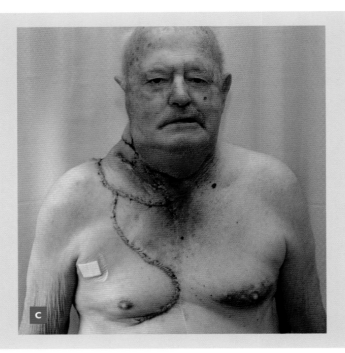

(c) Postoperative appearance showing direct closure of the pectoralis donor site. The posterior and anterior borders of the keystone flap underwent superficial necrosis during radiotherapy, which coincided with an exacerbation of his CLL, necessitating debridement and further advancement of the neck skin. This was well-tolerated by the patient.

TLC

Time (operation/cost)
150 minutes
Life quality (and aesthetics)
Excellent healing with minor flap necrosis developing after 2 weeks as an indicator of local recurrence in the setting of existing CLL
Complications
Immediate local recurrence, additional local flap for repair

Keystone island flaps for closure of defects in this region are principally raised on branches of the facial, superior thyroid and occipital vessels. The cervicosubmental keystone flap is a workhorse of reconstruction for large defects in this region (Ariyan 1979, Behan et al. 2011), with keystone flaps raised using cheek tissue and based on the facial artery most commonly used for smaller and anterior defects. Figures 4.6 to 4.10 show some typical defects in this region and demonstrate keystone elevation and closure of these defects. Figure 4.13 shows a free-flap closure of a similar defect. With time, free flaps in this region undergo pin-cushioning and ptosis of the flap, with poor cosmesis. Buried free-tissue transfer to this region has been described recently but this is principally for contour correction following parotidectomy rather than for fasciocutaneous closure (Cannady et al. 2010).

FIGURE 4.13 A 45-year-old man with multiple basal cell carcinomas of the right temple. The tumour developed basi-squamous differentiation with metastatic spread to the preauricular region. This figure (shown as Figure 2.9) is re-presented here now that our flap classification scheme has been described and to aid discussion of the relative merits of forms of flap reconstruction in the head and neck region

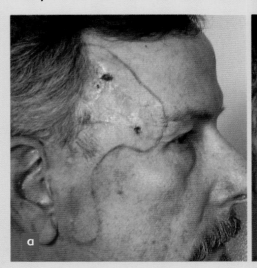

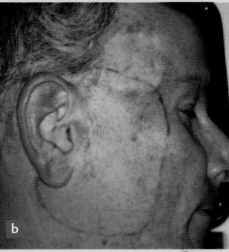

(a) Appearance at presentation with lesions of the right temple and small area of cutaneous involvement in front of the ear.

(b) Following excision of the primary lesion in the temple with skin graft reconstruction, lymphatic spread to the parotid became evident.

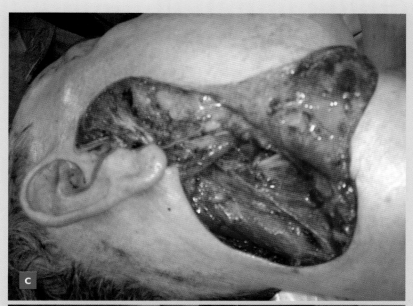

(c) Surgical defect following superficial parotidectomy with an anterior, undermined flap.

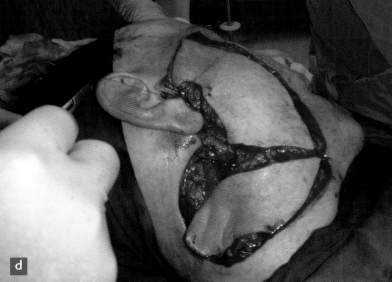

(d) SMAS keystone flap of the cheek is raised anterior to the defect and the undermined region has its perfusion augmented by incorporation within a larger, posterior cervicosubmental island keystone variant using IVAC.

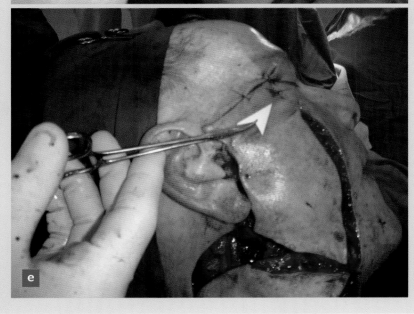

(e) A *red dot sign* of the SMAS cheek keystone flap demonstrates reliable perfusion of the flap.

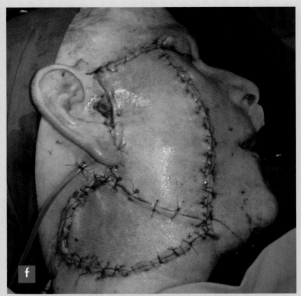

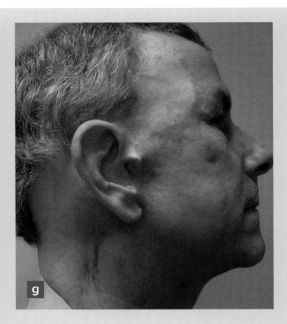

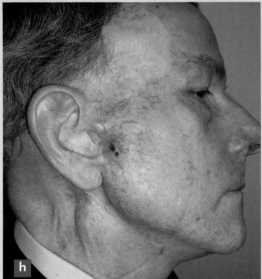

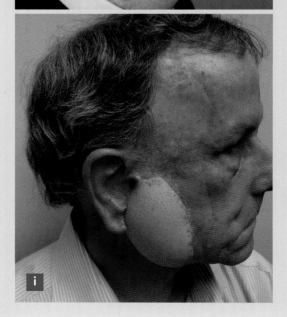

(f) Upon closure of both keystone flaps, excellent cutaneous vascularity is evident with good physiological tension.

(g) Appearance after 5 years before recurrence.

(h) Five years later, recurrent disease developed in the preauricular region.

(i) A free anterolateral thigh flap reconstruction of the preauricular region performed by another surgeon for recurrent disease. The anterior border of the previous SMAS keystone flap is visible approximately 2 cm anterior to the free flap. This highlights the differences between the postoperative appearances of free-flap reconstructions versus keystone flap reconstructions. The patient feels very self-conscious due to the poor colour match of the skin and significant ptosis of the flap. Revisional surgery is planned to improve his appearance.

TLC: Free-flap reconstruction

Time (operation/cost)		
360 minutes		
Life quality (and aesthetics)		
Poor with some social isolation, poor colour match and obvious ptosis		
Complications		
Needs revision		

CHEEK AND TEMPLE DEFECTS

Defects of the cheek and temple are two of the next most common large fasciocutaneous defects in the facial region. Skin graft reconstruction of these defects offers a poor contour restoration and cannot be undertaken for through-and-through defects into the oral cavity or over exposed bone. Local flap reconstruction can be plagued by distortion of important surrounding structures, such as the lower lid of the eye (ectropion or scleral show), the alar of the nose and the corner of the mouth (asymmetry). The unusual shape of the keystone flap drapes over this region well and, following wound healing, the aesthetics are generally very good. Care must be taken during blunt dissection of the deeper tissues so as to avoid facial nerve and parotid duct injury, but significant mobilisation of flaps in this region can be undertaken safely with this approach. Local neurovascular bases for keystone flaps include the facial/angular and infraorbital pedicles medially, zygomaticofacial, superficial temporal and transverse facial arteries superoposteriorly and the superior thyroid vessels inferiorly. The cervicosubmental flap can be used for larger defects and is particularly useful for reconstructing regions of hair-bearing skin in males, despite a mild difference in skin volume and colour. The cervicosubmental flap can be continued across the midline in the neck to permit coverage of defects extending beyond the zygomatic arch. Figure 3.7 demonstrates a representative clinical case of keystone reconstruction of defects in this region.

PERIORBITAL REGION

Few regions of the face are as sensitive in terms of the requirements of both aesthetic and functional reconstruction as the region immediately around the eye. Here, eyelid closure with the appropriate vector of contact between the lids and globe is paramount, but closely followed by the need to provide acceptable aesthetics. Such a specialised region has a very large number of described flaps for its reconstruction. Full-thickness eyelid reconstruction is based upon reconstruction of the two lamellae of the lids. The superficial lamella is composed of the orbicularis oculi muscle and skin. The deep lamella is formed by the tarsal plate and conjunctiva. A review of the available approaches for eyelid reconstruction is beyond the scope of this text, but keystone island flaps can be used for superficial lamella reconstruction, particularly in the lower lid, and truly come into their own in fasciocutaneous reconstruction near the inner and outer canthi. In this region, some of the benefits of using keystone island flaps include: they are curved to suit the local crease lines and curvature of the periorbital region; their islanding and multiple methods of movement into defects makes it easier to inset them without distorting the eyelids; and their reliable perfusion allows undermining and thinning of the flap at the time of the primary surgery to allow as close a match to the thin superficial lamella as possible. Multiple neurovascular and vascular pedicles are present in this region as the basis for keystone flaps, including the infraorbital, supratrochlear and supraorbital nerves and arteries and the angular, external nasal, infratrochlear, zygomaticofacial, zygomaticotemporal and superficial temporal arteries and their branches. Figure 4.14 demonstrates closure of a periorbital defect through the use of a keystone island flap. We hope that surgeons experienced in periorbital reconstruction may consider the use of the keystone island flap to augment their existing reconstructive techniques.

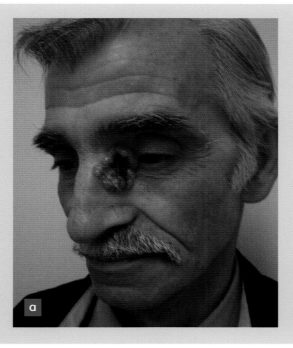

FIGURE 4.14 Periorbital reconstruction involving the inner canthus and bridge of the nose. A 56-year-old man with advanced basal cell carcinoma involving the underlying bone

(**a**) Preoperative view demonstrating large inner canthal lesion involving the canalicular system.

(Reproduced with permission from Behan F, Sizeland A, Gilmour F, Hui A, Seel M, Lo CH 2010 Use of the keystone island flap for advanced head and neck cancer in the elderly—a principle of amelioration. J Plast Reconstr Aesthet Surg 63(5):739–45.)

FIGURE 4.14

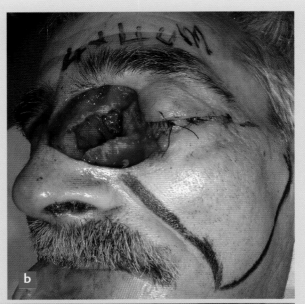

(b) A 4 × 4 cm defect following surgical excision, including the medial third of both eyelids, caruncle, nasal bones and part of the ethmoid complex. A cheek-based keystone flap, respecting natural skin creases, is designed with the infraorbital vessels at its base.

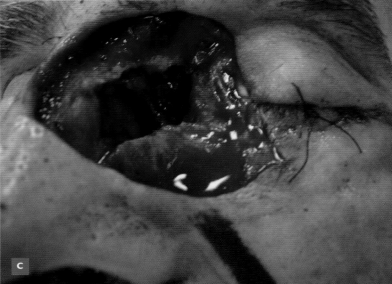

(c) Close-up view of the defect showing the bony defect.

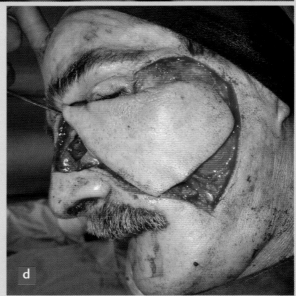

(d) Flap mobilised and advanced into the defect.

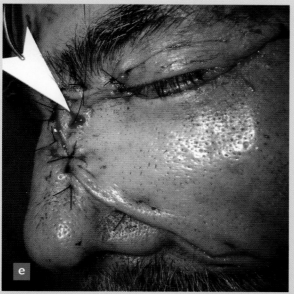

(e) A *red dot sign* indicating good blood supply to the tip of the flap. The inner aspect of the defect was allowed to mucosalise. The upward sweep of the flap provides support for the lower eyelid to minimise the risk of ectropion.

(f) Overview of the closure showing good eversion and lid support.

(g) Appearance at 5 days as swelling is starting to reduce.

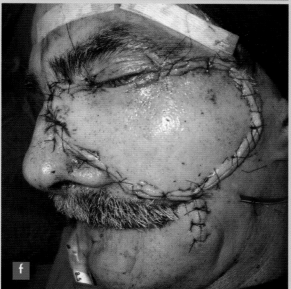

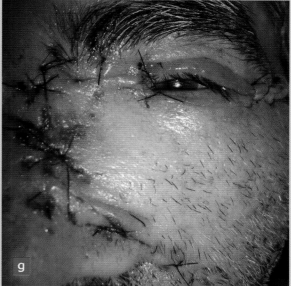

(h) At 12 months following surgery, there is no epiphora. Nasal drainage allowed through mucosalisation of the deep surface of the flap.

See video for Figure 4.14

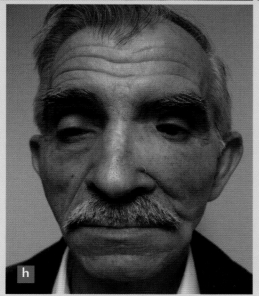

TLC

Time (operation/cost)
90 minutes
Life quality (and aesthetics)
Good with acceptable aesthetics—patient returned to social interaction
Complications
Mild epiphora that resolved without intervention

PERIORAL REGION

A number of parallels can be drawn between reconstruction of the periorbital region and perioral reconstruction. Both have orbicularis muscles (oculi and oris, respectively). Reconstruction of lip defects includes consideration of myocutaneous coverage, as well as mucosal lining. The fact that functional reconstruction must be undertaken in as aesthetic a manner as possible deserves repetition. The goals of reconstruction include maintenance of oral competence, sufficient opening to allow deglutition, oral care and insertion and removal of dental prostheses where required, and facilitation of speech, with sufficient aesthetics (including vermilion reconstruction where required) to permit positive social interaction. Again, this specialised region has had multiple flaps described for its reconstruction (Strauch et al. 2009). The flaps can be divided into vermilion and skin flaps, those containing skin only, and mucosal/tongue flaps. Each has its own advantages and limitations, particularly vermilion containing flaps, which can result in microstomia with larger defects.

Keystone reconstruction of the perioral region adds to existing approaches by providing reliable fasciocutaneous reconstruction in this region through the importation of closely matching local tissue while maximising mouth opening. Keystone flaps can be raised to include muscle for myocutaneous reconstruction and can be combined with mucosal advancement for vermilion and commissure reconstruction with mucosalisation of secondary intraoral defects if required. The facial artery and its branches, including the superior and inferior labial vessels and the mental neurovascular pedicles, are all useful for reconstruction in this region. Larger defects can be reconstructed by a combination of local cheek/lip keystone advancement flaps and a cervicosubmental flap from the commissure to the most lateral part of the defect. The robust vascularity of these flaps allows them to be split in the primary setting in combination with a commissuroplasty to widen the oral vestibule. Such an approach with other forms of non-islanded flap could lead to flap loss. The new tissue they import minimises distortion of the mouth and contributes to the postoperative aesthetics. Figures 4.15 and 4.16 demonstrate cases of perioral defects closed through the use of keystone island flaps.

FIGURE 4.15

FIGURE 4.15 Perioral defect in a 78-year-old female

(Reproduced with permission from Behan F, Sizeland A, Gilmour F, Hui A, Seel M, Lo CH 2010 Use of the keystone island flap for advanced head and neck cancer in the elderly—a principle of amelioration. J Plast Reconstr Aesthet Surg 63(5):739–45.)

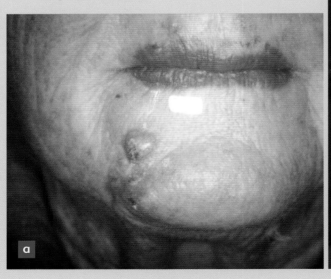

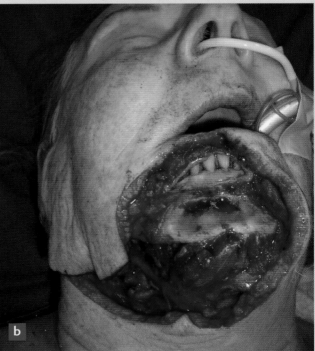

(a) A recurrent squamous cell carcinoma over the mental foramen, fixed to the underlying bone.

(b) The 8 × 8 cm surgical defect with preservation of a margin of vermilion, but half of the lower lip at the vermilion border is missing and two-thirds is missing at the gingivolabial sulcus. The mandible is exposed due to removal of the periosteum and a small amount of cortical bone.

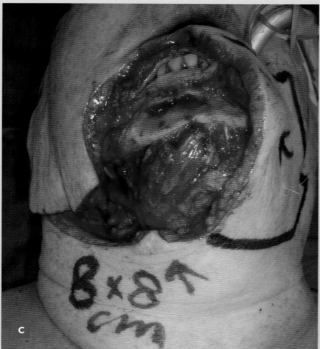

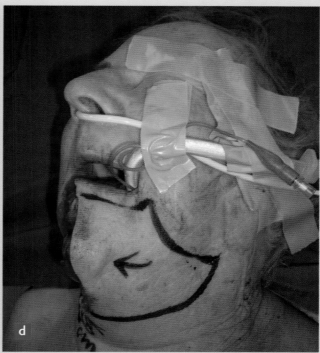

(c) Vascularised soft tissue cover is necessary and sought from the contralateral lower lip and cheek.

(d) Design of a contralateral asymmetrical keystone island flap based on the left mental neurovascular pedicle and the facial artery. A small V–Y point is present at the left labial commissure and a larger V–Y point inferolaterally.

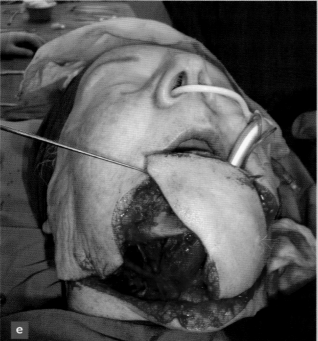

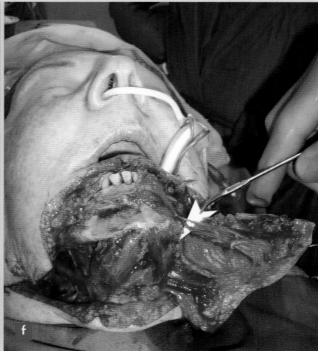

(e) Following elevation, the flap is advanced into the defect.

(f) The arrow indicates the mental neurovascular pedicle that supplies both sensation and vascularity to the flap.

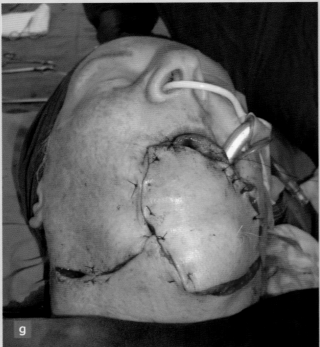

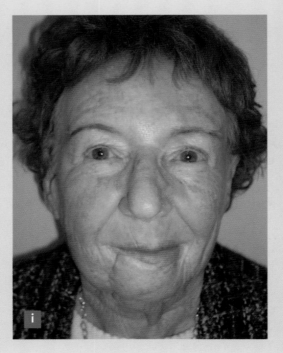

(g) Strategic mattress suturing provides approximation followed by subsequent hemming sutures. Note the increased vascularity with islanding (IVAC).

(h) Swollen but healthy appearance of the flap at 5 days.

(i) Appearance of the patient at 2 years.

See video for Figure 4.15

TLC

Time (operation/cost)		
90 minutes		
Life quality (and aesthetics)		
Good, with acceptable aesthetics		
Complications		
Occasional drooling, and uses straw for drinking		

FIGURE 4.16

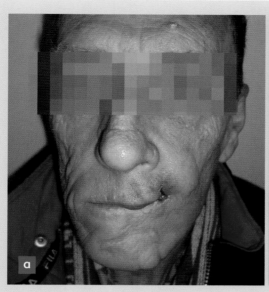

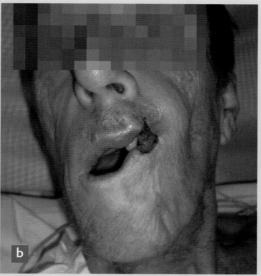

FIGURE 4.16 Perioral defect in 56-year-old male with radio-recurrent squamous cell carcinoma of the left oral commissure following previous excision and Abbe flap

(a) Extent of the defect is not apparent by direct visualisation.

(b) Trismus limits visibility of the lesion, but intraoral examination identifies attachment to the maxilla.

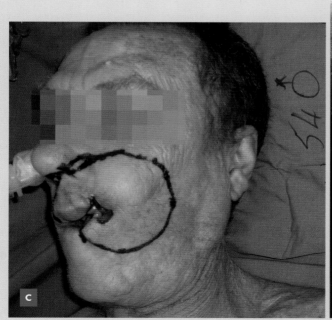

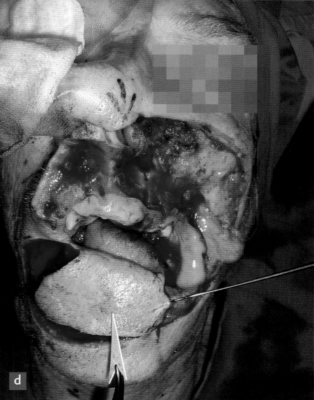

(c) Mark-out of the surgical excision.

(d) The defect is evident, crossing the midline of the upper lip and the left third of the lower lip. The arrow indicates a mental neurovascular pedicle-based flap with preservation of the mucosa of the vermilion, but mobilisation of the underlying orbicularis. This flap is advanced towards the site of the planned new left oral commissure.

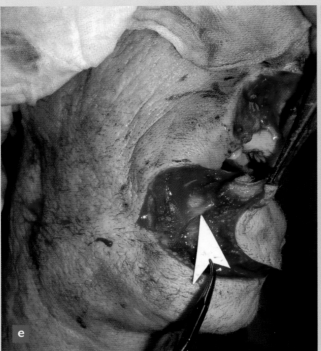

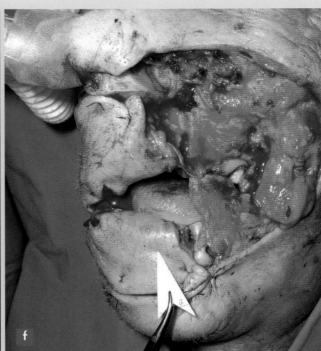

(e) The arrow indicates the inferior labial artery feeding into the upper part of the flap to augment its supply.

(f) The buccal mucosa is advanced to close the defect during lateral closure. Erythema of the lower flap (arrow) is evident. An upper lip flap has been raised in an analogous manner.

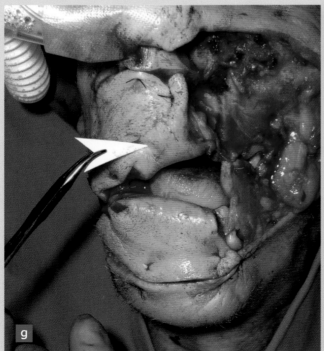

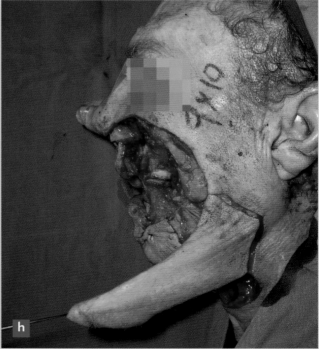

(g) Final position of the upper and lower lip flaps prior to closure of the lateral defect and left oral commissure reconstruction.

(h) A cervicosubmental (CSM) island flap is raised in irradiated tissue.

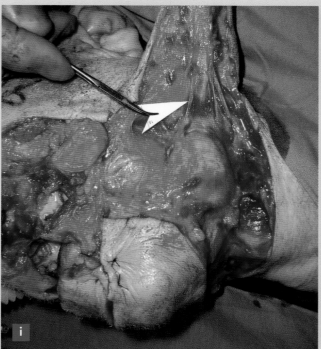

(i) This CSM island flap is based on direct branches from the facial artery (arrow) along with preservation of the cervical plexus branches by blunt dissection.

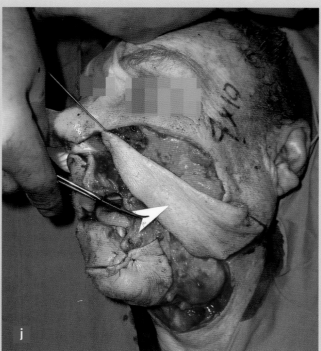

(j) Initial white lines of tension with single point fixation prior to definitive closure.

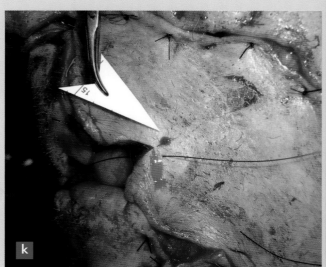

(k) Despite these lines, a *red dot sign* (arrow) is obvious during suturing of the new left oral commissure formed by division of the leading edge of the flap to form the commissure.

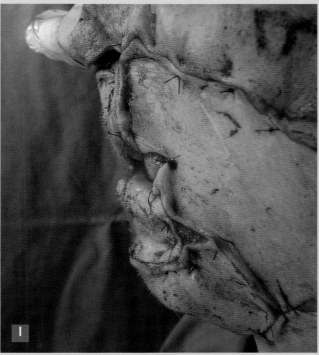

(l) Further suturing evens the tension across the flap, leading to the development of a vascular flare.

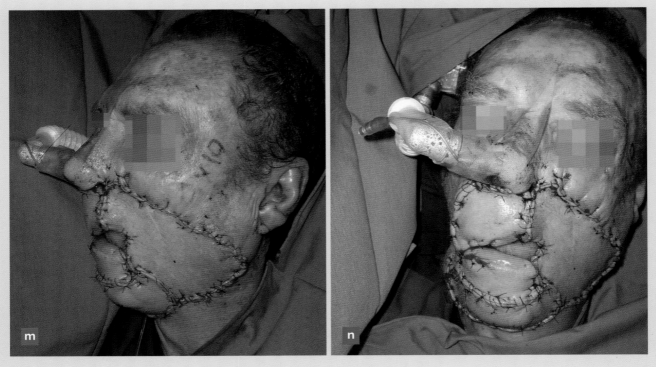

(m) Lateral appearance on completion of defect closure with direct closure of the CSI flap donor.

(n) Anterior view.

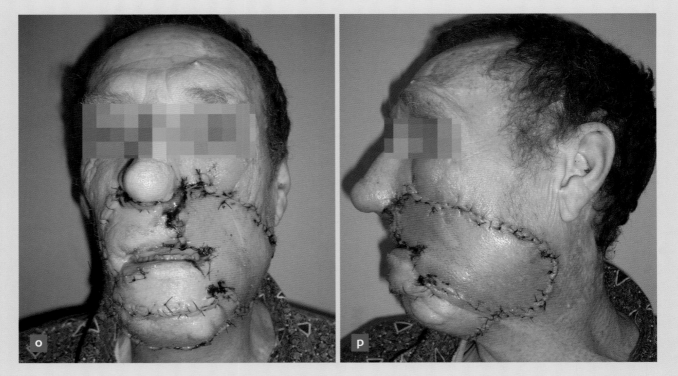

(o) & **(p)** Appearance at 2 days with noticeable redness towards the tip of the CSI flap consistent with previous irradiation and prolonged flap length.

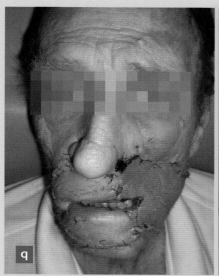
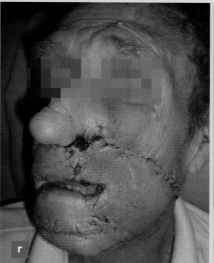
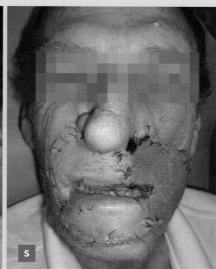

(q)–(s) Appearance at 5 days.

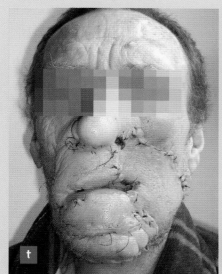
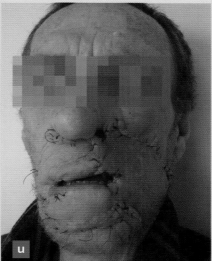
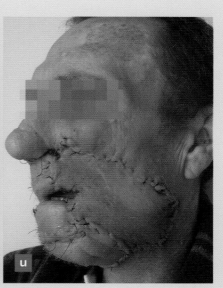

(t)–(v) Appearance at 10 days showing resolution of the redness and reliable healing.

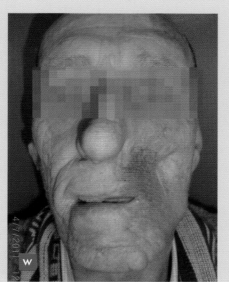

(w) The appearance at 9 months with no recurrence.

See video for Figure 4.16

TLC

Time (operation/cost)
130 minutes
Life quality (and aesthetics)
Good, but with early return to smoking, reasonable aesthetics
Complications
Oral commissure asymmetry corrected surgically at 8 weeks, non-compliant

THE SCALP

Locoregional flaps provide the ideal form of reconstruction for defects of the scalp due to the need to be suitably hair-bearing. Unfortunately, the convex nature of the scalp makes it difficult to provide sufficient tissue for reconstruction without the presence of significant dog ears or large, near-circumferential incisions for closure of scalp defects. This convexity of the scalp necessitates the use of flap variants that reproduce this convexity, including the omega (Ω) variant keystone and goblet island flaps. As with keystone island flaps in other regions, it is advisable to incorporate the equivalent of the panniculus carnosus layer within the flap base. In the scalp, this is the galea aponeurotica and/or occipitofrontalis. Use of the goblet island flap variant is demonstrated for fasciocutaneous reconstruction of a scalp defect in Figure 4.17.

FIGURE 4.17

FIGURE 4.17 Scalp defect in a 51-year-old woman with atypical fibroxanthoma of the vertex of the scalp. Keystone principles are utilised on the scalp as opposed to a strict keystone design

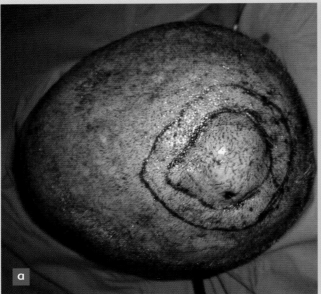

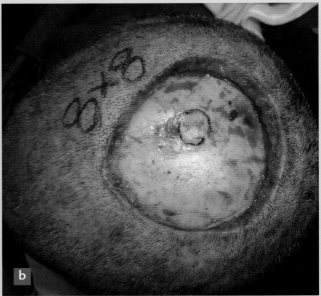

(a) Mark-out of the lesion and margins.

(b) The surgical defect (8 × 8 cm) following excision, with exposed cranium.

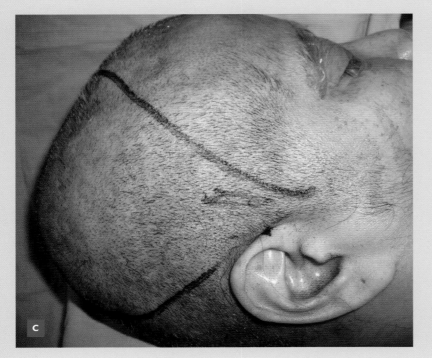

(c) A right superficial temporal artery-based goblet island flap is designed with a major V–Y point inferiorly.

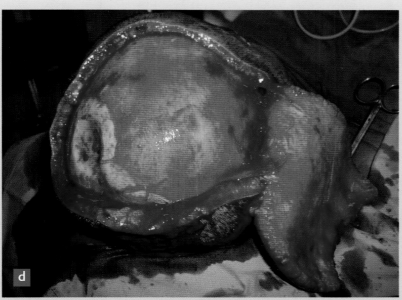

(d) The flap is bluntly dissected in the subgaleal plane with sharp elevation at the temporal lines.

(e) Inset of the flap over the defect.

(f) V–Y flap undertaken above the ear to facilitate closure.

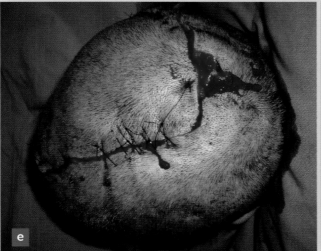

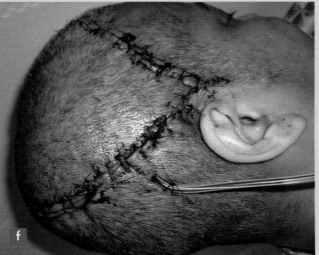

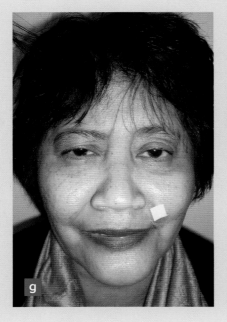

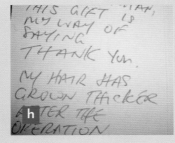

THIS GIFT ___ ___, MY WAY OF SAYING THANK You. MY HAIR HAS GROWN THICKER AFTER THE OPERATION

(h) A copy of her Christmas card where she has independently noted this increased hair growth.

(g) Postoperative appearance with full hair growth that is thicker in the island flap region than in the non-islanded hair-bearing scalp (a common clinical finding for islanded flaps in the scalp in our experience).

TLC

Time (operation/cost)	
100 minutes	
Life quality (and aesthetics)	
Good, hair quality improved in thickness and texture within flap (characteristic of scalp island flaps)	
Complications	
Nil	

FIGURE 4.18

NOSE

Some of the earliest flaps ever described were for nasal reconstruction. Therefore, the forehead flap has a long history of use in total and subtotal (subunit) reconstruction of the nose. Numerous variants have been described, including central or paramedian designs, with or without tissue expansion and with or without vascular delay. The keystone island flap has been used for nasal reconstruction using a transverse supraorbital donor site with survival of the flap due to its good perforator supply and islanding that incorporates the frontalis muscle within the flap. Also, cheek-based keystone island flaps (based on the infraorbital neurovascular bundle or facial artery branches) are of great use for lateral and alar subunit reconstructions. An example of the transverse forehead keystone island flap for nasal reconstruction is presented in Figure 4.18.

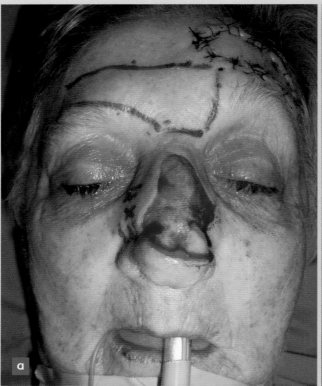

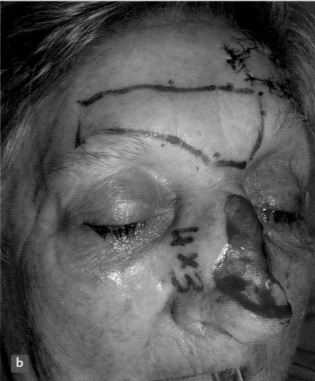

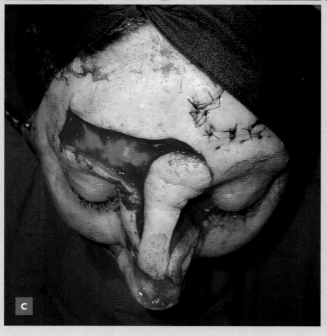

FIGURE 4.18 Nasal defect in a 75-year-old woman with multiple squamous cell carcinomas of the dorsum of her nose excised using the DRAPE procedure—delayed reconstruction after pathological evaluation—to establish adequate clearance

(a) In conjunction with a supraorbital keystone island flap to close the excision of an incompletely excised lesion above the left eyebrow, a transversely oriented keystone island flap is planned over the right brow (to assist symmetry of brow elevation).

(b) The defect (4 × 3 cm) permits planning of the dimensions of the flap. (*Note:* Caution should be exercised with unilateral supra-brow flap elevation due to the risk of postoperative brow asymmetry; this case is used to illustrate good survival of a transversely oriented flap.)

(c) Superior view following flap transposition on the supratrochlear vessels.

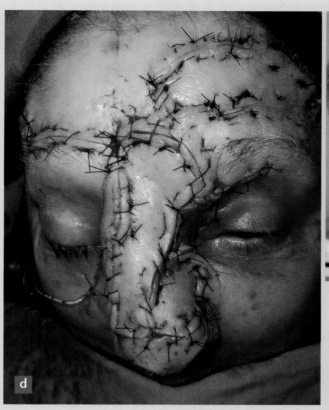

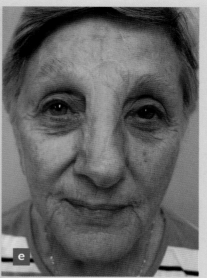

(e) Appearance at 7 months.

(d) The donor site is closed directly and the cheek skin is advanced up the left lateral nasal wall to facilitate closure.

See video for Figure 4.18

TLC

Time (operation/cost)
65 minutes
Life quality (and aesthetics)
Good, with acceptable aesthetics
Complications
Slow healing on left side of nose—resolved without intervention

NECK

Patients with lymphatic spread of cutaneous or mucosal malignancies to the cervical lymph nodes are a common presentation in head and neck units, and often have skin involvement or tumour fungation. Oncological clearance necessitates removal of the tumour, the involved integument and other potentially involved nodal basins. This produces a fasciocutaneous defect (often with exposed major vessels) with widely undermined skin flaps as part of the access for the resective surgeon. Regional flaps (e.g. pectoralis major flap) or free flaps (e.g. anterolateral thigh flap) have become the preferred form of reconstruction for these defects in many centres due to the degree of undermining involved with the neck dissection and the ligation of multiple branches of the external carotid artery during dissection. The keystone island flap has changed this clinical and reconstructive practice for the majority of neck defects in our centre. The use of locoregional flaps such as the keystone island flap has permitted the preservation of flaps such as the pectoralis major flap for salvage should recurrence occur. Islanding of the undermined skin can be performed as long as there is a minimum of one-third to one-half attachment to the underlying tissues to allow advancement, rotation or transposition while maintaining sufficient neurovascular supply and venous drainage. As described above, a platysma or fascial base is kept in the flap to ensure the integrity of the vascular plexuses within the flaps, as evidenced by the *red dot sign*, and islanding is undertaken to improve vascular perfusion to the undermined regions of the flap (for reasons discussed in Chapter 2). Even when many of the external carotid artery branches have been ligated, there are often still a number of vessels capable of supplying flaps in this region, including the facial (anterograde or retrograde), superior thyroid, occipital, transverse cervical and superficial cervical vessels, among others. The laxity (and sometimes elasticity) of the neck tissues in this region in the elderly is of benefit and tissue can even be recruited from the upper chest if necessary without significantly affecting head or neck movement after the immediate postoperative period. The most common sites for cutaneous defects in the neck are directly over major draining lymph nodes, including the submental, submandibular, jugular chain (upper third most common), posterior triangle and occipital nodes. Skin involvement overlying the postauricular nodes is also reasonably common, but has previously been described in the postauricular defects section of this chapter. A representative case is shown in Figure 4.19.

FIGURE 4.19

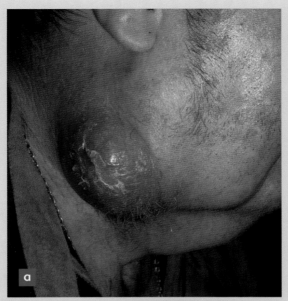

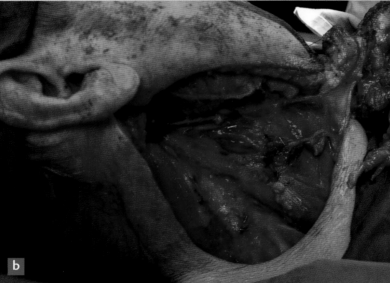

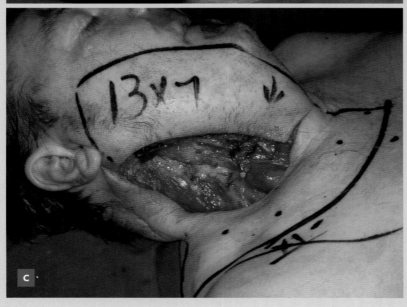

FIGURE 4.19 Neck defect in a 51-year-old man with a massive secondary deposit of squamous cell carcinoma involving the lower parotid and overlying skin (Australian disease)

(a) Lateral view of the tumour mass.

(b) A 13 × 7 cm defect is produced following tumour extirpation, including the lower parotid gland and neck levels II–V.

(c) A supraclavicular keystone island flap extending just beyond the midline closes the lower two-thirds of the defect, with a cheek (facial artery)-based flap planned for closure of the upper one-third (Yin Yang principle).

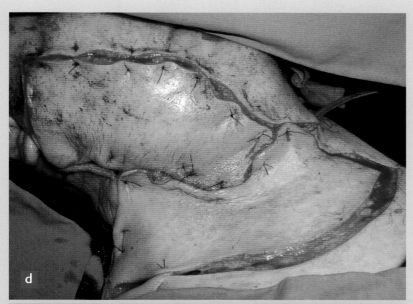

(d) Strategic mattress suturing of the flaps demonstrates good approximation and sound vascularity of the flaps despite undermining of the previous dissection.

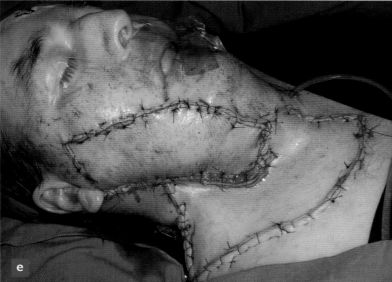

(e) Appearance following definitive closure.

(f) Appearance at 3 weeks showing reasonable healing despite postoperative radiotherapy.

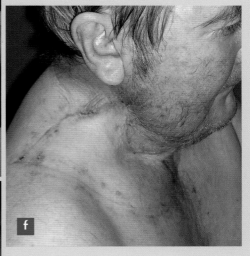

(g) Small area of epidermal loss near the right mastoid as a consequence of radiotherapy healed well without incident.

See video for Figure 4.19

TLC

Time (operation/cost)		
80 minutes		
Life quality (and aesthetics)		
Good with no delay in radiotherapy, acceptable aesthetics		
Complications		
Nil		

FIGURE 4.20

MULTIPLE SUBUNIT RECONSTRUCTION

Improved results in facial reconstruction are achieved where facial aesthetic units are respected. If a defect straddles multiple facial aesthetic units (e.g. cheek and temple), reconstruction of whole units results in a massive defect. Locoregional reconstruction of these types of defects is difficult by use of a single flap. Free-tissue transfer for these defects is commonplace; however, its poor tissue match can destroy the benefit of subunit reconstruction, and the added morbidity must be given consideration, especially in the elderly. An alternative approach is to use locoregional reconstruction (like for like) irrespective of facial subunits in select cases and, thereby, maximise benefit and minimise morbidity.

Figure 4.20 demonstrates multiple subunit reconstruction in an elderly patient through the use of a single locoregional flap, with minimal morbidity.

FIGURE 4.20 Multiple subunit reconstruction through the use of a single locoregional flap

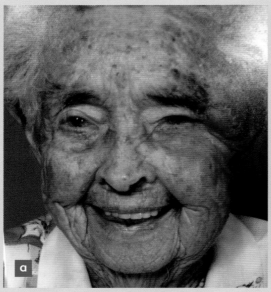 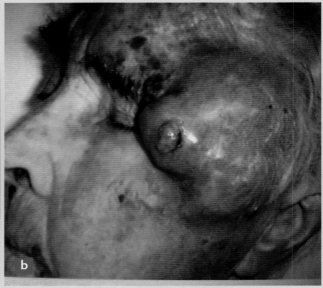

(a) A 96-year-old woman presented with a rapidly enlarging squamous cell carcinoma of the left temple.

(b) At operation, the tumour is now fungating and extends from the lateral orbital margin to the preauricular groove posteriorly and up into the temple and mid-cheek below.

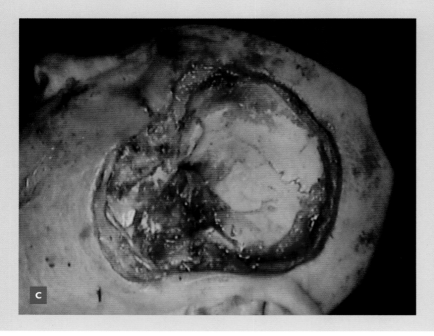

(c) The surgical defect is large and spans multiple aesthetic facial units—the temple and cheek with exposed bone of the temple, zygomatic arch and orbital rim.

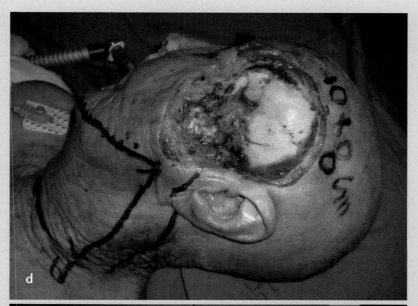

(d) Loss of the upper branches of the facial nerve is apparent within the defect and a cervicosubmental (CSM) flap is designed to make use of the neck skin laxity.

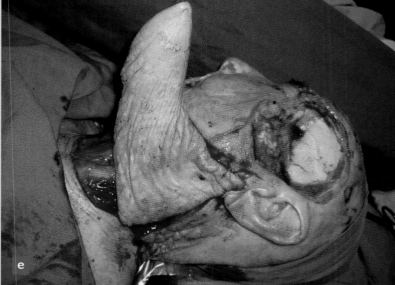

(e) The CSM flap is elevated over the midline of the neck to reach the upper border of the defect, preserving neurovascular structures where possible.

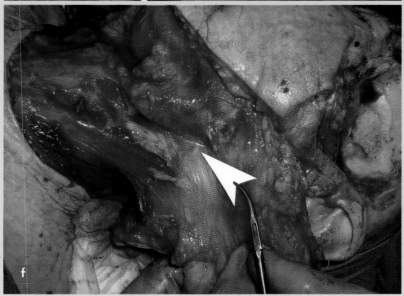

(f) The arrow indicates a perforator entering the undersurface of the flap, raised to include the platysma within its base. Care is taken to preserve these perforators where possible and where permitted by the degree of mobilisation required for flap inset.

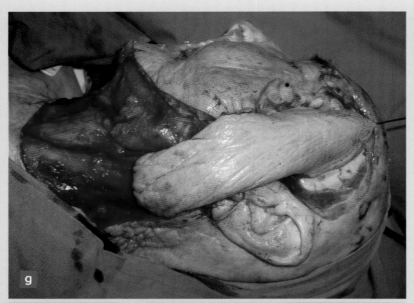

(g) Teasing of these perforators and the flap tissue can maximise flap mobility and stretch without additional risk and is stopped once the flap mobility is sufficient for defect closure. Although large, the secondary defect in the CSM technique is closed by direct apposition.

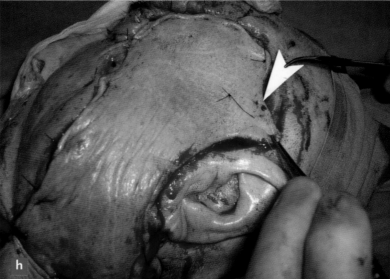

(h) A *red dot sign* during the insertion of strategic mattress sutures indicates reliable flap perfusion.

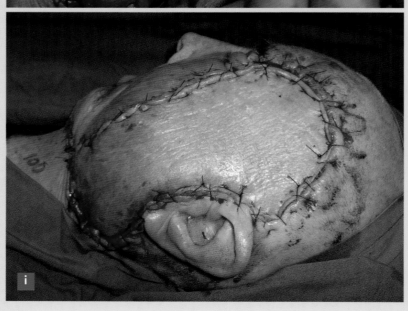

(i) At completion the donor defect is closed primarily, the vascular flare is slowly emerging and the total reconstructive time of 105 minutes was tolerated well by the elderly patient (and the anaesthetist).

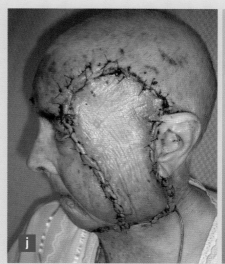

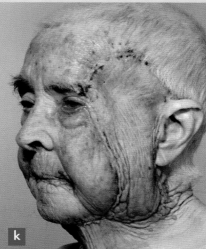

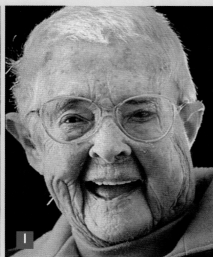

(j) At day 7 reliable wound healing is evident as the vascular flare is subsiding. A lower lid ectropion has developed as a result of her facial nerve resection and was to be reconstructed at a later stage, following radiotherapy.

(k) Appearance at 6 weeks showing good wound healing, but residual ectropion for correction. Otherwise she had good quality of life.

(l) Final appearance prior to her death from unrelated comorbidities reaffirms the usefulness of locoregional reconstruction in such cases.

(Reproduced with permission from Behan F, Sizeland A, Gilmour F, Hui A, Seel M, Lo CH 2010 Use of the keystone island flap for advanced head and neck cancer in the elderly—a principle of amelioration. J Plast Reconstr Aesthet Surg 63(5):739–45.)

TLC

Time (operation/cost)
105 minutes
Life quality (and aesthetics)
Good except for mild eye irritation. No delay in radiotherapy, acceptable aesthetics with static facial resuspension via the flap.
Complications
Lower lid ectropion (from facial nerve resection)

SUMMARY

The keystone island flap has changed reconstructive practice for fasciocutaneous head and neck defects in our centre. Fasciocutaneous defects are the most common form of defect following oncological surgery of the head and neck, which predominantly affects the elderly. Patients in this group often have multiple comorbidities, making complex forms of reconstruction suboptimal. Locoregional reconstruction (using the keystone island flap and its variants) offers a useful alternative to more complex forms of reconstruction because it is better tolerated, produces better aesthetics and improves the quality of life in head and neck patients compared with other approaches. Locoregional reconstruction should, therefore, be considered the ideal form of reconstruction in the majority of cases, with more complex reconstructions used in specific circumstances (e.g. bony/composite reconstruction).

BIBLIOGRAPHY

Ariyan S 1979 The pectoralis major myocutaneous flap. A versatile flap for reconstruction in the head and neck. Plast Reconstr Surg 63(1):73–81.

Bakamjian V Y, Long M, Rigg B 1971 Experience with the medially based deltopectoral flap in reconstructive surgery of the head and neck. Br J Plast Surg 24(2):174–83.

Behan F C, Rozen W M, Findlay M W, Gavriel H, Sizeland A 2011 The cervico-submental keystone island flap: a new locoregional flap in head and neck reconstruction. Plast Reconstr Surg (in press).

Cannady S B, Seth R, Fritz M A, Alam D S, Wax M K 2010 Total parotidectomy defect reconstruction using the buried flap. Otolaryngol Head Neck Surg 143(5):637–43.

Raasch B A, Buettner P G, Garbe C 2006 Basal cell carcinoma: histological classification and body-site distribution. Br J Dermatol 155(2):401–7.

Strauch B, Vasconez L O, Hall-Findlay E J, Lee B T 2009 Grabb's encyclopedia of flaps: volume 1: head and neck. Lippincott Williams & Wilkins, Philadelphia.

Chapter 5
The upper limb

Where observation is concerned, chance favours only the prepared mind.
Louis Pasteur (1822–1895)

The keystone island flap represents a single and simple flap solution that increases the available options for vascularised soft tissue cover in the upper limb with good functional and aesthetic results.

INTRODUCTION

Upper limb and hand injuries are the most common work-related injury type in Australia and represent a common presentation of non-work related injuries (ASAC 2008). Sun exposure, particularly to the dorsum of the hand and forearm, also results in high rates of skin cancer in this region (Raasch et al. 2006). As a consequence of these two causes (trauma and tumours), upper limb defects are very common.

Reconstruction of these defects seeks to optimise function, encompassing not only sensate prehension, but also the facilitation of social interaction through hand gestures and aesthetics. Proper upper limb function relies upon the synergistic action of a multitude of structures (tendons, vessels, nerves, etc.), often with complex interrelationships. These require protection by locally specialised sensate skin (including glabrous skin), soft tissue and fascia that facilitate this function. Soft tissue defects of the upper limb can, therefore, have a more significant impact than similar defects in other regions of the body and the long-term effects of scar shortening, skin graft contracture and stiffness from prolonged immobilisation must be considered when planning any soft tissue reconstruction in this region.

Locoregional flaps are well-suited to the reconstruction of soft tissue defects in the upper limb. They provide vascularised, locally matched fasciocutaneous coverage of vital structures with minimal long-term morbidity and improved aesthetics relative to skin graft and/or free-flap reconstructions. The use of random pattern flaps in the upper limb is problematic because of the suboptimal length to breadth ratios in this region (1:1) comparative to other areas, such as the face (6:1). In contrast, the keystone island flap overcomes these restrictions by deriving its blood supply from the numerous neurovascular and locoregional perforators present in the upper limb. In addition, following islanding, the flap displays a sanguine phase of hypervascularity (immediate vascular augmentation concept, IVAC) that provides additional safety to the use of flaps in this region. It is uncommon for vessels of the upper limb to be affected by vascular disease, and developmental differences in arterial and venous anatomy rarely affect local flaps, unlike pedicled flaps (e.g. radial forearm flap). Pedicled flaps sacrifice a major vessel supplying the hand and their use removes a potential donor vessel for later use in bypass surgery. Planning and raising island flaps in the upper (and lower) limb is relatively easy and it is at these sites that experience may be developed. We will discuss the principles specific to the elevation of keystone island flaps in the upper limb, then divide the upper limb into various subregions to assist discussion of the relevant neurovascular anatomy before moving to demonstrate the principles of keystone island flap elevation in these various subregions with clinical cases.

PRINCIPLES OF FLAP ELEVATION IN THE UPPER LIMB

Most of the cutaneous vascular supply in the upper limb perforates the deep fascia, either via fascial septae or as muscular perforators. This fact constrains the manner in which fasciocutaneous flaps can be raised in this region. The integral association of the perforators with underlying longitudinal structures results in greater flap movement perpendicular to the long axis of the limb rather than advancement proximally or distally. This pattern coincides with that of the dermatomes of the upper limb, which again are a useful aide-mémoire to the axis of flap design in this region. The specific flap orientation can be modified to run more obliquely to lie in skin folds, particularly around the extensor wad and volar wrist, where maximal skin laxity is present in this modified direction (the pinch test). Keystone transposition flaps must be planned in areas where direct closure of the donor defect can be undertaken; otherwise, skin grafts may be necessary.

NEUROVASCULAR ANATOMY AND ZONES IN UPPER LIMB RECONSTRUCTION

The blood supply to the skin of the upper limb is derived from the subclavian artery and its branches. It is possible to simplify the discussion of this anatomy by dealing with specific regions. The regions are as follows: the deltoid; lateral and medial arm; cubital fossa; the olecranon and extensor surface of the elbow; extensor and flexor surface of the forearm; dorsum of the hand; dorsum of the fingers; the palm; and the volar aspect of the digits.

Deltoid region

The deltoid region (Fig 5.1) includes supply from the deltoid branch of the thoracoacromial axis, in addition to supply from the posterior (and anterior) circumflex humeral vessels, whose branches reach the overlying skin via septocutaneous perforators on the anterior and posterior borders of the muscle or directly through the muscle. Flaps in this area should, therefore, either maintain the branch from the thoracoacromial axis or be oriented in the line of the deltoid fibres to permit maximum advancement of flaps perpendicular to the deltoid fibres, thereby maximising advancement. As an additional note, the use of keystone island flaps within the deltoid region appears to be less affected by hypertrophic scarring than is the use of other techniques in this area in our experience. This may be related to a combination of rapid healing and the even tension on the flap rather than the uneven tension achieved with elliptical excision alone.

The arm is characterised by medial and lateral intermuscular septae, which not only separate the flexor and extensor compartments, but are the source of numerous perforators for supply to the overlying skin (see Fig 5.1). The marked laxity of the medial arm skin readily permits direct closure of many upper arm defects but may result in significant contour deformity ('shark bite effect'). Keystone island flaps oriented along the longitudinal axis of the limb make full use of this laxity and can minimise contour deformity. The region around the elbow has numerous anastomosing vessels between the brachial supply in the arm and the radial and ulnar vessels in the forearm. This provides numerous vessels upon which flaps can be based, with the major limitation of flaps raised in this region being donor site laxity. Therefore, flaps raised in this region are either of limited transverse diameter or require skin grafting of the

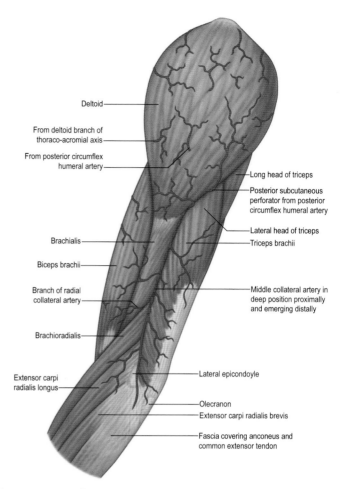

▲ FIGURE 5.1 Cutaneous arterial anatomy of the lateral aspect of the arm

This demonstrates numerous muscular perforators in the region of the deltoid muscle, along with additional septocutaneous vessels, particularly at its posterior border (posterior subcutaneous perforator from posterior circumflex humeral artery, PCHA). Further down in the arm, the major perforators are mostly septocutaneous, although numerous smaller muscular perforators are present from both the flexor and extensor compartments. In addition to the above vessels, neurovascular supply to the skin that is of use for inclusion within island flaps includes the axillary nerve over the deltoid, the superior lateral cutaneous nerve of the arm at the posterior border of the deltoid (from axillary nerve), the inferior lateral cutaneous nerve of arm (from radial nerve), and the intercostobrachial and medial cutaneous nerve of the arm medially.

(Reproduced with permission from Gray H, Standring S 2005 Gray's anatomy: the anatomical basis of clinical practice, 39th edn. Churchill Livingstone, New York, Fig 47.2.)

secondary defect. The lateral arm flap is a well-described flap in this region and can be raised either as a pedicled or free flap. In general, the cubital fossa should be avoided as a donor site for flaps despite significant laxity in some elbow positions and the presence of the inferior cubital artery within this region. Flaps raised here can have a significant impact on elbow movement and may be plagued by scar contracture in the longer term. The dorsal aspect of the elbow can be used more readily, but again, skin grafting of the donor defect may be necessary. Reconstruction of the lateral and medial aspects of the elbow should take into consideration the convex nature of these surfaces and, therefore, flap designs that recreate this convexity are to be encouraged (goblet and omega (Ω) variants; see Figs 4.17 and 4.10, respectively).

The forearm

There is relative laxity of skin over the convex muscle bellies in the extensor and flexor compartments of the forearm. This laxity may be utilised for the elevation of keystone island flaps and is well-suited as a site for developing surgical experience with keystone flaps. The blood supply of the forearm is dominated by two vessels, namely, the radial and ulnar arteries, with a more modest supply from the posterior interosseous artery (Fig 5.2). Numerous perforators of each of these vessels come to the undersurface of the skin via the deep fascia, and flaps elevated on perforators from these vessels tend to be relatively reliable since there are multiple perforator territories (Fig 5.3). Proximally in the forearm, the perforators are often fewer and have greater transverse reach. The perforators increase in number and decrease in size more distally in the forearm. Muscular perforators can be common in the proximal forearm but are rare distally, with most vessels passing from deep to superficial within fascia septae between tendons. Again, the greater ease of movement of perforators within septae perpendicular to the long axis of the limb promotes flaps oriented with this axis. Of important note, the venous drainage of the forearm is via the superficial venous system; therefore, it is important to preserve these as much as possible. In addition to the vascular supply from these perforators, a longitudinal system of vessels running with cutaneous nerves is well-developed. Preservation of these nerves (with their vessels) within flaps (including as flow-through configurations) augments the perforator supply without significant additional restriction of flap movement. This conjoint vascular supply makes flaps raised in this region very reliable without the express need for preoperative vascular imaging or Doppler ultrasound identification of perforators.

Dorsum of hand and fingers

The dorsum of the hand is characterised by multiple longitudinal structures passing immediately deep to the skin (depending on the relative adiposity of the patient). These include superficial veins, dorsal cutaneous nerve branches (with their associated vessels) and the long

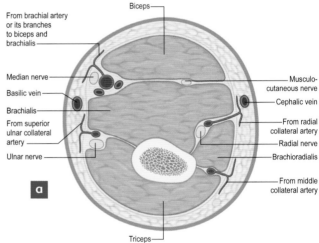

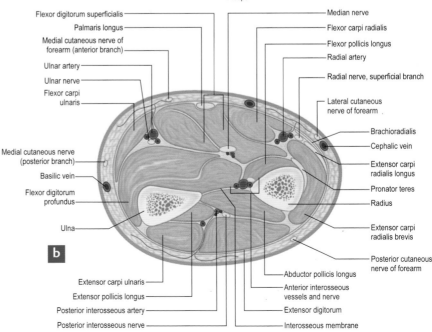

> **FIGURE 5.2 Cross-sections of the arm demonstrating the septocutaneous nature of major perforators to the skin**

(a) In the proximal forearm, the septocutaneous perforators of the radial, ulnar and posterior interosseous vessels are noted.

(b) In the distal forearm, most of the muscle bellies are now tendons with septae in-between through which the perforators pass. In addition to these vessels, smaller numerous muscular perforators and vessels travelling with the medial, lateral, posterior and superficial branches of the radial nerve supply blood to the overlying skin.

(Reproduced with permission from Gray H, Standring S 2005 Gray's anatomy: the anatomical basis of clinical practice, 39th edn. Churchill Livingstone, New York, Figs 47.1, 49.17.)

extensor tendons. Deep to these structures, branches of the radial (and ulnar) arteries course and send perforators superficially between the tendon sheaths to supply the overlying skin (Fig 5.4). Dorsal metacarpal arteries either branching off the radial artery (first dorsal metacarpal artery) or perforating from the volar deep vasculature of the palmar aspect provide additional deep branches to the overlying skin that extend roughly to the level of the distal crease of the proximal interphalangeal joint crease. These perforators have a reliable position just

proximal to web spaces 2–4 and more proximally in the first web space (Fig 5.5). Beyond this point on the digits, the major supply is via the dorsal branches of the digital vessels with smaller secondary supply from the vessels accompanying dorsal longitudinal structures, such as the veins and extensor expansion.

The vessels to the skin of the dorsum of the hand (with exceptions such as the first dorsal metacarpal artery) usually look very small during dissection and do not normally inspire confidence. However, when flaps are raised in

> **FIGURE 5.3 Cutaneous vascular territories of the elbow and forearm**

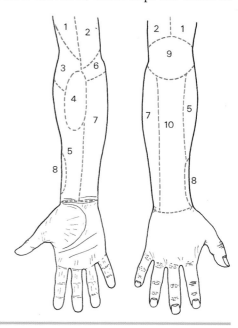

Key: 1 – middle and radial collateral arteries; 2 – superior ulnar collateral and brachial arteries; 3 – radial recurrent artery; 4 – inferior cubital perforator; 5 – radial artery; 6 – anterior ulnar recurrent artery; 7 – ulnar artery; 8 – anterior interosseous artery; 9 – olecranon anastomosis; 10 – posterior interosseous artery.

As seen in the diagram, there are numerous cutaneous vascular territories in the forearm. The importance of this is that no matter where the defect is, adjacent tissue of at least the same diameter as the defect will usually capture perforators from the adjacent vascular territory. This makes island flap elevation along the long axis of the limb with advancements perpendicular to this axis very reliable without the need for preoperative imaging or Doppler ultrasound/surgical identification of perforators during surgery.

(Reproduced with permission from Cormack GC lamberty BC 1994 The arterial anatomy of skin flaps, 2nd edn. Churchill Livingstone, New York, Fig 6.66.)

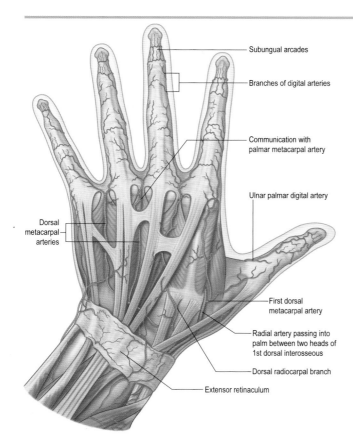

- Subungual arcades
- Branches of digital arteries
- Communication with palmar metacarpal artery
- Ulnar palmar digital artery
- Dorsal metacarpal arteries
- First dorsal metacarpal artery
- Radial artery passing into palm between two heads of 1st dorsal interosseous
- Dorsal radiocarpal branch
- Extensor retinaculum

◀ **FIGURE 5.4 Cutaneous blood supply to the dorsum of the hand and fingers**

Note the radial artery passing deep to the tendons in the anatomical snuffbox and giving off multiple branches that run from deep to superficial between the tendon sheaths. Similarly, the ulnar artery provides a similar supply to the ulnar side of the hand. At the level of the web spaces, dorsal metacarpal arteries come from the deep tissues to supply the skin in these regions. In addition to these vessels, the neurocutaneous supply via the superficial branch of the radial nerve and the dorsal branch of the ulnar nerve provides a more superficial and axially oriented blood supply for inclusion within dorsal island flaps.

(Reproduced with permission from Gray H, Standring S 2005 Gray's anatomy: the anatomical basis of clinical practice, 39th edn. Churchill Livingstone, New York, Fig 50.2B.)

> **FIGURE 5.5 Major sites of cutaneous perforators within the hand**

Note the prominent number of perforators along the axes of the radial and ulnar dorsal vessels and a prominence of dorsal metacarpal artery perforators to the skin. These perforators provide a rich cutaneous blood supply for island flaps to the dorsum of the hand.

(Reproduced with permission from Cormack GC lamberty BC 1994 The arterial anatomy of skin flaps, 2nd edn. Churchill Livingstone, New York, Fig 6.70.)

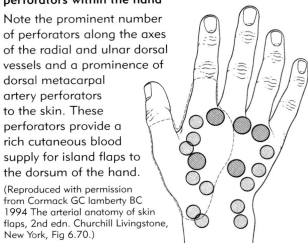

ligaments. Multiple vessels emerge from the digital vessels through their course, with a major branching pattern occurring at the trifurcation—a volar branch passes across to meet its counterpart from the other digital vessel, an intermediate branch to supply the pulp, and a smaller continuing vessel that arches up over the tip to meets its opposite number after giving off a branch to the nail bed. An extensive array of homodigital and heterodigital flaps, including digital artery perforator and flap-on-flap techniques, have been described but are beyond the scope of this text. Needless to say, maintenance of the deep perforating supply is vital to the success of volar digital flaps and the secondary defect usually requires grafting.

this region, it is usual to capture multiple perforators in this process, thereby improving the reliability of the flaps. Undermining is usually not necessary but can be performed to improve movement as long as these small perforators are preserved. If too much tension is present upon closure, it may be necessary to insert a discretional full-thickness skin graft into the donor side of the flap. A conjoint supply adds additional reliability via the maintenance of all longitudinal neurovascular structures passing through the flap, as these provide further blood supply to the skin and generally run in the plane between the long extensors and the overlying skin. A period of postoperative splintage facilitates wound healing and minimises possible dehiscence should the relatively pain-free nature of the recovery lead to overuse.

The palm

The palm is an area not classically associated with the elevation of fasciocutaneous flaps. This is because dense fibrous septae extend from the palmar aponeurosis to the overlying skin. Extensive mobilisation and division of these septae is necessary for adequate flap mobility. By the same token, the blood supply to the skin often reaches the surface via passage with (but not within) these septae (Fig 5.6). Therefore, flap elevation is achievable and islanding with maintenance of the maximum number of these perforators improves flap viability (IVAC) compared to dermal pedicle-based flaps that have undergone extensive undermining.

The use of palmar-based flaps permits closure of defects of the palm with like tissue. Blunt dissection of the subcutaneous tissue at the periphery of the flap preserves cutaneous nerve supply to these flaps, with eventual good return of sensation after an initial relatively pain-free postoperative period of neurapraxia. Within the fingers, the neurovascular bundles sit within the lateral digital fascia, with branches perforating volarly through Grayson's ligaments or dorsally through Cleland's

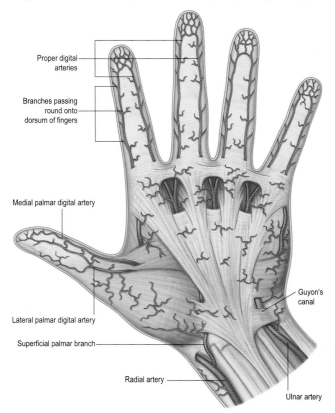

▲ FIGURE 5.6 Cutaneous blood supply to the volar aspect of the hand

Note the deep vessels derived from the radial and ulnar arteries that give rise to the superficial and deep palmar arches (not shown). The common digital arteries and direct cutaneous branches to the skin mainly come off the ulnar artery and its continuation as the superficial arch. Multiple perforators pass up between the flexor tendon sheaths, perforate the palmar fascia and supply the overlying skin. Mobilisation of island flaps in this area is supported by multiple perforators, but mobilisation requires division of dense septae running from the palmar fascia to the skin without division of these blood vessels.

(Reproduced with permission from Gray H, Standring S 2005 Gray's anatomy: the anatomical basis of clinical practice, 39th edn. Churchill Livingstone, New York, Fig 50.2A.)

CLINICAL CASES

The principles of keystone island flap elevation in the various subregions of the upper limb are demonstrated in the following clinical cases that are presented in Figures 5.7 to 5.11.

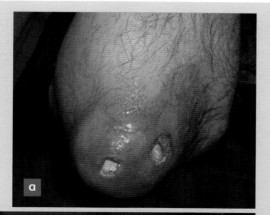

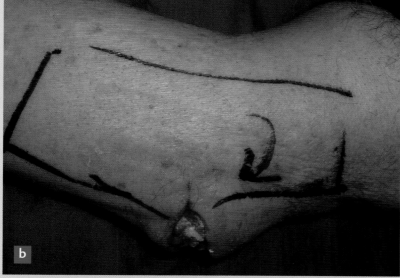

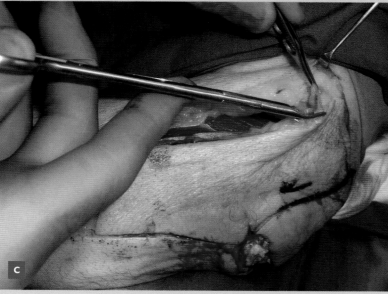

FIGURE 5.7 A 68-year old man with tophaceous gout extruding through the skin over the olecranon

(a) Two areas of skin breakdown with obvious tophi extruding through.

(b) The planning of a keystone island flap along the line of the lateral epicondyle to be transposed into the excisional defect.

(c) Elevation of the flap with inclusion of the deep fascia within the proximal half of the flap to ensure vascular patency. Clip ligation of vessels to assist haemostasis during flap elevation.

FIGURE 5.7

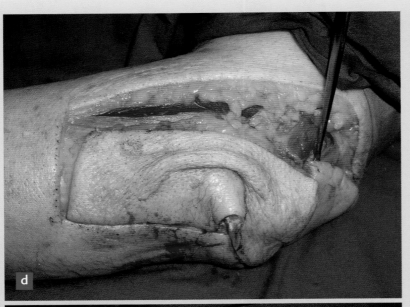

(d) Transposition permits coverage of the olecranon defect.

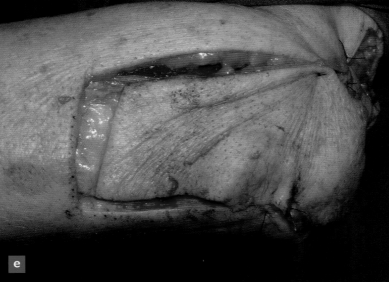

(e) The start of V–Y closure of the donor defect with strategic mattress sutures.

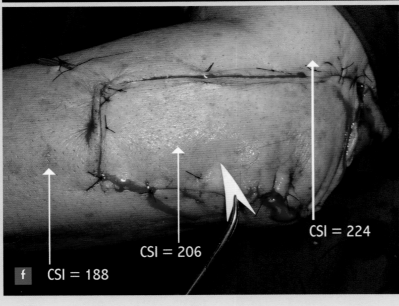

CSI = 224

CSI = 206

CSI = 188

(f) Upon release of the tourniquet, an initial flare is evident (arrow), demonstrating the most likely site of a perforator to the flap. This flare of hyperaemia then spreads throughout the flap.

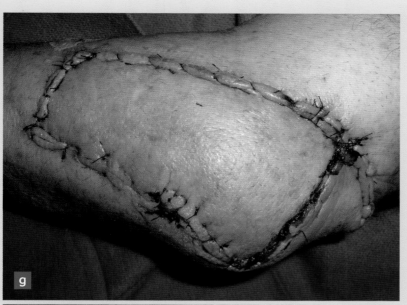

(g) Appearance after 1 week.

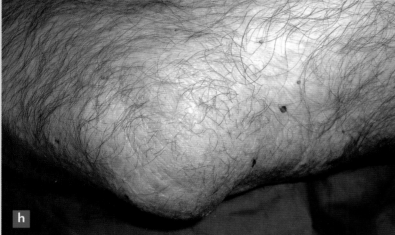

(h) Appearance at 18 months with no recurrence of gouty tophi.

See video for Figure 5.7

TLC

Time (operation/cost)		
45 minutes		
Life quality (and aesthetics)		
Good, no recurrence, acceptable aesthetics		
Complications		
Nil		

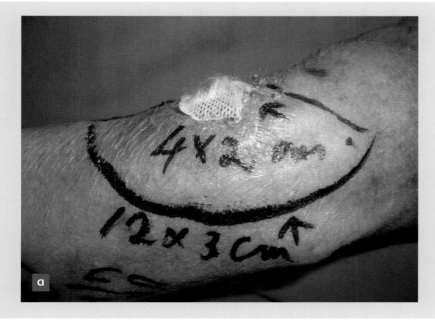

FIGURE 5.8

FIGURE 5.8 Elderly woman in intensive care with an ulcer due to a complication of intravenous therapy involving the cephalic vein on the radial aspect of the distal forearm

(a) Appearance after 1 week of dressings to the necrotic area (piece of dressing still present to minimise bleeding).

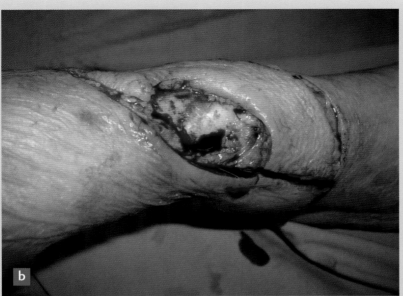

(b) Appearance following debridement down to the cephalic vein with protection of the lateral cutaneous nerve of the forearm branches.

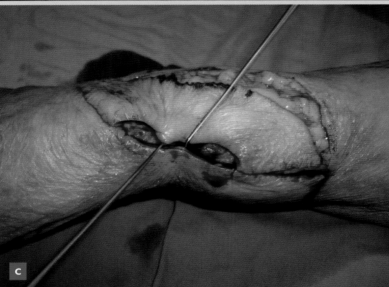

(c) Approximation of the wound margin creates a small secondary defect in the region of the ulnar styloid.

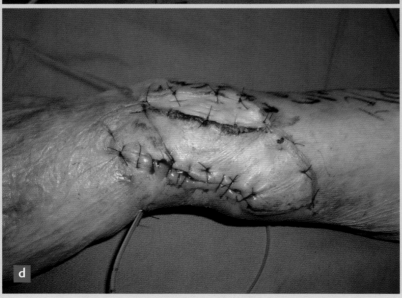

(d) A fenestrated full-thickness skin graft is used to cover the secondary defect.

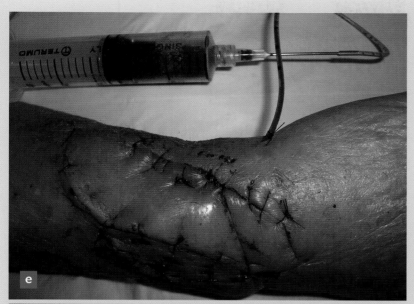

(e) A miniature vacuum drainage system is used under the flap, utilising a 20 mL Luer-Lok syringe, which is drawn to the required pressure and then blocked from returning to its starting position, thereby maintaining a vacuum.

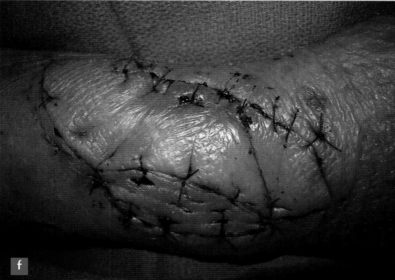

(f) Appearance at 3 days demonstrating early vascular changes within the graft consistent with revascularisation despite marked oedema of the wrist region.

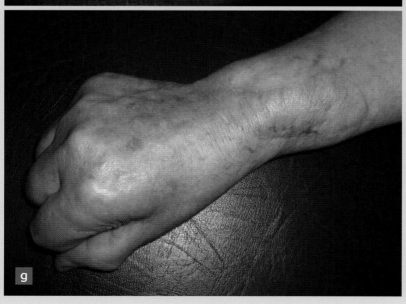

(g) Appearance following full healing with good function and acceptable aesthetics.

TLC

Time (operation/cost)
45 minutes
Life quality (and aesthetics)
Intensive care patient—performed under local anaesthetic without compromising patient, acceptable aesthetics
Complications
Nil

FIGURE 5.9

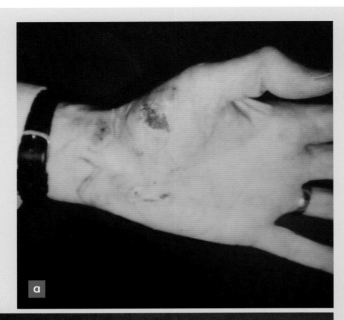

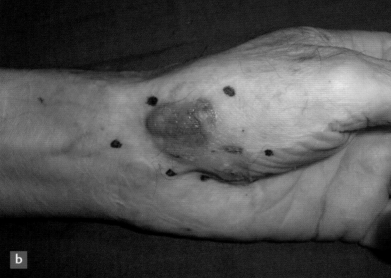

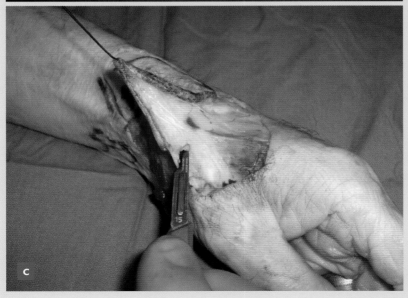

FIGURE 5.9 Elderly woman with multifocal squamous cell carcinoma of the thenar eminence leading to multiple procedures over 15 years

(a) Appearance 12 years before re-presentation.

(b) Appearance on re-presentation with dots indicating planned resection margin.

(c) Elevation of a keystone flap along the line of the second metacarpal.

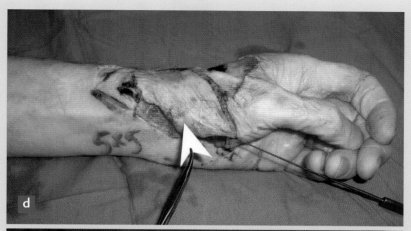

(d) Undermining of nearly half of the flap to permit transposition of the distal end of the flap and formation of an omega (Ω) flap variant to effect defect closure.

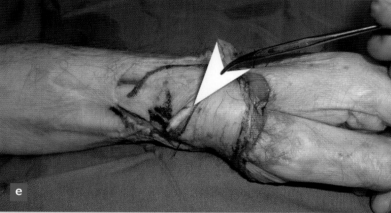

(e) The omega (Ω) flap variant of a keystone island flap is in place and shows a dog ear (arrow) centrally formed by the transposition of the distal end of the flap.

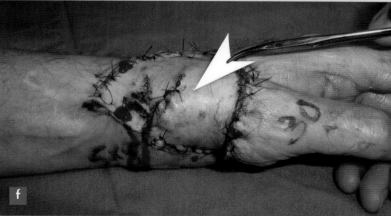

(f) The dog ear has been excised (skin only) without compromise to the flap (since the flap is based on perforators rather than a random skin pedicle). The donor site was closed primarily.

(g) Appearance 9 months after operation, with good function and acceptable aesthetics.

See video for Figure 5.9

TLC

Time (operation/cost)
30 minutes

Life quality (and aesthetics)
Good, early return of function; multiple skin cancers of the hand over 20 years; omega (Ω) variant flap allows twisting; the only postoperative recovery for the patient that was pain-free

Complications
Nil

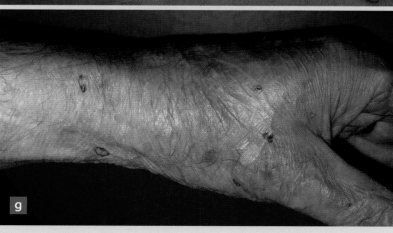

FIGURE 5.10

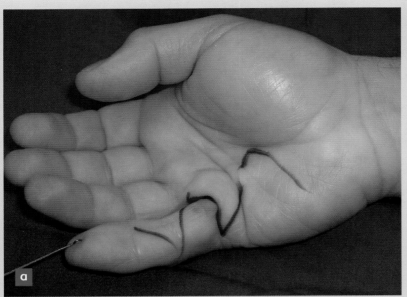

FIGURE 5.10 A 55-year-old diabetic man with recurrent Dupuytren's contracture of the right hand

(a) A Bruner's incision technique is used with modification to fit into the palmar and digital creases.

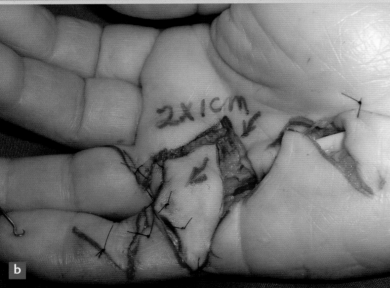

(b) Following completion of fasciectomy with full possible extension of the finger, there is a 2 × 1 cm palmar skin defect. A Bruner's island flap (an architectural variant of the keystone) is raised as a natural extension of an existing Bruner's incision. V–Y closure of this on its radial border permits Y–V closure of the 2 × 1 cm defect. This avoids the use of a skin graft, which can result in slow wound healing in diabetic patients.

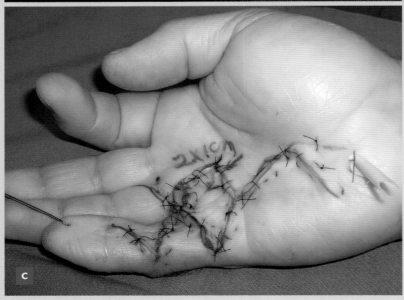

(c) Completion of closure prior to tourniquet release.

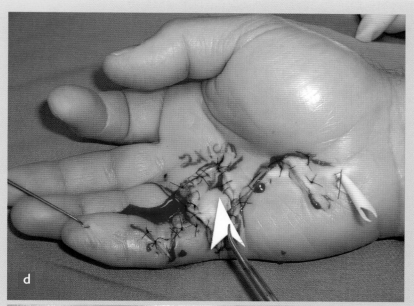

(d) On tourniquet release, the start of the vascular flare in the flap is seen at the radioproximal border spreading across the flap surface in the succeeding seconds.

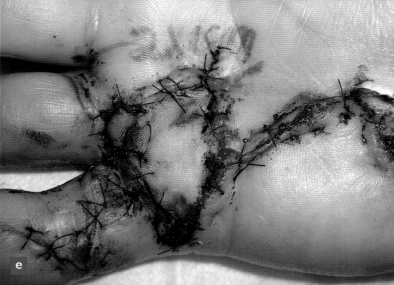

(e) Postoperative appearance at 11 days with some residual flexion of the little finger due to prolonged flexion preoperatively.

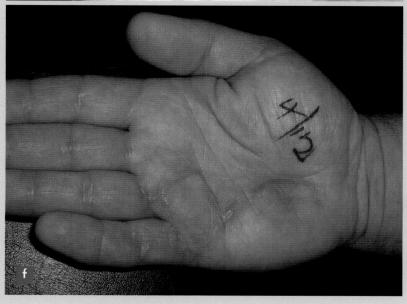

(f) Acceptable function and aesthetics almost 4 months after the operation.

See [video] for Figure 5.10

TLC

Time (operation/cost)
60 minutes
Life quality (and aesthetics)
Good, pain-free early mobilisation, acceptable aesthetics
Complications
Nil

FIGURE 5.11

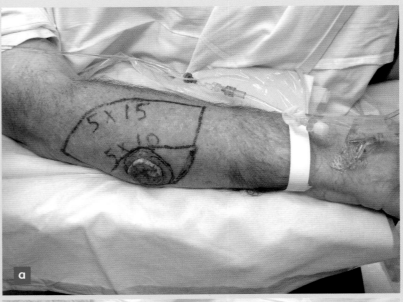

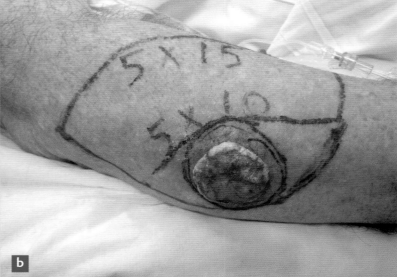

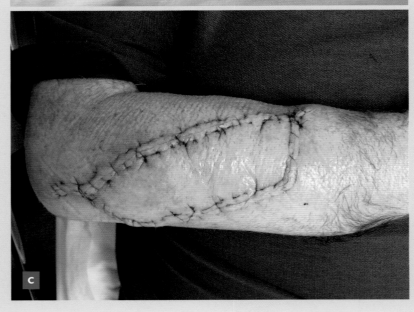

FIGURE 5.11 A direct comparison of the functional and aesthetic outcomes of fasciocutaneous island flap coverage versus skin grafting in the management of bilateral non-melanomatous skin cancer. A 50-year-old man presenting late with two advanced cutaneous lesions over the extensor aspect of both forearms. Both excisional defects were approximately 5 × 10 cm

(a) Position of the tumour on the extensor surface of the proximal forearm. A similar lesion was present on the contralateral forearm (not shown).

(b) Close-up of the lesion demonstrating a large exophytic tumour with the excision and keystone island flap designed slightly oblique to the longitudinal axis of the limb to fit in with the maximal skin laxity and relaxed skin tension lines.

(c) Appearance of the flap at 10 days post operation. The left arm was immobilised for 5 days to assist graft take. The patient retained full function of the right (dominant) hand (keystone flap side).

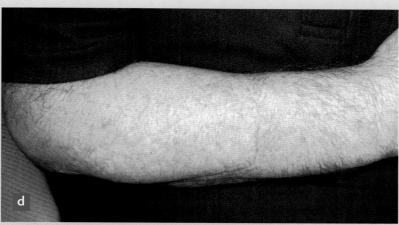

(d) Appearance of the keystone island flap reconstruction at 6 weeks post operation demonstrating acceptable aesthetics and no disruption of movement in the hand or forearm at any stage since the operation.

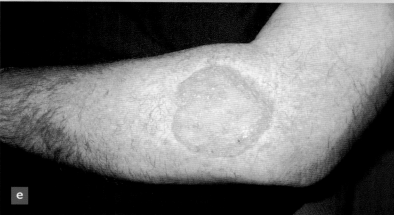

(e) The alternative appearance of the contralateral skin grafted defect demonstrating poorer aesthetics and some residual wrist stiffness secondary to his period of splintage. The skin donor site healed without incident but was reported by the patient as the most painful part of his postoperative recovery while his right forearm was relatively pain-free. The patient was adamant that any further surgery must utilise keystone island flap reconstruction, with avoidance of skin grafting in the future.

TLC: Keystone island flap in comparison to skin graft on contralateral side

Time (operation/cost)
50 minutes (versus 45 minutes)

Life quality (and aesthetics)
Good (versus poor—painful donor site—contracture and tightening with time), good aesthetics (patient unhappy with skin graft—poor)

Complications
Nil

SUMMARY

The use of keystone island flaps (and their variants) in the upper limb is very straightforward and reliable. The vascular anatomy of the upper limb is well-suited to the formation of these flaps, particularly oriented longitudinally to the long axis of the limb and over sites of skin laxity. The use of fasciocutaneous flaps in the upper limb has numerous benefits over other reconstructive approaches (see Fig 5.11) and is strongly recommended as a site where surgeons can develop proficiency with the use of this technique prior to moving on to other body regions.

BIBLIOGRAPHY

Australian Safety and Compensation (ASAC) Council 2008 Work-related hand and wrist injuries in Australia. ASAC Council, Canberra, http://safeworkaustralia.gov.au/AboutSafeWorkAustralia/WhatWeDo/Publications/Documents/202/WorkRelatedHandandWristInjuriesin Australia_2008_PDF.pdf.

Raasch B A, Buettner P G, Garbe C 2006 Basal cell carcinoma: histological classification and body-site distribution. Br J Dermatol 155(2):401–7.

Chapter 6

The trunk: the clavicles to the groin

Theory is all grey. And the golden tree of life is all green.
Goethe (1749–1832)

The trunk region is comprised of many specialised regions with specific needs. The keystone island flap is a single, simple tool that can be adapted for (multifunctional) reconstruction of small or large fasciocutaneous defects in these areas.

INTRODUCTION

Over one-third of the body surface area lies within the trunk. Tumours and trauma are again the most common cause of defects within this region, but other clinical causes can play a major role in specific areas. For example, infection, intra-abdominal pathology and previous or recent abdominal surgery can produce abdominal wall defects with significant implications for patients. Overall, the relative frequencies with which these types of defects occur depends on the site. In women, skin, breast and bowel cancer represent three of the four most frequent cancers worldwide. In men, they represent three of the top five most common cancers (IARC 2008). Significant fasciocutaneous defects can result from either oncological resection of these primary tumours (e.g. melanoma) or as a result of surgical complications (e.g. abdominal wall dehiscence) following oncological management. Some site-specific conditions are amenable to fasciocutaneous flap reconstruction, such as hidradenitis suppurativa (axillae or groin) and pilonidal sinuses (natal cleft).

The trunk is composed of a number of specialised areas with specific reconstructive needs. However, all have a number of similarities, including the way in which their cutaneous blood supply reaches the skin. Therefore, flap elevation undertaken in these regions has relative similarities when compared with flap elevation in other body regions (e.g. the limbs). Consequently, in this chapter we have subdivided the trunk into the following anatomical regions to facilitate discussion, with diagrams to illustrate the relevant vascular anatomy: back; chest wall and breast; abdominal wall; perineum; and buttock and perianal regions. As in all other regions of the body, it is essential to ensure that the defect site is clean, with appropriate haemostasis and clear of cancerous cells. Where there is uncertainty as to the preparedness of the defect site, dressings can be applied and reconstruction delayed until the defect site is ready for reconstruction (e.g. reconstruction of an infected pilonidal sinus wound should be delayed until the infection has settled and microbial swabs show minimal pathogens).

THE BACK

The back region covers a large amount (15%) of the surface of the body. It has the thickest non-glabrous skin (dermis) which provides protection from injury for the underlying bony structures from the spine, to the ribs and scapulae, as well as insulation from cold. Skin cancers (Chapter 8) are the most common malignancy in the world. Sun exposure to the back is also common. Unfortunately, the back is a difficult site for patients to visualise directly. Therefore, skin cancers of the back are often more advanced at the time of diagnosis compared with other body sites, leading to the need for surgical management more often. As a result of these factors, skin cancer is the major cause of fasciocutaneous defects of the back in ageing populations. Surgical excision of the full thickness of the skin, with or without underlying fat and/or fascia (depending on the nature and depth of the malignancy), results in often sizeable fasciocutaneous defects. The extensive surface area of the back usually permits direct closure of most small to medium-sized defects. Primary closure of larger defects may be possible but produces very long scars, with the increased risk of wound dehiscence and obvious contour irregularities. The keystone island flap permits simple closure of small to large defects through improved focal multiaxial (vectorial) recruitment of skin elasticity, with skin alignment for optimal aesthetics. This is superior to other recognised techniques that utilise tissue recruitment along a single axis (e.g. advancement) or direct closure that produces transverse recruitment alone. Multiaxial (vectorial) skin recruitment minimises pin-cushioning, wound dehiscence and wide or hypertrophic scarring, yet its simple geometry permits easy re-excision where margins are incomplete—all characteristics of the keystone design.

Capturing a blood supply

There are numerous segmental perforators in the paraspinal region that pass superficially to supply the skin, as well as a number of named and unnamed perforators passing to the skin from the parascapular muscles. Figure 6.1 shows the position of some of these perforators with corresponding vascular territories. In addition, previously named axial flaps, such as the scapular (Hamilton & Morrison 1982) and parascapular (Nassif et al. 1982) flaps, have well-described direct vessels (transverse and descending branches of the circumflex scapular artery, respectively) as their pedicle and these can be utilised for various skin patterns of flaps, including the keystone flap. Other reliable cutaneous vessels include a perforator near the inferior angle of the scapula that passes through the latissimus dorsi muscle, near its attachment to the scapula, before continuing on the skin. The latissimus dorsi muscle has numerous perforating vessels that are suitable as the basis for keystone flap elevation (Fig 6.2). As in other regions of the body, it is usually unnecessary to localise vessels pre- or intraoperatively by Doppler ultrasound for keystone elevation, but this approach may assist identification of the vessels supplying the flap over the latissimus dorsi muscle. Although these vessels can be traced back through the muscle, including mobilisation as thoracodorsal artery perforator flaps, this is rarely necessary due to the movement that can be gained by division of the deep fascia of the back and by avoiding skeletonisation of perforators, with the potential risk to the flap conjoint supply (including lymphatics and autonomics).

Principles of flap elevation in the back

The skin and subcutaneous fibrous structure in the back region is one of the thickest and least compliant in the body. Numerous random and axial pattern flaps can be raised in the back. Most of these flaps utilise a single modality (e.g. advancement or rotation) to effect wound closure. As a result, the dimensions of these flaps are often disproportionately large compared to the primary defect due to suboptimal cutaneous elasticity in regions of the back. One particular advantage of the keystone design for closure of back

defects is its capacity to use elements of advancement, rotation and transposition as a multiaxial (vectorial) utilisation of skin elasticity to effect closure. Even so, a considered approach to defects in the back provides the best results.

Dense fibrous septae from the skin to the spine provide midline support and minimise shear forces over the spinous processes of the vertebrae. This makes it difficult to move skin near the midline of

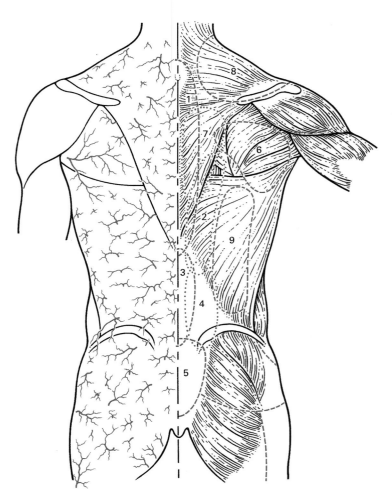

A FIGURE 6.1 Perforators and territories of cutaneous blood supply for the dorsal trunk suitable for keystone flap elevation

Key: 1 – medial dorsal cutaneous intercostal arteries; 2 – lateral dorsal cutaneous intercostal arteries; 3 – medial dorsal cutaneous lumbar arteries; 4 – lateral dorsal cutaneous lumbar arteries; 5 – sacral arteries; 6 – circumflex scapular artery including horizontal and vertical (parascapular) vessels; 7 – dorsal scapular/deep branch of transverse cervical artery; 8 – superficial cervical artery/deep branch of transverse cervical artery; 9 – musculocutaneous perforators through latissimus dorsi from intercostal and lumbar arteries.

(Reproduced with permission from Cormack & Lamberty 1994, Fig 6.24.)

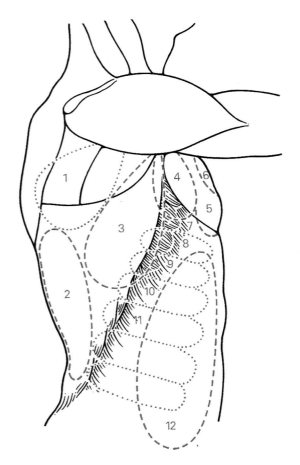

▲ **FIGURE 6.2 Perforators and territories of cutaneous blood supply for the lateral trunk suitable for keystone flap elevation**

Key: 1 – circumflex scapular artery; 2 – intercostal and lumbar perforators, 3 – thoracodorsal artery perforators; 4 – lateral thoracic and cutaneous branch from thoracodorsal artery; 5 – pectoral branch of thoracoacromial axis; 6 – internal thoracic artery perforators; 7–11 – lateral cutaneous branches of the intercostal arteries; 12 – intercostal perforators through the external oblique.

(Reproduced with permission from Cormack & Lamberty 1994, Fig 6.28.)

the back, particularly in a vertical axis. Flaps raised to incorporate the midline must extend to the paraspinous musculature so that the glide plane and improved transverse mobility of this region can be recruited. Alternatives for closure of midline defects include the use of transposition keystone flaps, with closure of the secondary defect positioned in a region of good laxity and glide, or double parallel keystone flaps closed in a Yin Yang manner.

Lateral to the midline there are suitable glide planes between the back skin (and underlying fat) and the fascia of the muscles of the back that permit robust and reliable flap movement. The longitudinal nature of the paraspinous musculature allows good movement transversely in this region but poor movement longitudinally, as seen in the upper limb. As we pass more laterally, the musculature is oriented so as to pass from the spine, upwards and laterally to the shoulder tip (see Fig 6.1). Again, the general rule that flap movement is best perpendicular to the long axis of muscles (therefore, the longitudinal axis of the flap runs with the underlying muscles) will facilitate the greatest movement. The deep fascia over the muscle limits further movement of flaps. Therefore, following islanding of a flap, further mobility can be gained by division of this deep fascia while preserving vascular support via avoidance of fascial undermining.

In the lumbar region, the skin is very thick and its underlying fascia is well-developed. Also, the latissimus dorsi muscle becomes more fibrous near its attachment in this region and, therefore, mobility of flaps in this region is more limited than in the upper back. As a result of this combination of features, flaps in this area must usually be planned to be much larger than the diameter that the defect would require in other body areas. Appropriate flap planning, patient selection and the use of deep absorbable sutures with strategic mattress suturing of the skin minimises the risk of dehiscence in the back, despite the forces placed on back skin as a result of movements such as bending. Figure 3.11 shows the synchronous elevation of two keystone flaps in the back following these principles with good results. Figure 8.8 demonstrates the use of the omega (Ω) variant for larger defects in the parascapular region. Large fasciocutaneous flaps in the back may require the use of suction drains to minimise the potential for seroma formation. Despite their use, seroma development can occur occasionally. Serial percutaneous drainage and compression usually resolves seromas of the back without further surgical intervention. Closure in the back is best undertaken with the support of deep absorbable sutures due to the thickness of the underlying dermis. Skin sutures can then be used to ensure adequate dermal-to-dermal apposition for reliable wound healing.

THE CHEST WALL AND BREAST

The three most common causes of fasciocutaneous defects in the chest wall and breast region are tumours, trauma and infection. Breast cancer is the most common cancer in women, excluding non-melanomatous skin cancer (IARC 2008). Although the keystone island flap can provide wound closure in non-skin-sparing mastectomy, its role is limited in the reconstruction of the majority of mastectomy defects (e.g. skin-sparing mastectomy), as it provides insufficient volume to reconstruct the breast contour. The keystone island flap is most useful in cases of advanced breast malignancy where vascularised skin coverage with rapid healing and minimal morbidity facilitates timely institution of adjuvant therapies. This preserves the latissimus dorsi and rectus-based flaps (where appropriate) for subsequent reconstruction should the patient demonstrate good disease-free survival without the potential donor site morbidity of these operations affecting the patient's oncological management or general health. Fasciocutaneous coverage for cardiothoracic surgery defects (including complications) can be undertaken using the keystone island flap where extensive dead-space obliteration is not necessary. In these settings, the reliable blood supply of the keystone island flap promotes healing and prompt recovery.

Cutaneous blood supply of the chest wall and breast

The chest wall area is very well-suited to the elevation of keystone island flaps due to its good tissue elasticity and predictable cutaneous blood supply. Figure 6.3 demonstrates how the segmental supply passes around the trunk, either in-between the ribs or in the neurovascular plane inferior to the costal margin. Along its course it gives off lateral and anterior perforators segmentally. This segmental supply can be seen in Figure 6.2, along with other direct cutaneous vessels contributing to territories higher up in the anterior chest (Figs 6.4, 6.5). These direct vessels include branches of the thoracoacromial, lateral and superficial pectoral vessels.

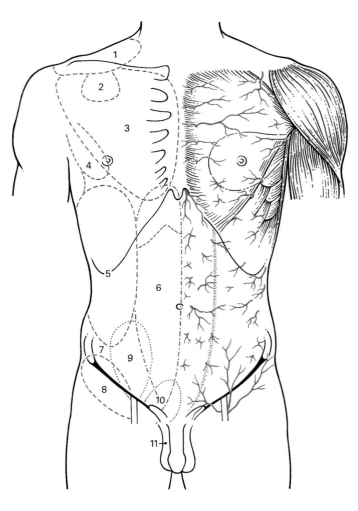

▲ **FIGURE 6.4 Perforators and territories of cutaneous blood supply for the anterior trunk suitable for keystone flap elevation**

Key: 1 – transverse cervical artery; 2 – direct cutaneous branch from thoracoacromial axis; 3 – internal thoracic artery perforators; 4 – superficial thoracic artery; 5 – intercostal perforators through external oblique; 6 – epigastric artery perforators (from the deep inferior and superior epigastric arteries) with occasional superficial superior epigastric artery in the upper region; 7 – small contribution from deep circumflex iliac artery (can be unreliable); 8 –superficial circumflex iliac artery; 9 – superficial inferior epigastric artery; 10 – superficial external pudendal artery; 11 – deep external pudendal artery.

(Reproduced with permission from Cormack & Lamberty 1994, Fig 6.32.)

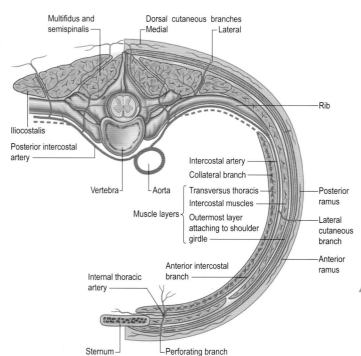

▲ **FIGURE 6.3 Oblique transverse section of the thorax demonstrating the passage of the intercostal arteries from the aorta around the intercostal space (and neurovascular plane in the abdomen) to anastomose with the internal thoracic (or epigastric) artery anteriorly**

Along this course it gives off numerous named perforators suitable as the basis for island (and free) flaps, such as the keystone flap.

(Reproduced with permission from Gray H, Standring S 2005 Gray's anatomy: the anatomical basis of clinical practice, 39th edn. Churchill Livingstone, New York, Fig 54.17.)

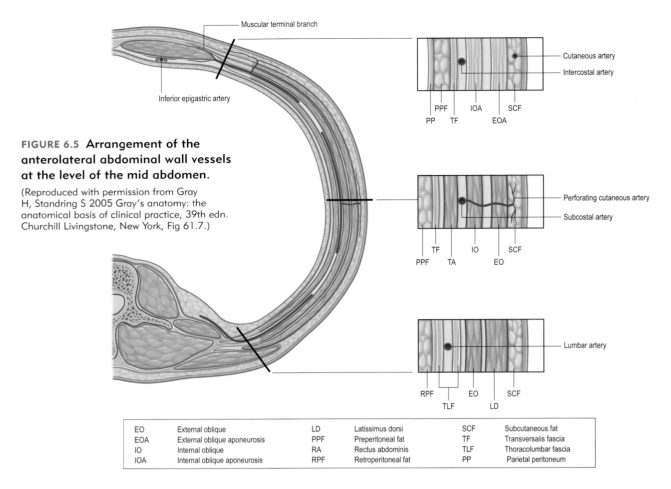

FIGURE 6.5 Arrangement of the anterolateral abdominal wall vessels at the level of the mid abdomen.

(Reproduced with permission from Gray H, Standring S 2005 Gray's anatomy: the anatomical basis of clinical practice, 39th edn. Churchill Livingstone, New York, Fig 61.7.)

EO	External oblique	LD	Latissimus dorsi	SCF	Subcutaneous fat
EOA	External oblique aponeurosis	PPF	Preperitoneal fat	TF	Transversalis fascia
IO	Internal oblique	RA	Rectus abdominis	TLF	Thoracolumbar fascia
IOA	Internal oblique aponeurosis	RPF	Retroperitoneal fat	PP	Parietal peritoneum

Principles of flap elevation in the chest wall and breast

The bucket-handle action of the ribs during inspiration relies upon the elasticity of the lateral chest wall to permit easy breathing. This region demonstrates some of the best skin elasticity in the trunk and, consequently, large defects may be closed here using locoregional reconstruction, particularly with the multiaxial (vectorial) tissue recruitment of keystone and similarly designed island flaps (Fig 6.6). As with other body sites, a few principles should be adhered to prior to reconstruction of fasciocutaneous defects of the chest wall and breast, including:

1 oncological clearance, elimination of significant tissue infection and removal of necrotic material
2 obliteration of dead space, particularly in infected wounds (e.g. post-cardiothoracic surgery defects) where the capacity to close the skin alone may be insufficient to manage the wound. Keystone flaps may be de-epithelialised to minimise dead space but are suboptimal for complex three-dimensional defects.

FIGURE 6.6

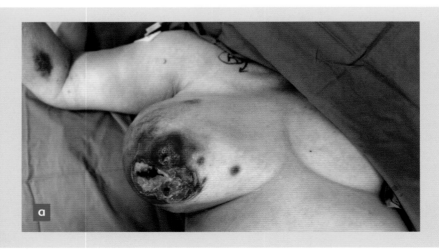

FIGURE 6.6 A 71-year-old woman with advanced fungating spindle cell tumour of the right breast

(a) Primary tumour with ulceration and skin loss mandating mastectomy with wide local skin excision.

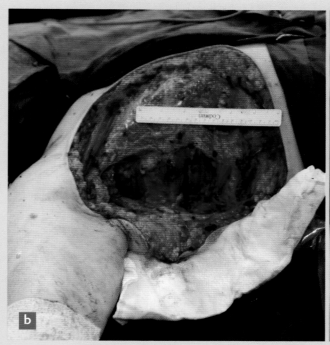

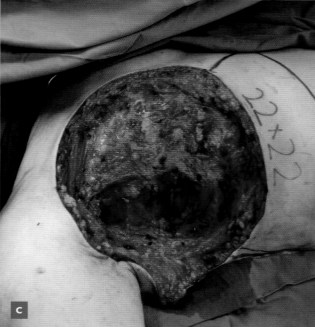

(b) Defect is 22 × 22 cm in size once the edges are pulled to their native position. The costal cartilages of three ribs are exposed.

(c) A keystone flap based upon intercostal artery perforators and incorporating the anterior abdominal wall fascia as its deepest layer is marked out. A line of perforators was obvious within the defect and the keystone flap planned to capture the continuation of this line into the intact skin inferior to the defect.

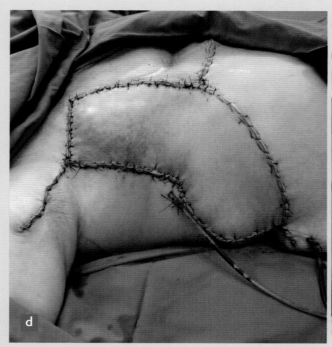

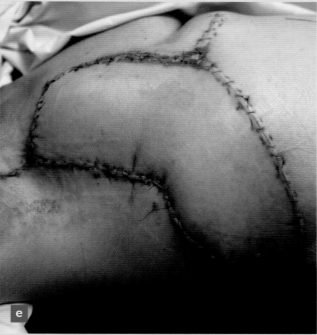

(d) The medial end of the keystone flap is transposed into the defect and the medial arm skin is advanced to permit closure without skin graft. Stretching of the keystone pedicle led to an initial purplish tinge to the tip of the flap, which returned to normal in recovery.

(e) At 3 weeks post operation, with a small superficial wound breakdown at the T-junction. Otherwise, the rest of the wounds have healed without problem. This did not delay radiotherapy.

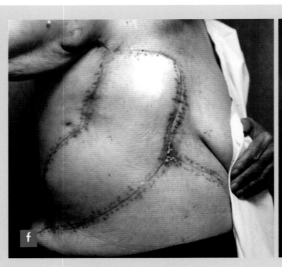

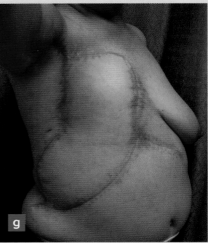

(f) Appearance during radiotherapy showing healing of the T-junction despite irradiation.

(g) Appearance at 3 months after chemotherapy. Patient comfortable with full shoulder abduction and no residual issues.

TLC

Time (operation/cost)
120 minutes
Life quality (and aesthetics)
Good once adjuvant therapies complete, flap not compromised
Complications
Delayed healing at T-junction not affecting commencement of adjuvant therapies; died of metastatic disease 18 months later

ABDOMINAL RECONSTRUCTION

The keystone flap is very useful in the anterior abdominal wall because the natural elasticity of this region combines well with the multiaxial (vectorial) tissue recruitment of the keystone flap. The abdominal wall is composed of two main layers. The skin and underlying fascial layers are superficial, with interposed adipose tissue of variable thickness depending on the body habitus. The anterior abdominal musculature lies deeper, with fascial coverings that have a bearing on the vascular integrity of the overlying skin. Acting together, these lamellae provide sufficient distensability so as to support full abdominal contents and deep diaphragmatic breathing. At the same time, the anterior abdominal wall maintains the abdominal contents within the abdominal cavity through a combination of dynamic muscles and static fascia while facilitating postural movements, bracing and forcible coughing.

Defects of the anterior abdominal wall may be skin alone or both of these layers. Adequate reconstitution of the deep lamella is necessary prior to the use of fasciocutaneous reconstruction in defects of both lamellae. Superficial defects alone can be managed in isolation. Therefore, adequate assessment of the integrity of the musculofascial anterior abdominal wall is vital in fasciocutaneous reconstruction of the abdomen. Previous attempts to reconstruct the deep layer may contribute to morbidity via infection of mesh or significant skin graft contracture and tethering, making reconstruction difficult. As with elsewhere in the trunk, skin cancer resection can result in large areas of fasciocutaneous loss, but as the abdomen is less exposed to the sun and readily visible to most patients, advanced cutaneous malignancies of the abdomen are uncommon. Local wound problems and complications from intra-abdominal pathology are a more common cause of anterior abdominal wall defects. These include surgical wound dehiscence and fistula formation. Adequate management of these conditions is facilitated by a two-team approach (duet surgery). An abdominal surgical team manages the bowel and minimises other contributing factors, such as intestinal secretions, and a reconstructive team focuses on closing the wounds once the aetiological agent (where able to be remedied) is removed. These patients may have multiple surgical scars on their abdomen, so a sound preoperative appreciation of normal and the altered cutaneous vascular anatomy is essential.

Cutaneous vascular anatomy of the anterior abdominal wall

The cutaneous vascular anatomy of the anterior abdominal wall has been one of the most intensively studied in whole body. From the pioneering work of Salmon and Manchot (Cormack & Lamberty 1994), through Behan's own cadaveric injection studies for the elevation of the abdominal angiotome (now encompassing the deep inferior epigastric perforator flap) (Behan & Wilson 1975), the understanding of the angiosomes of the rectus muscle (Taylor 2003) through to more recent developments in vital, real-time vascular perfusion and perforator studies using computerised tomographic angiography (CTA), this intensely studied region is now well-understood (Rozen et al. 2010).

The major contributions to the cutaneous blood supply of the abdomen are from two overlapping systems: the epigastric system and the segmental subcostal and lumbar vessels. The epigastric system is composed of three variably dominant and communicating vessels: the deep inferior epigastric, the superficial inferior epigastric and the superior epigastric vessels. These all supply cutaneous vessels. The deep vessels (superior epigastric and deep inferior epigastric) run deep to the rectus abdominis from superiorly and inferiorly, with their communication occurring at the level of the midpoint between the umbilicus and the xiphoid process. This vessel system sends a series of perforators through (or around) the rectus muscles to supply the overlying skin, with the potential to capture adjoining territories in the contralateral rectus and ipsilateral flank. The superficial inferior epigastric (SIE) vessels, where dominant, may be capable of supplying the entire anterior abdominal wall and run superiorly from the common femoral artery in the groin within the subcutaneous fat to supply the skin directly.

The other major system of vessels is segmental and can be considered a direct continuation of the intercostal vessels beyond and below the level of the costal cartilages. These vessels travel circumferentially in the neurovascular plane between the internal oblique and the transversus abdominis muscles, sending a number of perforators at intervals to the overlying skin before entering the lateral aspect of the rectus abdominis muscle. The vasculature of the abdominal integument demonstrates a very important point in regard to the difference between arterial and venous supply to regions. Just as with radial-artery-based flaps in the upper limb, the predominant venous drainage for the anterior abdominal wall may be to the superficial inferior epigastric system, even when the dominant arterial supply may be from the deep inferior epigastric artery. For this reason, keystone and similar island flaps should preserve all superficial veins and nerves where possible to facilitate this drainage. Previous abdominal surgery with potential for damage to one or more of these vessels may require preoperative Doppler ultrasound or CTA studies to identify the available perforators prior to the planning of major fasciocutaneous flaps in the abdomen.

Principles of flap elevation in the abdomen

There are two main forms of keystone island flap used in the anterior abdominal wall. The first is fasciocutaneous only but preserves the anterior abdominal wall. It is designed and elevated in a similar manner to elsewhere in the body. Islanding of the skin alone provides some movement, with division of successive deeper fascial layers providing even more movement. Avoidance of previous abdominal scars is helpful in assisting mobility of the flap, but not always essential as long as the flap's dimensions allow for the recruitment of reliable perforators. Superficial veins and all neurovascular structures are preserved where possible to ensure adequate venous drainage and provide conjoint blood supply where possible. Flaps can be oriented in almost any direction in this region. Those running obliquely along the line of the external oblique in the lateral abdomen or vertically with the rectus abdominis in the midline and paramedian areas seem to close with the greatest ease. Variants that maintain some convexity (e.g. omega (Ω), goblet or Yin Yang) are useful (Fig 6.7) but not mandatory, as the abdomen will take on its own shape with time. Care must be taken where previous or current stomas are present as distortion of these can have adverse consequences for the patient.

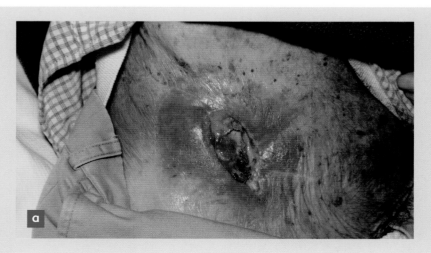

FIGURE 6.7 **An 88-year-old male with basal cell carcinoma of the right iliac fossa complicated by wound breakdown from radiotherapy. Importation of vascularised tissue is ideal for reconstruction in these cases**

(a) Initial presentation with infected ulcer with surrounding erythema.

FIGURE 6.7

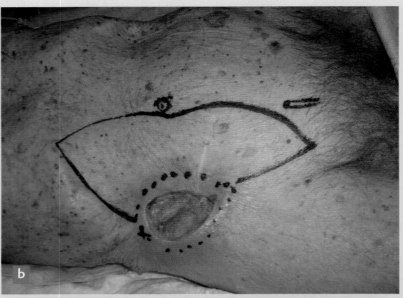

(b) Following surgical excision of the ulcer and antibiotic treatment, a keystone flap is designed based inferiorly on abdominal wall perforators.

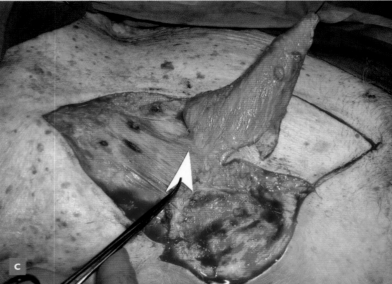

(c) The upper end of the keystone flap is elevated off the anterior abdominal wall (in this cachectic man), demonstrating one of these perforators (arrow).

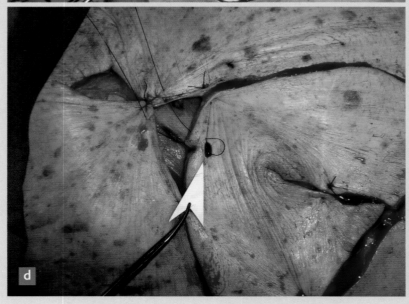

(d) The donor site is closed primarily and the flap displays a *red dot sign* (arrow).

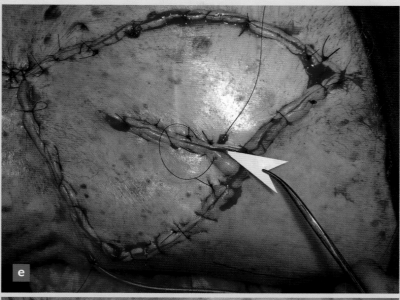

(e) Closure of the defect demonstrates a *red dot sign* on the flap once again (arrow).

(f) The wound has healed well and, by 3 weeks, is ready for suture removal.

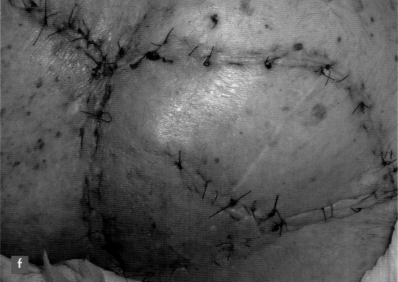

TLC

Time (operation/cost)		
60 minutes		
Life quality (and aesthetics)		
Good, with acceptable aesthetics		
Complications		
Nil		

This fasciocutaneous flap approach can be undertaken in conjunction with separate reconstruction of the anterior abdominal wall, including component separation or the use of mesh repair.

The other form of keystone flap used in the abdomen incorporates the anterior abdominal fascia in its base. In the lateral abdomen, this involves division of the fascia over the abdominal muscles. Vessels running in the neurovascular plane (between the internal oblique and transversus abdominis) are, therefore, preserved and movement of the flap with V–Y closure of the divided layers of the abdomen is undertaken at the donor site. Centrally, the rectus muscle itself may be mobilised in the base of the keystone flap to aid movement, but this does not usually require division of the muscle. As with all other abdominal wall closures, adjunctive procedures can help reconstruct the abdominal wall, including the use of mesh repairs if necessary, and keystone island flaps can be used to salvage infectious complication with such approaches. In large abdominal wall closures, the Yin Yang variant can be of great use because of its excellent tissue recruitment, maintenance of gentle convexity and the offset of its donor site closures (on opposite sides of the primary defect, one up, one down), spreading tension across a greater surface area. An example of this type of flap is shown in Figure 6.8.

FIGURE 6.8

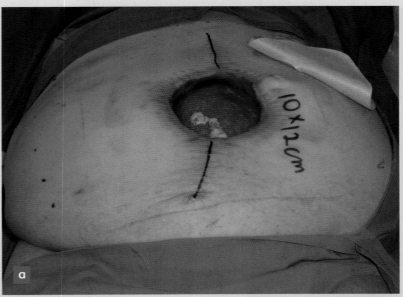

FIGURE 6.8 **A 70-year-old type-2 diabetic patient with a 10 × 12 cm defect of the anterior abdominal wall with left side paramedian stoma. This followed a wound dehiscence as a complication of a Hartmann's procedure and failure of mesh repair, vacuum-assisted (VAC) dressing and split-thickness skin grafting**

(a) Disc-shaped defect of the anterior abdominal wall (10 × 12 cm), with a further 10 cm of undermining from correct use of VAC dressing.

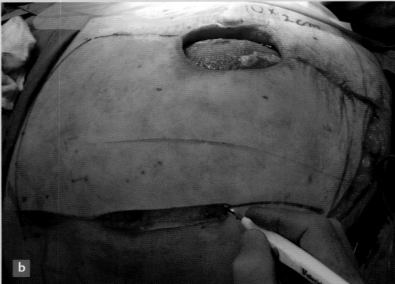

(b) Following revision of the edges of the defect, a right-sided keystone flap is raised using cutting diathermy, based upon the intact abdominal wall perforators more laterally.

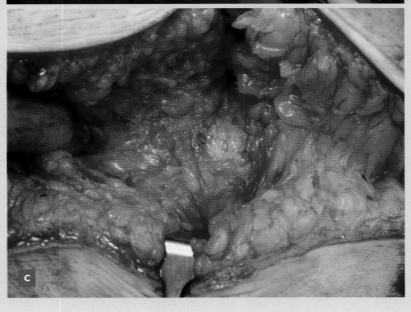

(c) Blunt dissection with the index finger to preserve the integrity of the superficial neurovascular structures, including superficial veins.

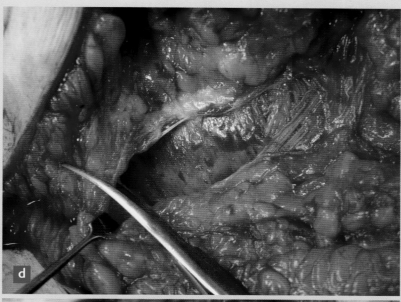

(d) The anterior abdominal fascia is divided to facilitate flap mobilisation while preserving the underlying external oblique muscle.

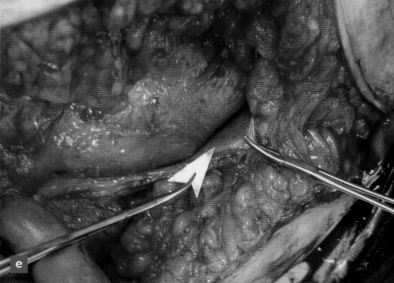

(e) A plane has now been developed between the deep fascia of the anterior abdominal wall (arrow) and the underlying tissues.

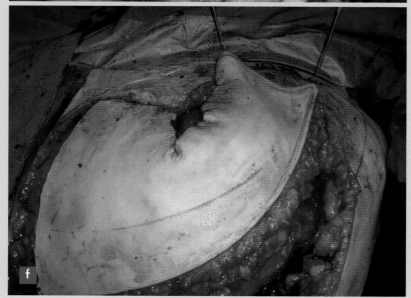

(f) The inferior end of the flap is elevated in this plane and transposed to cover the defect.

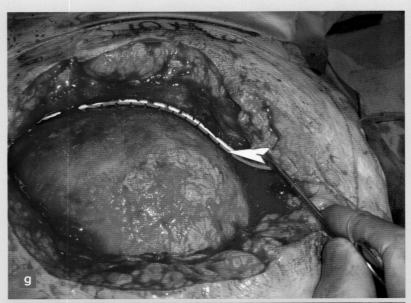

(g) Drains are inserted to minimise dead space during healing, with two in each lateral gutter of the defect and one for the donor site.

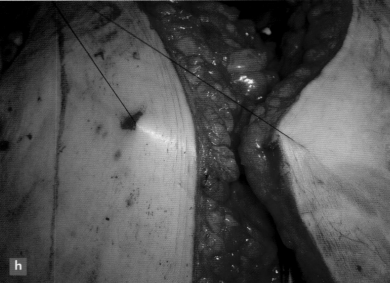

(h) A *red dot sign* confirms the increased vascular perfusion to the skin with islanding, as detailed in Chapter 2.

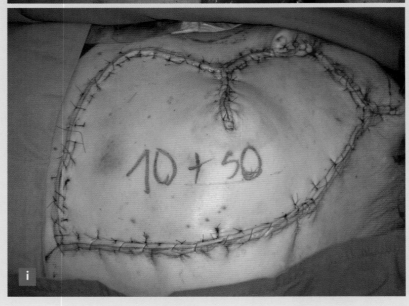

(i) Wound appearance following completion of closure with strategic mattress suturing and a continuous hemming suture. The total time for the reconstruction is 70 + 50 = 120 minutes.

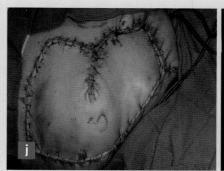 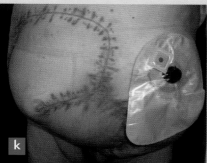 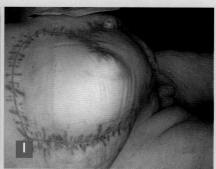

(j) Appearance at 5 days post operation showing no evidence of complications. Patient went home at day 10 after 6 months in hospital prior to referral for keystone surgery.

(k) Appearance at 6 weeks post operation showing good healing and no functional issues.

(l) A residual dog ear of the flap is evident and this can be revised under local anaesthetic.

TLC

Time (operation/cost)
120 minutes
Life quality (and aesthetics)
Good, patient initially concerned about dog ear despite previous appearance
Complications
Haematoma drained at 7 days; no sequelae

See video for Figure 6.8

THE PERINEUM

Oncological resection is the most common reason for the development of perineal defects. Reconstruction of these defects usually requires vascularised tissue coverage, particularly with radiotherapy (pre- or postoperatively). As in other areas, pathological clearance of the tumour is advisable before undertaking reconstruction. A number of flaps are existing workhorses for perineal reconstruction. These include myocutaneous flaps, such as the vertical (VRAM) (Shukla & Hughes 1984) and extended rectus abdominis muscle (Villa et al. 2011) flaps, and gracilis myocutaneous flaps (McCraw et al. 1976), as well as fasciocutaneous flaps, such as the Singapore (Wee & Joseph 1989) and lotus petal flaps (Yii & Niranjan 1996). All of these flaps require knowledge of their vascular anatomy and incorporation of specific named vessels within the flaps for their survival. Despite this, sometimes the distal ends of these flaps can be unreliable (e.g. VRAM and extended VRAM). One major benefit of keystone island flaps over the use of other flaps in this region is their reliability without specific incorporation of named vessels within the flap. Using the principles of keystone elevation, the reconstruction of small to moderate-sized defects can be achieved in a relatively straightforward manner. The reliable nature of the blood supply to keystone flaps (immediate vascular augmentation concept, IVAC)

also permits shaping and contouring of the flap with certainty (including the excision of any dog ears). These sorts of manoeuvres are not generally possible with other types of flap.

Cutaneous vascular anatomy of the perineum

The perineal vessels are the dominant neurovascular supply to the skin of the perineal region. They leave the pelvis and enter the posterolateral aspect of the perineum by passage through the greater and lesser sciatic notches, running forward to ramify in the base of the mons pubis after giving off multiple vessels along its course, including vessels extending down the upper, inner aspect of the thigh. These vessels are the basis for a number of flaps, including the lotus (Yii & Niranjan 1996, Warrier et al. 2004) and modified lotus petal flaps (Warrier et al. 2004), but can also supply keystone design flaps without their strict identification. The mons pubis is also supplied from its lateral aspect by the superficial external pudendal vessels (Figs 6.4, 6.9) as direct branches from the common femoral artery, but these are generally only of use when reconstructing mons defects specifically. The external genitalia are supplied by the deep external pudendal vessels with a small contribution from the superficial external pudendal vessels. The principles of keystone elevation are the same here as elsewhere and Figure 6.10 demonstrates a simple keystone island flap used for perineal reconstruction.

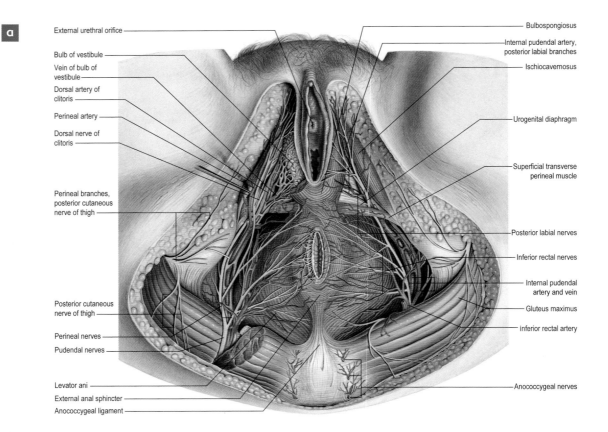

a

External urethral orifice
Bulb of vestibule
Vein of bulb of vestibule
Dorsal artery of clitoris
Perineal artery
Dorsal nerve of clitoris
Perineal branches, posterior cutaneous nerve of thigh
Posterior cutaneous nerve of thigh
Perineal nerves
Pudendal nerves
Levator ani
External anal sphincter
Anococcygeal ligament

Bulbospongiosus
Internal pudendal artery, posterior labial branches
Ischiocavernosus
Urogenital diaphragm
Superficial transverse perineal muscle
Posterior labial nerves
Inferior rectal nerves
Internal pudendal artery and vein
Gluteus maximus
Inferior rectal artery
Anococcygeal nerves

▲ **FIGURE 6.9** **Course, branches and perforators of the internal pudendal artery (and inferior rectal artery) in the (a) female and (b) male perineum. Note that the relationship between the perineal structures and the underlying vessels makes local flaps well suited for use in this region, depending on defect and size.**

Numerous perforators are present with extension from the perineum onto the inner aspect of the upper thigh. The inner groin crease skin is well-suited to perineal reconstruction due to its good blood supply, similar colour and texture to the perineum.

(Reproduced with permission from Gray H, Standring S 2005 Gray's anatomy: the anatomical basis of clinical practice, 39th edn. Churchill Livingstone, New York, Figs 76.20, 77.4.)

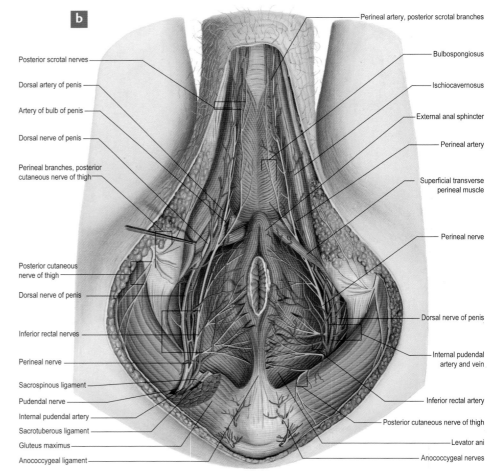

b

Posterior scrotal nerves
Dorsal artery of penis
Artery of bulb of penis
Dorsal nerve of penis
Perineal branches, posterior cutaneous nerve of thigh
Posterior cutaneous nerve of thigh
Dorsal nerve of penis
Inferior rectal nerves
Perineal nerve
Sacrospinous ligament
Pudendal nerve
Internal pudendal artery
Sacrotuberous ligament
Gluteus maximus
Anococcygeal ligament

Perineal artery, posterior scrotal branches
Bulbospongiosus
Ischiocavernosus
External anal sphincter
Perineal artery
Superficial transverse perineal muscle
Perineal nerve
Dorsal nerve of penis
Internal pudendal artery and vein
Inferior rectal artery
Posterior cutaneous nerve of thigh
Levator ani
Anococcygeal nerves

FIGURE 6.10 **A 42-year-old female with radio-recurrent squamous cell carcinoma of the posterior vaginal wall/vestibule**

FIGURE 6.10

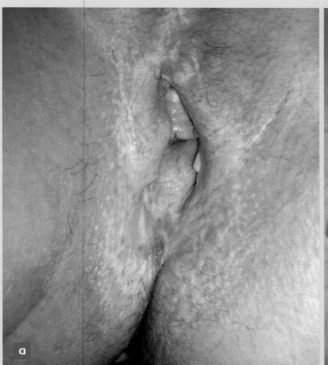

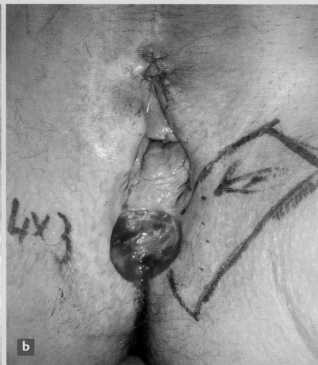

(a) Lesion following biopsy confirmation of diagnosis.

(b) A 4 × 3 cm defect is produced by surgical excision of the lesion.

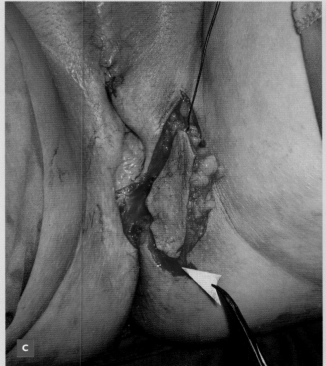

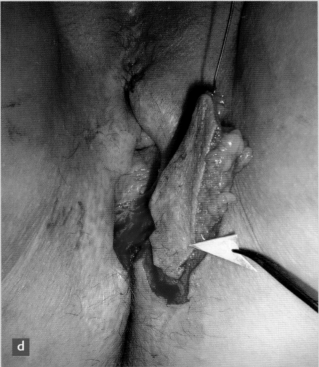

(c) A keystone flap posteriorly based on internal pudendal artery perforators is marked, then elevated.

(d) The flap is islanded and demonstrates good vascularity.

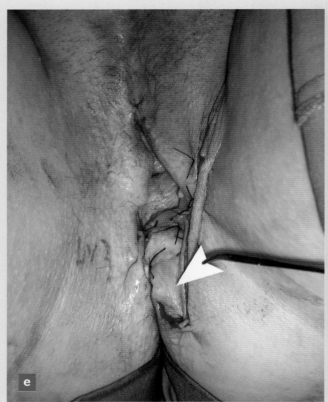

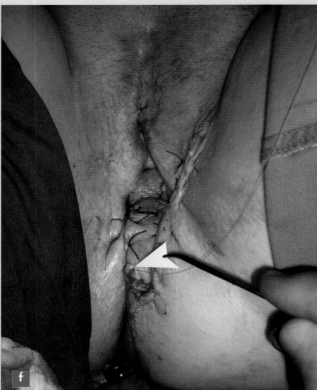

(e) Strategic mattress suturing of the flap into the defect permits approximation and direct closure of the donor site.

(f) Continuous suturing with an absorbable suture demonstrates a *red dot sign* consistent with increased cutaneous blood flow.

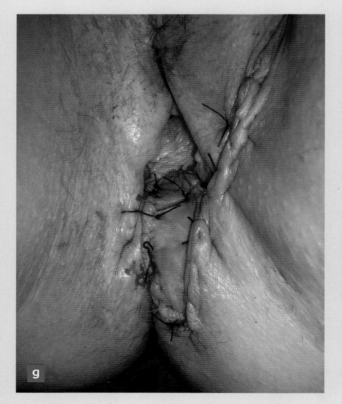

(g) A healthy flap upon completion of suturing.

TLC: Conjoint flap vascularity: pudendal artery branches and external pudendal nerve

Time (operation/cost)
60 minutes
Life quality (and aesthetics)
Good with normal function and acceptable appearance
Complications
Nil

BUTTOCK AND PERIANAL RECONSTRUCTION

The most common cause of perianal reconstruction is following excision of pilonidal sinuses. Appropriate clearance of the sinus(es) and their infected and inflammatory contents is necessary prior to surgical reconstruction, otherwise early recurrence will ensue. Obliteration of the acute natal cleft angle will also minimise late recurrence. The keystone flap can be a useful design to achieve this by bridging across the natal cleft, thereby providing a less acute angle. The Yin Yang variant (double keystone flaps) is particularly useful where large cutaneous defects are formed. Other common causes of perianal and buttock skin defects include pressure areas and oncological defects following abdominoperineal resection. The keystone island flap has its place among other flap types and designs in the reconstruction of these defects. The simplicity of this flap design and the ease of its application, particularly in the elderly, adds to its appeal.

Cutaneous vascular anatomy of the buttock region

As shown in Figures 6.1 and 6.11, numerous cutaneous perforators within the buttock region pass through the gluteus maximus muscle. They are derived from the superior and inferior gluteal arteries that run deep to this muscle. The perforators are sufficiently numerous that pre- or intraoperative Doppler ultrasound identification of perforators is not usually necessary.

Principles of flap elevation in the buttock region

The buttock region is composed of two large convex surfaces (the buttocks proper) with a midline flat plane over the sacrum superiorly and a deep natal cleft inferiorly. Mobilisation of flaps from the buttocks is relatively straightforward due to their convexity, which supplies additional surface area. There is usually a well-built adipose tissue layer immediately deep to the skin and then the gluteus muscles themselves. Island flaps such as the keystone maximise the reliability of flaps in this region and permit multiaxial (vectorial) recruitment of tissue. This multiaxial recruitment minimises contour deformity as a result of flap closure (scar is better tolerated than contour deformity in this region). Islanding may be of skin, fat and fascia or include all structures down (and occasionally including) the muscle layer, depending on the size and requirements of the defect. Figure 6.12 demonstrates the use of keystone closure for a moderate-sized fasciocutaneous defect of the natal cleft.

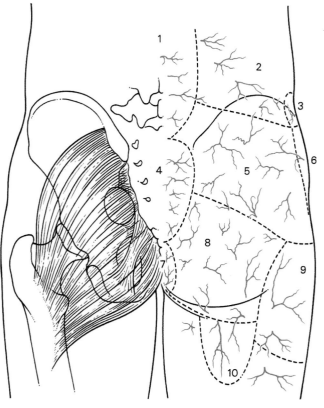

◄ **FIGURE 6.11 Perforators and territories of cutaneous blood supply for the buttock suitable for keystone flap elevation**

On the left is the outline for the course of the gluteus maximus muscle. On the right are the large number of cutaneous perforators that pass to the skin in this region, including the territories outlined in the key.

Key: 1 – medial dorsal cutaneous branches of lumbar arteries; 2 – lateral dorsal cutaneous branches of lumbar arteries and the iliolumbar artery; 3 – superficial circumflex iliac artery; 4 – lateral sacral arteries; 5 – superior gluteal artery; 6 – lateral circumflex femoral artery via the tensor fascia lata; 7 – internal pudendal artery; 8 – inferior gluteal artery; 9 – first profunda perforator; 10 – branch of the inferior gluteal artery travelling with the posterior cutaneous nerve of the thigh. All of these territories are suitable for keystone flap elevation, but caution should be exercised in the use of the sacral perforators since this area is not particularly mobile, therefore more laterally based flaps are advisable.

(Reproduced with permission from Cormack & Lamberty 1994, Fig 6.83.)

FIGURE 6.12

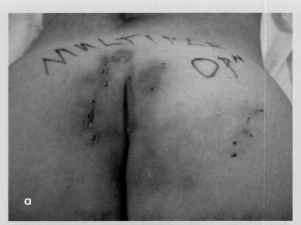

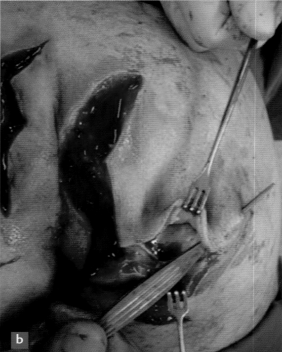

FIGURE 6.12 A 38-year-old male presents with a 20-year history of recurrent abscesses in the buttock region treated with multiple abscess drainage procedures but no surgical excision

(a) Site of numerous sinuses extended well beyond the midline, particularly on the right.

(b) Forceps demonstrate the epithelial lined sinuses.

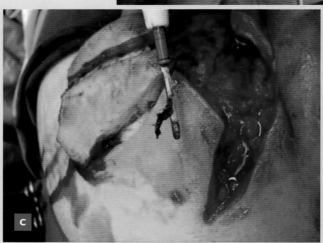

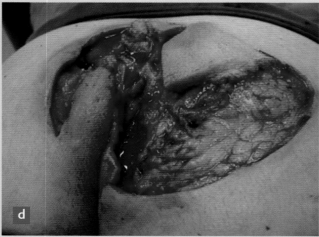

(c) Surgical excision of the tracts with some residual debris and hair.

(d) Appearance of the defect site following surgical excision (15 × 10 cm) of the sinuses.

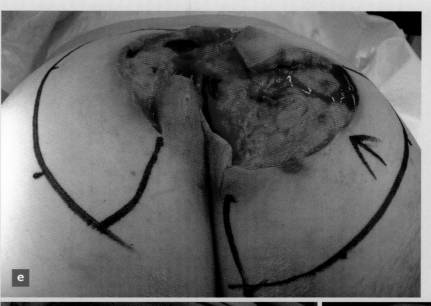

(e) Double lateral keystone flaps are designed for defect closure.

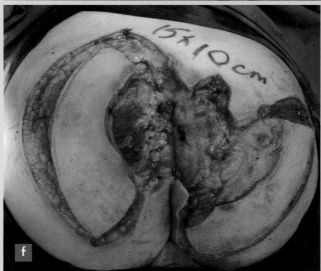

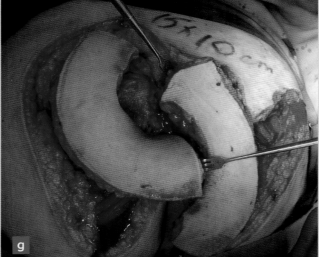

(f) Following islanding of the flaps.

(g) Closure of the flaps in a Yin Yang manner to equalise tension across the entire wound and obliterate the natal cleft to minimise recurrence.

(h) Initial apposition of the flaps using strategic mattress suturing with demonstration of two *red dot signs* in the left flap (lower).

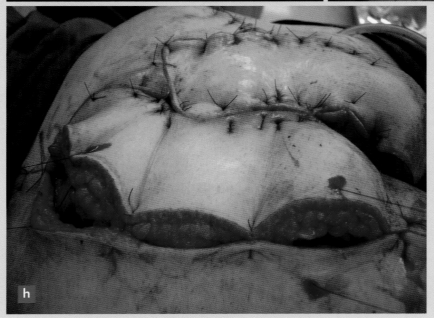

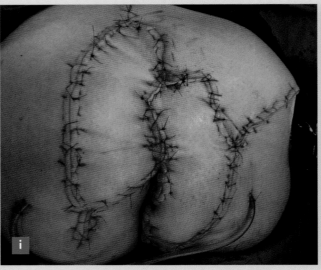

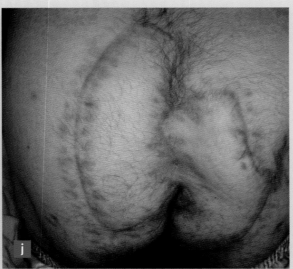

(i) Appearance following wound closure.

(j) Appearance 8 months later without recurrence.

TLC

Time (operation/cost)		
120 minutes		
Life quality (and aesthetics)		
Good with normal function and acceptable appearance		
Complications		
Nil		

(Reproduced with permission from Behan F, Rozen WM, Tan S 2011 Yin-Yang flaps: the mathematics of two keystone island flaps for reconstructing increasingly large defects. ANZ J Surg 81(7–8):574–5.)

SUMMARY

The trunk is large with diverse regions that share a number of similarities in terms of their cutaneous vascular supply. Numerous axial and random pattern flaps have been described in each of these regions. The keystone island flap offers the benefits of being a single, simple design with application in all of these body areas without the need for specific identification of vessels at its base. No other single flap provides this facility.

BIBLIOGRAPHY

Behan F C, Wilson J 1975 The principle of the angiotome, a system of linked axial pattern flaps. Sixth International Congress of Plastic and Reconstructive Surgery, Paris.

Cormack G C, Lamberty B G H 1994 The arterial anatomy of skin flaps, 2nd edn. Churchill Livingstone, Edinburgh.

Hamilton S G, Morrison W A 1982 The scapular free flap. Br J Plast Surg 35(1):2–7.

International Agency for Research on Cancer (IARC) 2008 GLOBOCAN 2008. Cancer incidence and mortality worldwide: IARC CancerBase no. 10. IARC, Lyon, http://globocan.iarc.fr/.

McCraw J B, Massey F M, Shanklin K D, Horton CE 1976 Vaginal reconstruction with gracilis myocutaneous flaps. Plast Reconstr Surg 58(2):176–83.

Nassif T M, Vidal L, Bovet J L, Baudet J 1982 The parascapular flap: a new cutaneous microsurgical free flap. Plast Reconstr Surg 69(4):591–600.

Rozen W M, Ashton M W, Le Roux C M, Pan W R, Corlett R J 2010 The perforator angiosome: a new concept in the design of deep inferior epigastric artery perforator flaps for breast reconstruction. Microsurgery 30(1):1–7.

Shukla H S, Hughes L E 1984 The rectus abdominis flap for perineal wounds. Ann R Coll Surg Engl 66(5):337–9.

Taylor G I 2003 The angiosomes of the body and their supply to perforator flaps. Clin Plast Surg 30(3):331–42.

Villa M, Saint-Cyr M, Wong C, Butler C E 2011 Extended vertical rectus abdominis myocutaneous flap for pelvic reconstruction: three-dimensional and four-dimensional computed tomography angiographic perfusion study and clinical outcome analysis. Plast Reconstr Surg 127(1):200–9.

Warrier S K, Kimble F W, Blomfield P 2004 Refinements in the lotus petal flap repair of the vulvo-perineum. Aust N Z J Surg 74(8):684–8.

Wee J T, Joseph V T 1989 A new technique of vaginal reconstruction using neurovascular pudendal-thigh flaps: a preliminary report. Plast Reconstr Surg 83(4):701–9.

Yii N W, Niranjan N S 1996 Lotus petal flaps in vulvo-vaginal reconstruction. Br J Plast Surg 49(8):547–54.

Chapter 7
The lower limb

The golden rule is, there are no golden rules.

George Bernard Shaw (1856–1950)

Loss of mobility can be devastating to the functional capacity of patients. The keystone island flap provides simple, reliable fasciocutaneous coverage of lower limb defects with minimal immobilisation.

INTRODUCTION

The lower limb is integral to walking and normal independence. As a result, injuries and defects to the lower limb can have a major impact on mobility and, thus, affect activities of daily living. Prolonged immobilisation through trauma or following surgery results in deconditioning, especially in the elderly. Rehabilitation may return patients to near pre-existing function but often at a substantial cost relative to similar injuries in other body regions (Hartholt et al. 2010). Where rehabilitation is unsuccessful or not practical, loss of independence and institutionalisation adversely affects quality of life and may even shorten life expectancy (Lee et al. 2009). The ideal lower limb reconstruction results in rapid, reliable defect coverage with minimal morbidity, early mobilisation and good aesthetics. Unlike most other reconstructive options, the keystone island flap (and variants) can achieve this outcome in suitable patients and defects by minimising operating time and maintaining quality of life and aesthetics, with minimal complications.

A vast array of reconstructive options has been described for lower limb reconstruction. This is indicative of the increased challenges of reconstruction in the lower limb compared with other body regions of the body and the fact that no single reconstruction is ideal in every situation. The lower limb has the longest arteries, veins and nerves in the body. Arterial disease manifests early within the lower limb (along with coronary and carotid disease), resulting in decreased blood supply, poorer healing, intermittent claudication, rest pain and arterial ulceration. These changes may be compounded by the presence of diabetes mellitus contributing both micro- and macroangiopathy. The dependent position of the limb requires functioning venous valves, appropriate movement for the action of deep venous return via muscle pumps and functional lymphatic drainage. Venous disease from incompetent venous valves causes venous stasis, lipodermatosclerosis and venous ulceration, and contributes to varicose veins. Neuropathies such as diabetic neuropathy affect the lower limb first because these are the longest sensory nerves in the body.

A proper assessment of any fasciocutaneous defect of the lower limb should include the identification of any pre-existing disease, particularly where it is reversible. Any intervention to optimise arterial inflow in patients with peripheral vascular disease can improve the success rate of locoregional reconstruction. If neglected, poor healing may result, with reconstructive failure worsening the morbidity for the patient (hence the maxim *primum non nocere*—first do no harm). Identification of the causative agent and any associated issues will also have a bearing on the reconstruction.

The two most common causes of fasciocutaneous defects in the lower limb are trauma and tumours. Minor trauma to the legs in elderly patients, particularly in the pretibial region, is associated with significant morbidity due to their thin skin and the relatively subcutaneous position of the bones in the leg. Skin grafting of this low-velocity trauma is usually effective in closing the defect, but the immobilisation necessary for major soft tissue defects to ensure graft take can decondition the elderly and frail. Where feasible, keystone flap closure of these major defects is associated with early mobilisation and minimal deconditioning, with significant benefits to the patient and health budgets. Trauma as a specific entity is covered further in Chapter 10, but it is worth mentioning that high-velocity trauma can cause extensive devascularisation and circulatory stasis. Locoregional reconstruction in this setting should be undertaken with caution. A brief delay in reconstruction to permit assessment of locoregional vascularity may permit reliable use of local tissue for reconstruction in these cases (Behan et al. 1994).

The other major cause of fasciocutaneous defects of the lower limb is tumours. Skin cancers are relatively common in the lower limb, particularly in ageing populations (UN Department of Economic and Social Affairs 2010). Primary skin cancers are quite frequent below the knee and secondary deposits in the groin are an additional surgical challenge, as often experienced in melanoma (see Chapter 8). Following appropriate surgical clearance, keystone island flaps (or variants, see Chapter 3) are effective in reconstructing fasciocutaneous defects of the lower limb due to the well-developed system of perforators in this region. Smaller defects can usually be closed directly with keystone flap coverage, and early mobilisation (the same day) undertaken. Occasionally, a small skin graft may be necessary for the secondary defect if tension is too great. Graft loss in these smaller skin grafts is relatively infrequent due to minimal shear and, therefore, they usually tolerate early mobilisation well. Early mobilisation provides significant benefits for elderly patients. Additional keystone flap benefits include reliable healing, the capacity to cover non-vascularised defects (e.g. exposed bone), improved contour reconstruction and aesthetics.

As was evident in the upper limb, the lower limb has many musculocutaneous and septocutaneous perforators supplying the skin, along with a few direct vessels and the vessels accompanying cutaneous nerves (augmenting blood supply in keystone flaps designed along the dermatomes). These form the basis of a very large number of described flaps for reconstruction, including regional arteriovenous, neurovascular and venous flaps, as well as free flaps. In addition, muscle flaps (e.g. gastrocnemius flaps) in the leg have been used successfully for the reconstruction of leg defects, particularly in the upper and middle thirds of the leg. However, the functional disability that results from defunctioning a muscle in an already injured limb can be significant and may bear medicolegal implications (Daigeler et al. 2009). This approach, particularly in the young, compares poorly to the use of fasciocutaneous reconstruction (locoregional or free) where the defect does not have complex three-dimensional geometry and where dead space can be obliterated appropriately.

Free-flap reconstruction remains the principal form of reconstruction in specific instances. Its application remains unchallenged in devascularising trauma of the lower limb or in reconstruction of whole compartments of the leg as free vascularised functional muscle, thereby providing both tissue coverage and reconstituting some muscle function. Large defects of the lower third of the leg form another classic indication for the use of free-tissue transfer in the lower limb. Free-tissue transfer

in appropriate patients has a very low failure rate in the hands of trained microsurgeons within dedicated specialised units (Wei et al. 2001). However, free-flap reconstruction involves very prolonged surgery with significant morbidity for patients, including the added morbidity from the flap donor site. Locoregional reconstructive expertise has suffered from the dominance of microsurgery in recent times, with an apparent de-emphasis within plastic and reconstructive surgical training. When free-flap reconstruction is undertaken for defects that might otherwise be suitable for locoregional reconstruction, patients may be placed at undue risk and health budgets may reflect this additional cost.

Locoregional reconstruction must be tailored specifically to the defect, the available tissues and blood supply. Where vascularised tissue is required, locoregional fasciocutaneous reconstruction represents a viable alternative that fulfils the objectives of minimising operating time and maintaining quality of life and aesthetics, with minimal complications. This is because it provides robust vascularised soft tissue cover using locally matched tissue, with improved aesthetics, minimises functional morbidity for the limb and avoids damaging other body regions in the process. Only where locoregional reconstruction is not applicable, or where a secondary goal of free-tissue transfer is sought (e.g. flow-through flap for peripheral revascularisation), should free-tissue transfer take precedence.

CUTANEOUS VASCULAR ANATOMY OF THE LOWER LIMB

The rich network of fasciocutaneous vessels in the lower limb provides a sound basis for the use of perforator-based fasciocutaneous flaps, such as the keystone island flap, in the lower limb. For descriptive purposes, we will examine the cutaneous vascular anatomy in the following regions of the lower limb: thigh; knee; leg; ankle and dorsum of foot; and plantar surface of the foot.

The thigh

The blood supply to the skin of the thigh is predominantly from the profunda femoris artery and its branches. This branches off the common femoral artery within the upper thigh and passes posterolaterally in the leg to supply the muscles of the anterior compartment before sending either direct septocutaneous or indirect musculocutaneous perforators to the skin. The vascular anatomy of this region is well understood due to the use of the profunda branches for various regional and free flaps, including the anterolateral thigh (ALT) flap, tensor fasciae lata (TFL) flap and anteromedial thigh flap, among others. These vessels may be imaged preoperatively via computerised tomographic angiography (CTA) or identified intraoperatively using Doppler ultrasound. These approaches have been developed for free-tissue transfer and are not necessary for keystone flap elevation as long as the dimensions of the flap are sufficiently large to capture at least one of these perforators. With many free flaps, a good-sized pedicle is vital, mainly for ensuring adequate venous drainage (the arterial supply from even small perforators is often sufficient for large tissue flaps). As McGregor* indicated, venous insufficiency is more of an impedance to flap success than is arterial input, which has been demonstrated in the keystone island flap. For these flaps, the preservation of multiple cutaneous veins is an important principle, as this removes venous restriction and, therefore, relatively small unnamed perforators can be used to support the flap without explicit dissection or skeletonisation. In fact, if inadvertent injury to venous structures occurs, repair of these is undertaken to avoid venous difficulties or arteriovenous mismatch. Figures 7.1 to 7.3 demonstrate the numerous perforators of the thigh and show how these perforators reach the skin for use as the basis for keystone flaps.

The knee

The cutaneous blood supply to the knee region is often neglected in surgical texts and in the minds of reconstructive microsurgeons. Since the development of musculocutaneous flaps and the popularity of texts such as that written by Mathes and Nahai (1997), cutaneous blood supply has been described in terms of musculoskeletal or septocutaneous perforators (and their muscular relations) or individual direct vessels to the skin of use in specific named flaps. The only reference to the geniculate vessels in microsurgery appears when considering free-vascularised bone transfer on the medial geniculate system. As a result, these vessels can easily be overlooked as a source of perforators to the overlying skin and as a basis for locoregional flaps. As illustrated in Figure 7.4, the geniculate anastomosis of vessels is a rich vascular network giving off numerous perforators to the skin. The middle geniculate artery is the only vessel of this group that does not supply perforators to the skin. Otherwise, the popliteal artery gives off the following vessels that provide perforators: the medial and lateral superior geniculate, the medial and lateral inferior geniculate, the anterior recurrent and the descending geniculate arteries. A number of local fasciocutaneous flaps have been described in this region based on geniculate vessel perforators, including the popliteo-thigh flap, the lateral genicula flap, the lower lateral thigh flap and the posterolateral thigh flap (Cormack & Lamberty 1994).

* Ian McGregor, a well-known surgeon from the famous Canniesburn Plastic & Reconstructive Surgery Unit in Scotland.

The leg

Three major vessels supply the skin of the leg. The popliteal artery gives off the anterior tibial artery and then bifurcates into the posterior tibial and peroneal arteries. Each of these vessels runs within a musculofascial compartment of the leg, namely the anterior, posterior and lateral compartments, respectively. From the vessels within these compartments, both musculocutaneous and fasciocutaneous perforators emerge to supply the overlying skin. The fasciocutaneous perforators are well-developed in the septa between the compartments of the leg. It is relatively easy to identify the site of these perforators intraoperatively using Doppler ultrasound but we have not found this to be necessary in the planning of most keystone island flaps in this region.

Other vessels provide additional cutaneous blood supply in this region. The sural vessels join to form the short saphenous artery (otherwise referred to as the median superficial sural artery) running with the sural nerve. The artery of the great saphenous vein (running with the saphenous nerve) is a continuation of the

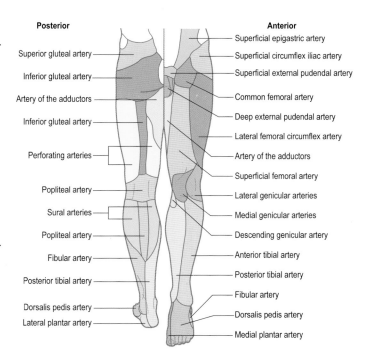

⋀ **FIGURE 7.1 Skin territories supplied via perforators from underlying named vessels show a predictable pattern in the lower limb. Designing flaps so as to capture these territories aids the reliable elevation and mobilisation of flaps in the lower limb. There are individual differences in the size of these territories and in the course of the perforators during their transit to the skin**

(Reproduced with permission from Gray H, Standring S 2005 Gray's anatomy: the anatomical basis of clinical practice, 39th edn. Churchill Livingstone, New York, Fig 79.5.)

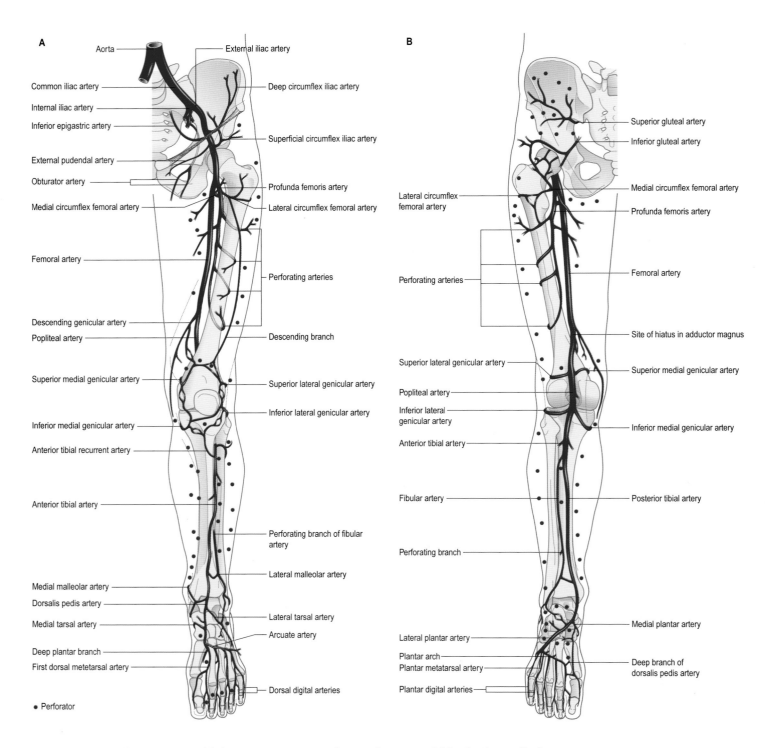

A

Aorta

Common iliac artery

Internal iliac artery

Inferior epigastric artery

External pudendal artery

Obturator artery

Medial circumflex femoral artery

Femoral artery

Descending genicular artery

Popliteal artery

Superior medial genicular artery

Inferior medial genicular artery

Anterior tibial recurrent artery

Anterior tibial artery

Medial malleolar artery

Dorsalis pedis artery

Medial tarsal artery

Deep plantar branch

First dorsal metetarsal artery

• Perforator

External iliac artery

Deep circumflex iliac artery

Superficial circumflex iliac artery

Profunda femoris artery

Lateral circumflex femoral artery

Perforating arteries

Descending branch

Superior lateral genicular artery

Inferior lateral genicular artery

Perforating branch of fibular artery

Lateral malleolar artery

Lateral tarsal artery

Arcuate artery

Dorsal digital arteries

B

Lateral circumflex femoral artery

Perforating arteries

Superior lateral genicular artery

Popliteal artery

Inferior lateral genicular artery

Anterior tibial artery

Fibular artery

Perforating branch

Lateral plantar artery

Plantar arch

Plantar metatarsal artery

Plantar digital arteries

Superior gluteal artery

Inferior gluteal artery

Medial circumflex femoral artery

Profunda femoris artery

Femoral artery

Site of hiatus in adductor magnus

Superior medial genicular artery

Inferior medial genicular artery

Posterior tibial artery

Medial plantar artery

Deep branch of dorsalis pedis artery

FIGURE 7.2 Major cutaneous vascular perforators within the lower limb are at regular intervals and run within septae (or through muscles directly) to reach the undersurface of the skin. Numerous smaller perforators are spaced in between these major perforators, depending on the size of their cutaneous territory. Dots mark the sites of these regular major cutaneous perforators

(Reproduced with permission from Gray H, Standring S 2005 Gray's anatomy: the anatomical basis of clinical practice, 39th edn. Churchill Livingstone, New York, Fig 79.7.)

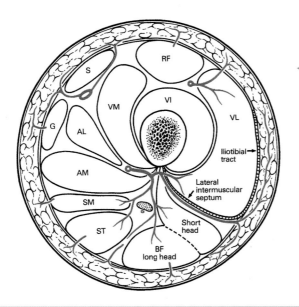

◄ **FIGURE 7.3** Transverse section of the mid thigh, showing the three principal vessels at this level and how their perforators reach the skin

(Reproduced with permission from Cormack & Lamberty 1994, Fig 6.85.)

▶ **FIGURE 7.4** The peripatellar plexus is a group of communicating vessels surrounding the knee. These provide for circulation during movement of the limb, where single end-vessels would likely be compressed during movement or prolonged postures. The majority of these vessels send vessels to supply the overlying skin, and these can be used as the basis for locoregional flaps

(Reproduced with permission from Gray H, Standring S 2005 Gray's anatomy: the anatomical basis of clinical practice, 39th edn. Churchill Livingstone, New York, Fig 113.3. p. 4072.)

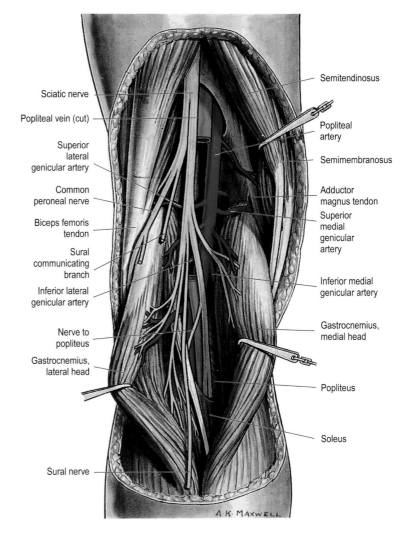

superficial femoral artery and contributes supply to the upper medial calf. These vessels, along with arteries following the other cutaneous nerves of the leg, provide additional (conjoint) supply for keystone and similar island flap designs. Figures 7.5 to 7.7 demonstrate these vessels and their cutaneous perforators.

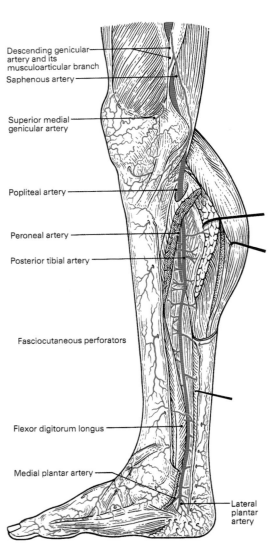

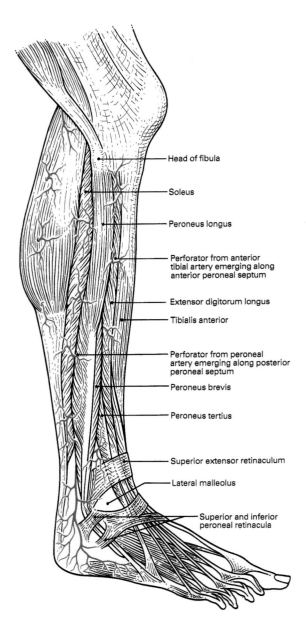

▲ **FIGURE 7.5 The posterior tibial artery of the medial aspect of the leg with numerous musculocutaneous and septocutaneous branches**

Cutaneous perforators can be readily identified using Doppler ultrasound but the ready availability of perforators means that this is usually not necessary during flap planning if the ratio of flap to defect size is appropriate.

(Reproduced with permission from Cormack & Lamberty 1994, Fig 6.111.)

▲ **FIGURE 7.6 Cutaneous perforators of the lateral aspect of the leg**

In addition to gastrocnemius muscle perforators, the main source of perforators for the lateral leg is the peroneal artery, with some of the largest perforators running within the posterior peroneal (intermuscular) septum. The lateral compartment of the leg contributes only a small amount of the circumference of the leg and, therefore, keystone island flaps that require division of the deep fascia may be limited by this longitudinal septum. For this reason, transverse movement is more effective than longitudinal flap movement.

(Reproduced with permission from Cormack & Lamberty 1994, Fig 6.109.)

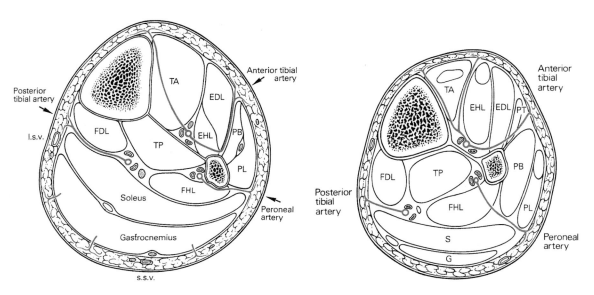

▲ FIGURE 7.7 Cross-sectional anatomy of the upper third and lower third of the leg, demonstrating the passage of perforating vessels from the three major vessels of the lower limb to the overlying skin

These vessels can be traced, if required, and a number of skeletonised perforator-based flaps have been described.

(Reproduced with permission from Cormack & Lamberty 1994, Figs 6.104 and 6.105.)

The ankle and dorsum of the foot

In the region of the ankle, the vessels of each of the three compartments of the leg continue down immediately deep to the deep fascia and tendons where present and, therefore, maintain a relatively superficial course relative to their positions in the upper leg. At this point, they continue to supply the overlying skin, along with the vessels accompanying the cutaneous nerves in this region (including the saphenous nerve and superficial peroneal nerve branches). Despite a significant number of perforators, the distal third of the leg and ankle region have little skin laxity; therefore, island flap elevation can be undertaken but may require skin grafting of any secondary defect. As we move to the dorsum of the foot, the same vessels supply the skin but the skin laxity increases, making fasciocutaneous flaps easier to elevate. In this region, the predominant vascular supply is derived from the dorsalis pedis artery, and sizeable flaps can be raised on its perforators. Figures 7.8 to 7.10 demonstrate the pertinent cutaneous vascular anatomy of this region.

❯ FIGURE 7.8 The deep course of the anterior tibial and dorsalis pedis arteries in the anterior ankle region

These give rise to cutaneous perforators that pass between the overlying tendons and around or through the extensor retinaculum of the ankle. Despite this good blood supply, there is often insufficient skin laxity to permit flap elevation without secondary skin grafting in this region.

(Reproduced with permission from Gray H, Standring S 2005 Gray's anatomy: the anatomical basis of clinical practice, 39th edn. Churchill Livingstone, New York, Fig 84.1.)

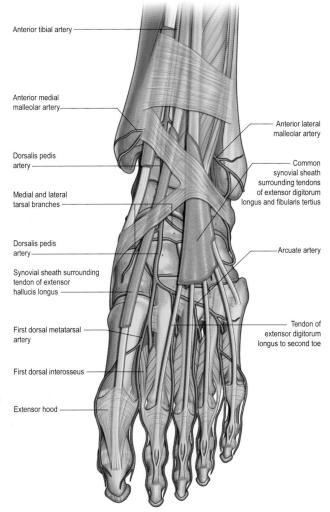

> **FIGURE 7.9** **Numerous intercommunications between the vessels passing across the ankle provide a reliable source of perforating vessels to the overlying skin. These perforators pass around tendons, particularly the Achilles tendon, to supply the overlying skin and, therefore, as elsewhere in the limbs, flaps designed to run in the long axis of the limb are preferred. The limited skin excess in this region results in a skin graft often becoming necessary for closure of the secondary defect. Caution should be used in this region in patients with diabetes and peripheral vascular disease as macro- and microvessel disease often adversely affect wound healing and flap survival in this region**

(Reproduced with permission from Gray H, Standring S 2005 Gray's anatomy: the anatomical basis of clinical practice, 39th edn. Churchill Livingstone, New York, Fig 84.9.)

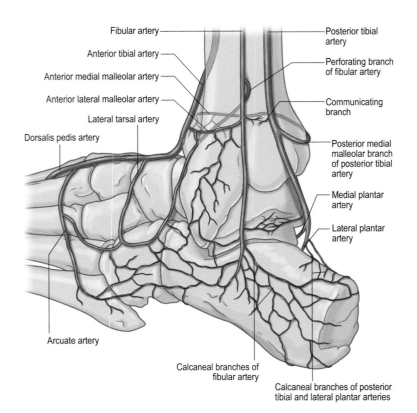

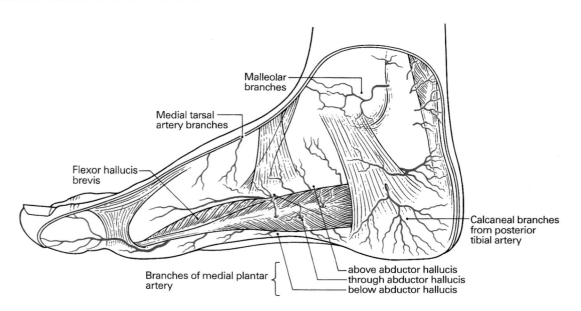

▲ **FIGURE 7.10** **Cutaneous perforators to the medial aspect of the foot**

A number of musculocutaneous and fasciocutaneous perforators supply the skin of the medial aspect of the foot. In the region of the ankle, the dense medial collateral ligament can limit advancement and, therefore, flaps in this region have to utilise transposition more frequently. The septocutaneous perforators in the midfoot can be traced to their parent vessels if additional movement is required, but this is not generally advisable for musculocutaneous perforators due to the increased morbidity of this approach. The medial plantar flap is a good example of an existing flap described within the literature that utilises these principles.

(Reproduced with permission from Cormack & Lamberty 1994, Figure 6.124.)

The plantar surface of the foot

The plantar surface of the foot can be a challenging region in which to operate. It has a tough fibrous structure with glabrous skin tethered to the underlying plantar fascia and via deeper connections; this anchors the tissue to the underlying bones. In between are well-innervated lobules of fat for cushioning, and deep to the plantar aponeurosis are the tendons and intrinsic muscles of the foot. The mobilisation of flaps on the plantar aspect of the foot can be undertaken reliably due to the rich number of perforators in this region. Deep vessels provide the rich perforator supply to the skin. Named flaps, like the medial plantar flap, are based upon perforators traced and skeletonised back to the parent vessels (medial plantar vessels), but non-named perforators can be used with significant mobilisation possible by division of the plantar aponeurosis, while maintaining the perforating vessels entering the undersurface of the flap.

FLAP ELEVATION IN THE LOWER LIMB

There are remarkable similarities in the techniques used for flap elevation in the lower limb and the analogous regions of the upper limb. As discussed in Chapter 5 with the upper limb, the predominant blood supply to the lower limb is the septo- and musculocutaneous perforators. The muscles and septa they perforate are oriented longitudinally within the limb. As a result, movement transverse to the long axis of the limb is relatively easy but proximodistal movement is difficult. The skin incisions can be modified to suit the relaxed skin tension lines and maximal tissue elasticity of each region; however, the components of flap movement are relatively transverse.

Flap elevation in the groin and thigh

The skin of the groin is relatively thin and elastic comparative to other regions in the lower limb. This makes it well-suited to fasciocutaneous flap closures where direct wound apposition is not possible. However, the more common groin defects encountered in reconstructive practice arise from groin dissection for lymph node metastases. Where this involves the overlying skin, defects can be large and have exposed large vessels, including the femoral artery and vein. The strong need for adjuvant radiotherapy in these cases makes reliable robust fasciocutaneous coverage mandatory. Numerous approaches have been used to effect coverage of these defects, including the importation of tissue from the abdomen (e.g. rectus abdominis myocutaneous flaps). A less invasive approach is the use of a quadriceps keystone flap based on the perforators of the lateral circumflex femoral

vessels, along with neurovascular supply via the anterior and lateral cutaneous nerves of the thigh. The area of this flap can be very large, with V–Y closures undertaken inferiorly at the lateral aspect of the knee and superiorly at the lateral aspect of the anterior superior iliac spine. This approach is frequently used for closure of groin dissections for melanoma without the need for sartorius transfer. The application of the keystone flap in melanoma will, therefore, be discussed in further detail in Chapter 8, with Figure 8.7 demonstrating a clinical case of groin defect closure.

Anterior and posterior thigh reconstructions can be undertaken in a straightforward manner, with the long axis of the keystone flap (or variants) oriented parallel to the long axis of the limb. As with other areas, division of the skin will permit some movement, with greater movement gained on sequential division of the deep fascia on the secondary defect side and then circumferentially around the flap for larger defects. Preservation of subcutaneous neurovascular structures provides eventual return of sensation and good venous drainage from these flaps. It is uncommon to need a skin graft for the secondary defect in this region as long as the flap dimensions are suitably large. Where a defect cannot be oriented longitudinally, transversely oriented keystone flaps can be raised, but their advancement may be difficult and two flaps may be required (on either side of the defect) to effect closure directly or by asymmetrical movement of opposing ends of the flaps (Yin Yang variant). Figure 7.11 demonstrates the use of a double keystone flap in a non-advantageously oriented defect with good results, but it is advisable to avoid transversely oriented flaps where possible.

Flap elevation around the knee

As discussed previously, the knee has a rich vascular network with numerous vessels contributing perforators to supply the overlying skin. As with other convex areas of the body, flap designs that try to recreate a convexity do well over the surface of the knee. These include transposition, omega (Ω), goblet and Yin Yang variants of the keystone flap. The tethered nature of the deep fascia in this region makes longitudinal advancement difficult and, therefore, recruitment of flaps from the lateral aspect medially are often more effective in fasciocutaneous closure in this region. Skin grafting of a small area of secondary defect may be necessary if flap closure is under more than physiological tension. A period of supported mobilisation in a Zimmer (or similar) knee splint is useful in these cases, as long as the straps for the splint do not place direct pressure over the flap. Figure 7.12 illustrates the transposition of a keystone flap to effect knee reconstruction.

FIGURE 7.11

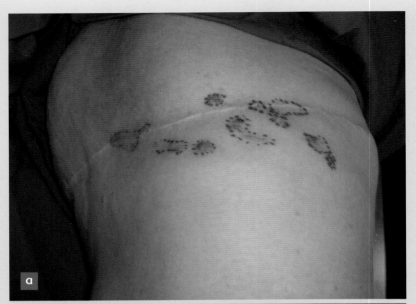

FIGURE 7.11 **A 68-year-old female who developed melanoma in a congenital melanocytic naevus of the thigh**

(a) Congenital melanocytic naevus present since birth was excised, along with the melanomatous component, 12 months previously. Patient presents with multiple sites of recurrence along a transversely oriented scar.

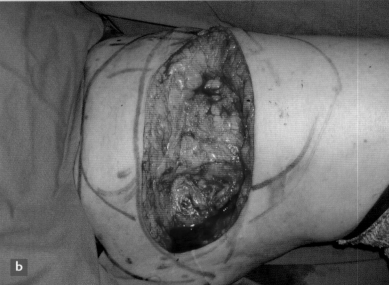

(b) Following defect excision, a 20 × 7 cm defect is produced down to the deep fascia over the quadriceps, with removal of the great saphenous vein.

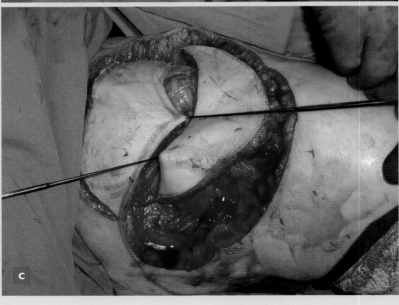

(c) Keystone flaps raised above and below the defect due to the transverse orientation (non-ideal) and size of the primary defect.

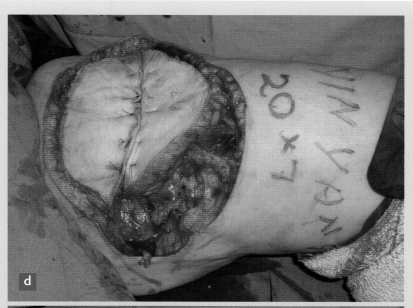

(d) Direct appositional closure of the defect by suturing the flaps together.

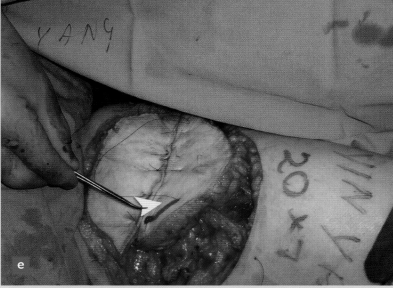

(e) A *red dot sign*, indicating increased perfusion of the flap side of the wound compared with the surrounding non-islanded skin.

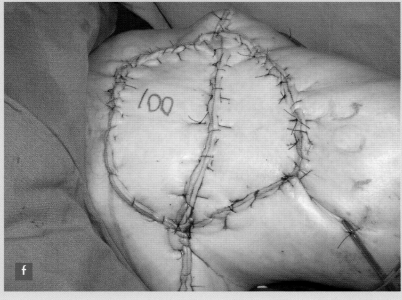

(f) Appearance at closure with minor dog ears at either end of the wound that were allowed to settle with time.

See video for Figure 7.11

TLC: Conjoint flap vascularity

Time (operation/cost)
100 minutes
Life quality (and aesthetics)
Good with normal function and medial and lateral dog ears resolved without additional surgery
Complications
Nil

FIGURE 7.12

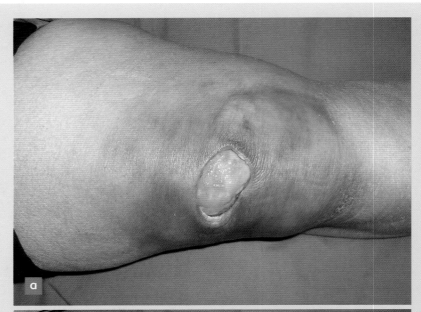

FIGURE 7.12 A middle-aged woman with an infected prepatellar bursa of the knee with skin breakdown and loss

(a) The defect prior to excision of the bursa, showing significant undermining.

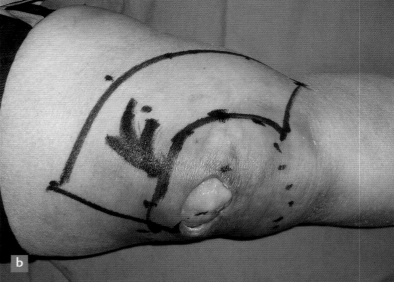

(b) The flap is designed to utilise the perforators from the perigenicular circulation on the medial aspect of the knee (see Fig 7.4) to support a keystone flap for transposition from above the bursa.

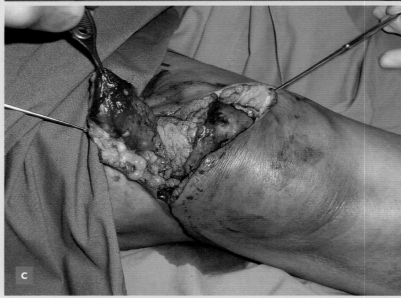

(c) Excision of the prepatellar bursa, stained with methylene blue to ensure complete removal.

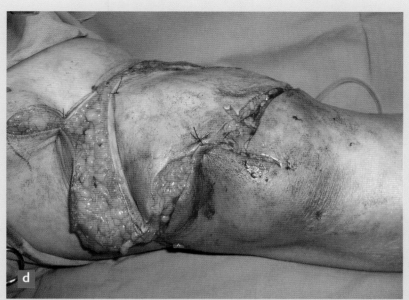

(d) Initial transposition of the flap and closure of the secondary defect.

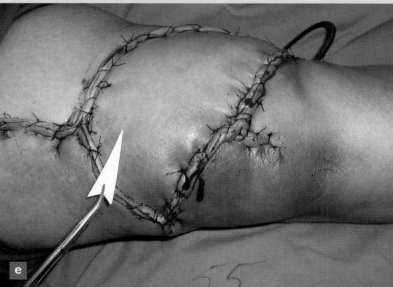

(e) Appearance following closure of the wound and donor site.

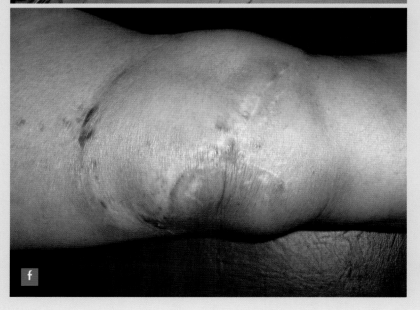

(f) Appearance 10 months later without recurrence and with no issues with mobility.

See video for Figure 7.12

TLC: Conjoint flap vascularity

Time (operation/cost)
40 minutes
Life quality (and aesthetics)
Good with normal function and acceptable aesthetics
Complications
Nil

Flap elevation in the leg

Fasciocutaneous closure is relatively simple in the upper two-thirds of the leg, with the exception of flaps that must pass over the subcutaneous border of the tibia. Flaps in this upper region are performed in a region of relative elasticity of skin, and good tissue mobility can be gained by incising skin followed by the deep fascia. This is a very suitable region for gaining experience with keystone flap reconstruction and, hence, avoiding skin grafting with its associated postoperative immobilisation and potential for deconditioning. Keystone island flaps for suitable defects in the lower limb can be undertaken in the ambulatory setting as long as the patient will be compliant with avoiding prolonged dependency of the operative limb during the first 1–2 postoperative weeks. Defects of the lower third of the leg can still be reconstructed using keystone and similarly designed island flaps but, as there is less donor skin elasticity, a small skin graft for the secondary defect may be necessary. As in other areas, preoperative Doppler ultrasound may be used to isolate specific perforators. This is not our practice as a routine but may be useful where orthopaedic appliances, such as external fixators, limit the normal flap dimensions or design and, therefore, identification of a perforator may permit a smaller flap to be elevated in specific areas.

The pretibial border warrants special note. In this region, there are no perforating vessels passing up from the periosteum directly to the skin. Therefore, the blood supply to the overlying skin enters from the adjoining skin that overlies the fascial septa and musculature. Advancement from laterally or medially over the subcutaneous border of the tibia occurs up and over a convex, often sharp, bony prominence. Keystone flap closure in this region should be undertaken with caution. Where it is used, the flap raised should be significantly larger than closure of similar defects in more advantageous positions. Figure 7.13 demonstrates a standard closure of a large defect for primary melanoma of the leg using a keystone flap without the need for secondary skin grafting. Additional cases include Figure 2.8 and Figure 8.1.

FIGURE 7.13

FIGURE 7.13 Elderly woman with a T4b melanoma of the posterior aspect of her calf for wide local excision and flap closure to aid early mobilisation due to her advanced age

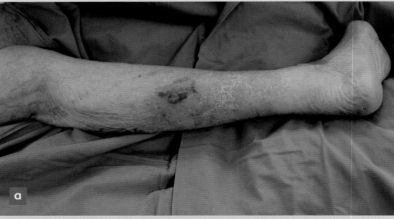

(a) The ulcerated exophytic nodules of melanoma are demonstrated rising from a flat pigmented lesion.

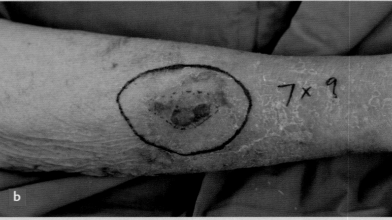

(b) Following inclusion of a minimum of 2 cm margin, a defect of 7 × 9 cm is to be produced.

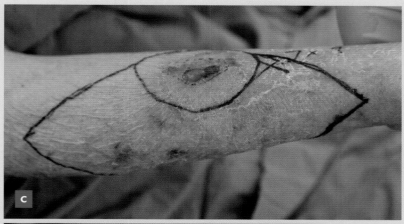

(c) & **(d)** A single keystone flap is planned out to be significantly wider than the defect width due to her thin skin.

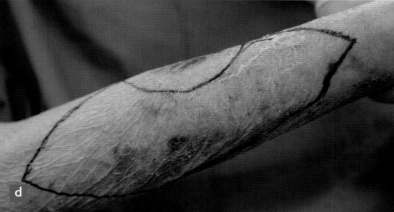

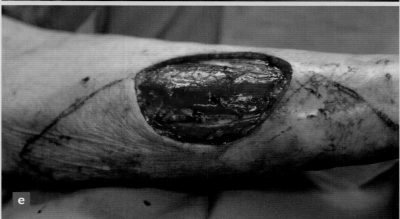

(e) The defect following excision of the tumour, including the deep fascia.

(f) Closure of the defect, with a single area of skin tear from an initial tension suture. This did not affect wound healing and no secondary skin graft was necessary. Fine crease lines can be seen radiating from the primary defect side of the flap with maximal creep in this direction, while laxity is present by V–Y advancement at right angles to this plane.

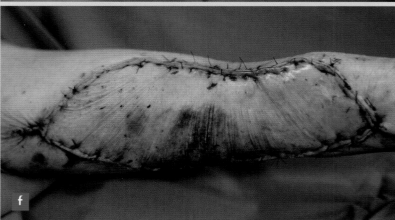

TLC: Conjoint flap vascularity

Time (operation/cost)
50 minutes
Life quality (and aesthetics)
Good with early mobilisation and acceptable appearance
Complications
Nil

Flap elevation in the ankle and dorsum of the foot

In an analogous manner to the wrist and dorsum of the hand, the ankle and dorsum of the foot share similar characteristics. There is little tissue redundancy immediately around the ankle and, therefore, local flaps in this region need careful planning. Despite this, numerous perforators are present and flaps can be raised to incorporate neurovascular structures to improve their reliability (see Fig 2.6). Transposition flaps with skin grafting of the secondary defect are often necessary to supplement keystone flap use in this region.

On the dorsum of the foot there is usually excellent tissue elasticity and mobility. Numerous perforators arise from the dorsalis pedis artery and pass in between the long (and short) extensors of the toes to supply the overlying skin. The superficial peroneal nerve divides into multiple branches over the dorsum of the foot and these can contribute additional blood supply to dorsal plantar flaps. Longitudinally oriented flaps have the best movement, as in other areas. The distal ends of the flaps can be extended just into the web spaces to utilise the extra tissue laxity of these regions to effect V–Y closure. Figures 7.14 and 7.15 show simple keystone flaps for the lateral ankle and the dorsum of the foot using this laxity in the web space.

FIGURE 7.14

FIGURE 7.14 A traumatic sinus of the lateral aspect of the right ankle in a young woman where stable soft tissue coverage is necessary for wearing footwear

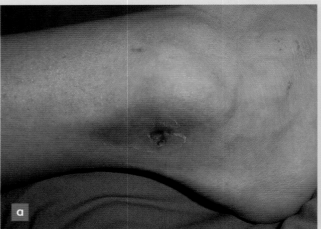
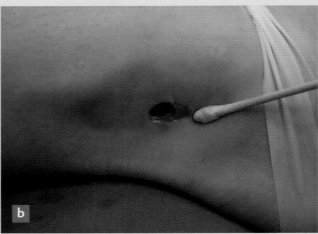

(a) The opening of the sinus is evident posterior to the lateral malleolus.

(b) Probing of the sinus demonstrates significant undermining posterior to the fibula above and below the sinus.

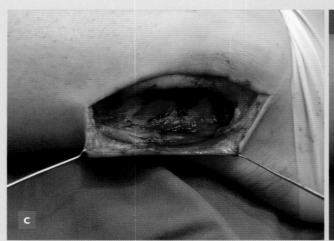
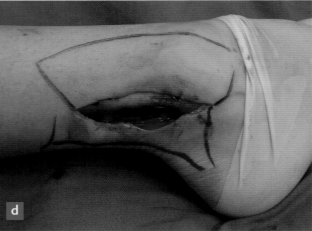

(c) Excision of the sinus, with methylene blue dye to assist clearance of the lining, results in a defect as shown but the wound is no longer able to be closed primarily.

(d) A keystone flap is designed based on the anterior tissue so as to capture the lower peroneal perforators in the region of the inferior aspect of the lateral compartment.

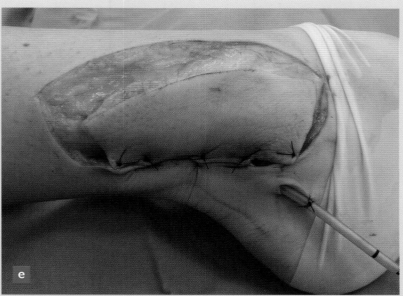

(e) Appearance after closure of the primary defect and

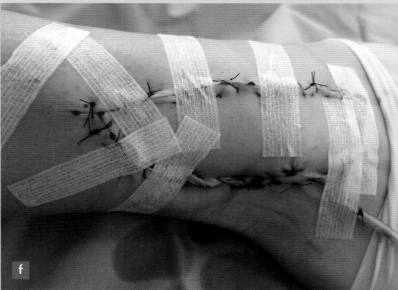

(f) following complete closure with V–Y advancements to assist transverse skin recruitment and wound closure.

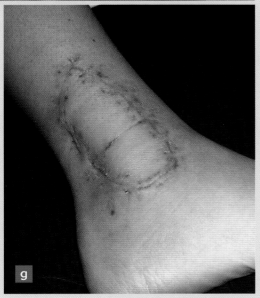

(g) Appearance at 2 months postoperatively with good healing and function. The scars are yet to mature and fade. The same principle may be used to cover exposed metalware.

TLC: Conjoint flap vascularity

Time (operation/cost)
40 minutes
Life quality (and aesthetics)
Good, with normal function and acceptable appearance
Complications
Nil

FIGURE 7.15

FIGURE 7.15 Simple case of the use of the (Ω) keystone flap for closure of defects on the dorsum of the foot

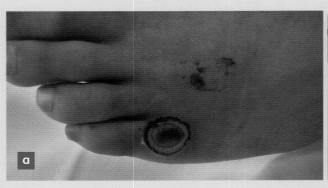

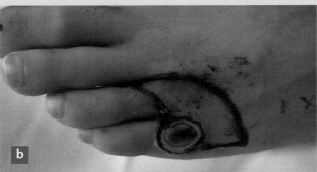

(a) A full-thickness burn of the dorsum of the left little toe, including involvement of the paratenon.

(b) A simple keystone flap is planned so that one end is sited within a web space to facilitate V–Y closure in this region. Following excision of the burn, a non-graftable wound bed is present with uncovered extensor tendon to the small toe.

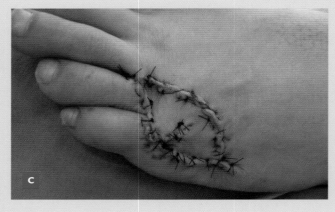

(c) Following flap closure over the defect, the wound is sealed with minimal tension and little effect on foot or toe movement.

TLC: Conjoint flap vascularity		
Time (operation/cost)		
20 minutes		
Life quality (and aesthetics)		
Good, with normal function and acceptable appearance		
Complications		
Nil		

Flap elevation in the plantar foot

Locoregional flaps in the foot are characterised by difficulty with flap mobilisation and some donor site morbidity in the short term. However, the maxim of 'the next best skin is the next best skin' still applies. More simple options, such as skin grafting, lead to unacceptable long-term morbidity due to instability of the skin and recurrent breakdown. There are limitations in the use of free-flap reconstruction (despite some neurotisation), with shear relative to the surrounding normal plantar skin. Therefore, despite the short-term morbidity of plantar flaps for closure of plantar defects, the long-term results are often more favourable than with other approaches.

The technique of plantar flap elevation involves division of the skin and blunt dissection of the underlying fat, with additional sharp division of any fascia septa around the circumference of the flap. Once the plantar aponeurosis is reached, it may be left in place or divided to gain further mobility. Care must be taken deep to this layer as the neurovascular bundles of the digits are within one muscle layer deeper in the foot. This layer provides the movement for flaps in this region, with the best movement transverse to the long axis of the foot, but dissection back to the perforators themselves provides additional movement. In the heel region, the fascia joining the skin to the underlying structures gains anchorage to the calcaneum directly. These fascial attachments can be sharply divided while maintaining the neurovascular supply to the flap by focused sharp dissection with scissors. Figure 7.16 shows how plantar keystone flap elevation can be performed, even near the heel region.

FIGURE 7.16

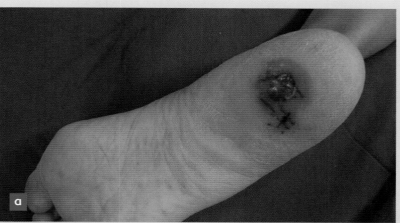

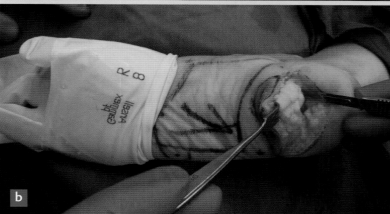

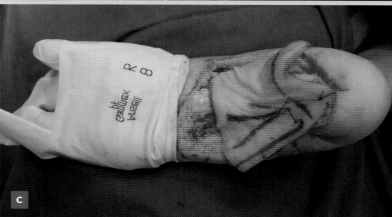

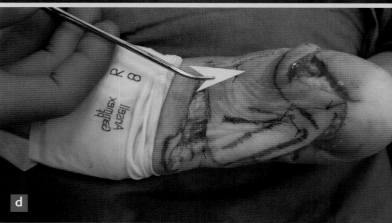

FIGURE 7.16 An 82-year-old woman with ulcerated acral lentiginous melanoma of the heel, 2.2 mm Breslow thickness

(a) The primary lesion shows previous scar from a recent confirmatory biopsy. The brown discolouration is antiseptic ointment, not in-situ disease.

(b) The DRAPE (delayed reconstruction after pathology evaluation) procedure is used, with excision of the primary tumour undertaken with a 2 cm margin down to the plantar aponeurosis and a plantar flap planned (defect size 5 × 4 cm).

(c) The medial perforators are retained as the pedicle for the plantar arch keystone flap and the lateral aspect of the flap is elevated and transposed to close the defect.

(d) Initial V–Y closure is undertaken at the donor site and the tourniquet is released, showing an early blush of reperfusion from the medial aspect of the flap (arrow).

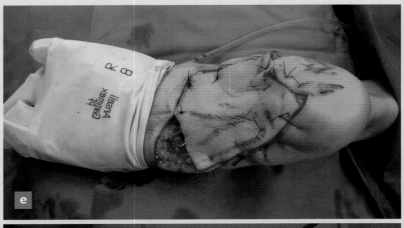

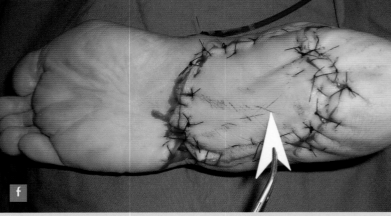

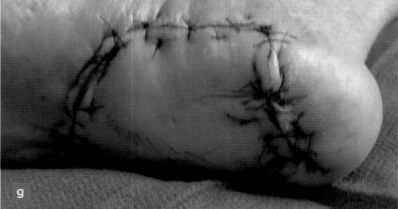

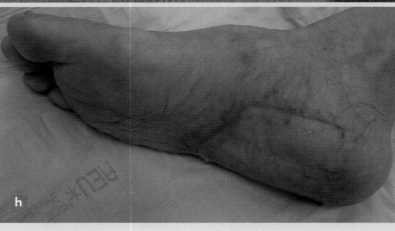

(e) & **(f)** Progressive closure of the defect with a marked vascular blush evident (consistent with the immediate vascular augmentation concept, IVAC).

(g) Appearance at 4 days.

(h) Appearance at 2 months with normal weight-bearing with her walking frame and with full tactile sensation.

See for Figure 7.16

TLC: Conjoint flap vascularity

Time (operation/cost)
45 minutes
Life quality (and aesthetics)
Good walking with frame by 6 weeks (elderly++), acceptable aesthetics
Complications
Developed pneumonia 4 months postoperative (not related) and died

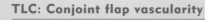

SUMMARY

The lower limb shares many similarities with the upper limb in terms of its vascularity and regional specificity of flap elevation. However, it has additional challenges, particularly due to its weight-bearing, dependent position during walking and sitting, which places additional demands on reconstructive techniques used in this region. The keystone island flap is well-suited to meet these additional challenges by providing reliable vascularised soft tissue cover that permits early mobilisation and good restoration of function and aesthetics.

BIBLIOGRAPHY

Behan F C, Terrill P J, Ashton M W 1994 Fasciocutaneous island flaps for orthopaedic management in lower limb reconstruction using dermatomal precincts. Aust N Z J Surg 64(3):155–66.

Cormack G L, Lamberty B G H 1994 The arterial anatomy of skin flaps, 2nd edn. Churchill Livingstone, Edinburgh.

Daigeler A, Drücke D, Tatar K, Homann H H, Goertz O, Tilkorn D, Lehnhardt M, Steinau H U 2009 The pedicled gastrocnemius muscle flap: a review of 218 cases. Plast Reconstr Surg 123(1):250–7.

Hartholt K A, van Beeck E F, Polinder S, van der Velde N, van Lieshout E M, Panneman M J, van der Cammen T J, Patka P 2011 Societal consequences of falls in the older population: injuries, healthcare costs, and long-term reduced quality of life. J Trauma 71(3): 74–53.

Lee J S, Chau P P, Hui E, Chan F, Woo J 2009 Survival prediction in nursing home residents using the Minimum Data Set subscales: ADL Self-Performance Hierarchy, Cognitive Performance and the Changes in Health, End-stage disease and Symptoms and Signs scales. Eur J Public Health 19(3):308–12.

Mathes S J, Nahai F 1997 Reconstructive surgery: principles, anatomy and technique. Churchill Livingstone, Edinburgh.

United Nations Department of Economic and Social Affairs, Population Division 2010 Population ageing and development 2009. United Nations, New York.

Wei F C, Demirkan F, Chen H C, Chuang D C, Chen S H, Lin C H, Cheng S L, Cheng M H, Lin Y T 2001 The outcome of failed free flaps in head and neck and extremity reconstruction: what is next in the reconstructive ladder? Plast Reconstr Surg 108(5):1154–60; discussion 1161–2.

Section 3

Special Applications of Keystone Island Flaps

Chapter 8
Melanoma

Advice is sought to confirm a position already taken.

Sir William Osler (1849–1919)

Melanoma excision results in sizeable fasciocutaneous defects. Of those that cannot be closed primarily, the keystone flap provides closure in the majority of these cases with improved reliability, healing, mobility and quality of life for patients compared to other approaches.

INTRODUCTION

Melanoma is a malignant tumour of the skin and mucosal surfaces that has a proclivity for early local and lymphovascular spread (perineural spread in neurotropic/desmoplastic forms) relative to other cutaneous malignancies (Petersson et al. 2009). Its aetiology is multifactorial but genetic clustering within families (Goldstein & Tucker 2001) and increased incidence with sun exposure are two major factors implicated in its pathogenesis (Whiteman et al. 2001). The incidence of primary melanoma in Australia is significantly higher than in other developed countries, representing the fourth most common cancer (excluding non-melanomatous skin cancer) (IARC 2008). This relates to both cultural factors and to the mismatch between skin pigmentation (fairer skinned, Fitzgerald type 1 & 2) and climatic conditions (high sun exposure). As a result, melanoma and its management are a greater burden on the health sector than in other countries. This creates significant expertise in the management of melanoma in dedicated centres within Australia.

The management of melanoma is best undertaken by a multidisciplinary team. Such an approach combines patient education (including their families), surveillance, surgical and non-surgical management modalities, and both clinical and basic science research in a coordinated manner. Once the diagnosis of melanoma has been confirmed by biopsy, appropriate staging must be undertaken to establish the grade of tumour, as well as nodal and distant metastases, to determine the appropriate treatment regimen (Balch et al. 2009). The keystone flap has evolved as an invaluable tool in the surgical reconstruction of primary and secondary melanoma (and other cutaneous malignancies) due to the sizeable fasciocutaneous defects that can be produced by melanoma excision. In primary melanoma, adequate surgical margins are vital to minimise the risk of locally recurrent disease. These begin with 5 mm margins for lentigo maligna, through to a minimum of 1–2 cm margins for invasive melanoma (ACN 2008). This results in surgical defects that are 1–4 cm larger in diameter than the primary lesion. This range is usually well within the capacity of keystone flaps (see below) to effect closure of defects under physiological wound tension, with reliable healing and with minimal immobilisation (including the quaternary response, see Chapter 2). The depth of melanoma excision is usually to at least one anatomical plane deeper than the tumour. In invasive disease, this may include all subcutaneous fat and the deep fascia. As a result, not only is there a fasciocutaneous defect created, but a significant contour deformity. Skin grafting is a reliable form of wound closure for vascularised wound beds, such as the majority of melanoma excisions, but is associated with significant donor site discomfort for the patient and does not provide any significant reconstruction of contour deformity ('shark-bite' deformity). The use of the keystone flap (including its variants) provides not only skin coverage with locally matched skin, but reconstructs contour, thereby optimising aesthetics and postoperative quality of life (an important consideration in melanoma patients). Early, pain-free mobilisation with keystone flap reconstruction provides additional benefits compared to skin grafts. Its simple geometrical design permits re-excision, should inadequate margins occur, in a relatively straightforward manner.

Surgical management of clinical nodal metastases is relatively straightforward. However, when the overlying skin is involved with disease, a large oncological defect may result, with exposed neurovascular structures. For this reason, reliable, vascularised soft tissue coverage is essential. The keystone flap is well-suited to provide such coverage, especially in the groin (Behan et al. 2010, quadriceps keystone flap), where local wound complications from groin dissection are common. As a result of this usefulness in both primary and secondary disease, the keystone island flap has become widely used in the closure of melanoma (and other cutaneous malignant) defects within Australia.

IMPORTANT PRINCIPLES IN KEYSTONE FLAP CLOSURE OF MELANOMA DEFECTS

We have covered the principles of keystone flap design and its variants in Chapter 3, but some important points are worth reiterating in relation to the specific management of melanoma. These principles include the following:

1 Correct pathology with estimation of staging (Balch et al. 2009).
2 Planning for the management of potential nodal disease via consideration of sentinel lymph node biopsy (SLNBx) at the time of wide local excision.
3 Establishment of adequate surgical margins where possible prior to reconstruction—consideration of the delayed reconstruction after pathology evaluation (DRAPE) procedure.
4 Appropriate and timely healing so as to facilitate the commencement of adjuvant therapies where indicated.
5 Low morbidity surgery concentrating on early return to normal activities of daily living, good aesthetics and optimal quality of life.

These points deserve some further explanation.

Correct pathology and staging

Correct diagnosis is essential. Misdiagnosis of melanoma can result in dire consequences for patients. Under the microscope, melanoma can look like many other poorly differentiated tumours (from spindle cell tumours to Spitz naevi) and, therefore, many pathologists keep it as a differential diagnosis for poorly differentiated tumours. Specific tumour markers and immunohistochemical labelling can aid in the diagnosis, but a combination of markers can make the diagnosis of melanoma more likely even though none has true specificity. Thus, we rely on both expert pathologist opinion and specific tumour markers/immunohistochemical labelling in combination to confirm the diagnosis. A secondary pathological review, particularly by a pathologist specialising in melanoma diagnosis, is often very useful.

Furthermore, the pathological staging criteria have changed every few years in recent history as further information comes to light on the most important prognostic factors. As a result, the primary pathology report may not include sufficient information, such as the presence of micro- or macro-ulceration, number of mitoses per millimetre square (mm^2) and so on (see Tables 8.1 and 8.2 for American Joint Committee on Cancer [AJCC] criteria, Balch et al. 2009). These are important in determining the adequacy of current margins or in planning wide local excision. Flap reconstruction should be avoided until wide local excision is undertaken (with consideration of SLNBx, see below). Despite being based on the same evidence, the guidelines for excision margin differ in various countries. In general, the excision of invasive melanoma requires a minimum of a 1 cm margin. Once the thickness of the tumour, or other features, such as ulceration or high mitotic count per mm^2 are known, a 2 cm margin may be recommended. There is no evidence that more than a 2 cm margin for any melanoma provides a significant enough benefit in terms of decreased local recurrence when compared with the morbidity of patients with wider excisions. The current AJCC melanoma staging and classification scheme is presented in Tables 8.1 and 8.2 (Balch et al. 2009). The keystone island flap can also be used for other similar poorly differentiated tumours that can be difficult to distinguish from melanoma, such as spindle cell tumours (see Fig 8.8).

The role of sentinel lymph node biopsy at the time of keystone reconstruction

The role of SLNBx in melanoma is currently under intense investigation via the Multicenter Selective Lymphadenectomy Trial-II (MSLT-II). At this time, its principal role is in providing additional prognostic information (Morton et al. 2005) but further research is required to determine whether it can provide an unequivocal survival benefit (Thomas 2009). It is beyond the scope of this text to cover the relevant arguments for or against the use of SLNBx in specific cases. However, two important points should be emphasised. First, the appropriate timing for SLNBx is at the time of wide local excision of the primary tumour (unless a recent flap reconstruction of the primary tumour has been undertaken). Therefore, consideration of SLNBx should be undertaken at the time of wide local excision and keystone flap reconstruction. Failure to do so will remove this as an option for the patient. Second, SLNBx is used as a selection criterion for inclusion within some clinical trials of potentially beneficial treatments for advanced disease. Even if patients have a relatively thin tumour (e.g. T1b, see Table 8.1), they still have the potential to develop more advanced disease in the future, and failure to perform SLNBx in these

TABLE 8.1 TNM staging from the revised AJCC guidelines for melanoma, 2009

Classification	Thickness (mm)	Ulceration status/mitoses
T		
Tis	NA	NA
T1	≤1.00	a: Without ulceration and mitosis <1/mm^2
		b: With ulceration or mitoses ≥1/mm^2
T2	1.01–2.00	a: Without ulceration
		b: With ulceration
T3	2.01–4.00	a: Without ulceration
		b: With ulceration
T4	>4.00	a: Without ulceration
		b: With ulceration
	No. of metastatic nodes	**Nodal metastatic burden**
N		
N0	0	NA
N1	1	a: Micrometastasis*
		b: Macrometastasis†
N2	2–3	a: Micrometastasis*
		b: Macrometastasis†
		c: In-transit metastases/satellites without metastatic nodes
N3	4+ metastatic nodes, or matted nodes, or in transit metastases/satellites with metastases nodes	
	Site	**Serum LDH**
M		
M0	No distant metastases	NA
M1a	Distant skin, subcutaneous or nodal metastases	Normal
M1b	Lung metastases	Normal
M1c	All other visceral metastases	Normal
	Any distant metastasis	Elevated

Abbreviations: NA, not applicable; LDH, lactate dehydrogenase.
*Micrometastases are diagnosed after sentinel lymph node biopsy.
†Macrometastases are defined as clinically detectable nodal metastases confirmed pathologically.
(Reproduced with permission from Balch et al. 2009.)

cases will remove the option of possible beneficial treatments. Obviously, this discussion needs to be undertaken in a centre with melanoma expertise and surgeons experienced in SLNBx, and weighed against the additional morbidity of the procedure. SLNBx does not affect the capacity to undertake keystone flap reconstruction.

Use of DRAPE in keystone closure

DRAPE, or *delayed reconstruction after pathology evaluation*, is a useful approach in melanoma and other malignant tumours. It involves excision of the primary tumour with an appropriate clinical margin and then dressing of the defect while awaiting reconstruction. A formal histopathology report can

TABLE 8.2 **Combined TNM staging for melanoma—revised AJCC guidelines for melanoma, 2009**

	Pathological staging*				Clinical staging**		
	T	**N**	**M**		**T**	**N**	**M**
0	Tis	N0	M0	0	Tis	N0	M0
IA	T1a	N0	M0	1A	T1a	N0	M0
IB	T1b	N0	M0	IB	T1b	N0	M0
	T2a	N0	M0		T2a	N0	M0
IIA	T2b	N0	M0	IIA	T2b	N0	M0
	T3a	N0	M0		T3a	N0	M0
IIB	T3b	N0	M0	IIB	T3b	N0	M0
	T4a	N0	M0		T4a	N0	M0
IIC	T4b	N0	M0	IIC	T4b	N0	M0
III	Any T	N > N0	M0	IIIA	T1–4a	N1a	M0
					T1–4a	N2a	M0
				IIIB	T1–4b	N1a	M0
					T1–4b	N2a	M0
					T1–4a	N1b	M0
					T1–4a	N2b	M0
					T1–4a	N2c	M0
				IIIC	T1-4b	N1b	M0
					T1-4b	N2b	M0
					T1-4b	N2c	M0
					Any T	N3	M0
IV	Any T	Any N	M1	IV	Any T	Any N	M1

*Pathological staging includes microstaging of the primary melanoma and pathological information about the regional lymph nodes after partial (i.e. SLNBx) or complete lymphadenectomy. Pathological stage 0 or IA patients are the exception; they do not require pathological evaluation of their lymph nodes.

**Clinical staging includes microstaging of the primary melanoma and clinical/radiological evaluation for metastases. By convention, it should be used after complete excision of the primary melanoma with clinical assessment for regional and distant metastases.

(Reproduced with permission from Balch et al. 2009.)

usually be generated within as little as 2–3 days and avoids reliance on the accuracy (or otherwise) of frozen sections intraoperatively. If clearance has been achieved, the patient can then undergo a second stage involving keystone flap reconstruction of the defect. Alternatively, where clear margins have not been achieved, a second excision of the relevant positive margin can be undertaken and either reconstruction performed at that time or delayed again until the formal pathology result is received. This approach is achievable in most patients using modern dressings (e.g. alginates or hydrocolloids) without compromising local tissues, the subsequent

reconstructive result or increasing the risk of wound infection. It significantly reduces the risk of re-excision, with encroachment on the keystone flap reconstruction. While the simple geometry of keystone flaps permits further excision where margins are incomplete, this is not ideal as it reduces the size of the original flap, increases wound tension and risks local wound complications.

Timely commencement of adjuvant therapies in keystone flap closures

As with any advanced malignancy, high-grade melanomas often benefit from multimodal therapy combining surgical excision with radiotherapy, chemotherapy and/or immunomodulation (e.g. interferon). Prompt wound healing and avoidance of complications permit the timely institution of these therapies, possibly maximising disease-free and overall survival. The robust vascular supply of the keystone flap assists prompt wound healing even where physiological tension is present. Any excessive tension should prompt the prudent use of a small skin graft to the secondary defect. The healing time will be similar to the overall wound healing and minimal immobilisation is necessary due to the small size of the skin graft.

Quality of life and early functional recovery with low morbidity surgery

The aggressive nature of melanoma and dissemination at the time of diagnosis can significantly reduce life expectancy. For this reason, reconstructive approaches that are relatively simple, minimally morbid and facilitate early return to activities of daily living are important. A strong focus on good postoperative patient quality of life as a primary goal in melanoma reconstruction is vital. The keystone flap is well-suited to meet these criteria. Timely healing minimises the period of dressings and return appointments. Division of superficial cutaneous nerves and neurapraxia of deeper cutaneous nerves leads to a relatively pain-free postoperative recovery, thereby improving patient comfort. The reconstruction of contour with the use of locally matched skin and soft tissues improves aesthetics and early mobilisation maintains function. For these reasons, the keystone island flap has been adopted in many specialised melanoma units in Australasia as the reconstruction method of choice where primary closure is not possible.

USE OF KEYSTONE FLAPS FOR NODAL METASTASES

In advanced melanoma, tumour cells can spread to regional lymphatics, lodging in the sentinel node and surrounding lymph nodes as the disease progresses. Extracapsular extension in these cases can lead to involvement of the overlying skin. In-transit cutaneous metastases may also be present in the region. Complex reconstructions of these defects following skin excision and nodal clearance may add unreasonable morbidity in these instances, and delay healing and commencement of adjuvant therapies. Local wound complications are relatively common following nodal clearances, especially in the groin; therefore, simple but effective strategies are to be encouraged.

The keystone island flap provides robust vascularised fasciocutaneous coverage of these defects with minimal morbidity and timely wound healing. We have already seen examples of its use in closures following nodal dissections and parotidectomies in the head and neck in Chapter 4. The quadriceps keystone flap has been used by Behan for almost a decade and, recently, the cutaneous vascularity to this flap was described by Saint-Cyr and colleagues (2009). Almost the entire anterior surface of the thigh can be elevated to utilise the entire elasticity of skin in this region for closure of groin defects and to maximise perforator input. Comparative to other regional flaps, such as the use of the rectus abdominis myocutaneous flap, the avoidance of muscle dissection lowers donor site morbidity and ensures increased patient comfort postoperatively.

Figures 8.1–8.8 demonstrate many of these principles through clinical cases of keystone closure for both primary and secondary defects.

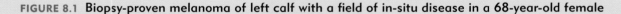

FIGURE 8.1 **Biopsy-proven melanoma of left calf with a field of in-situ disease in a 68-year-old female**

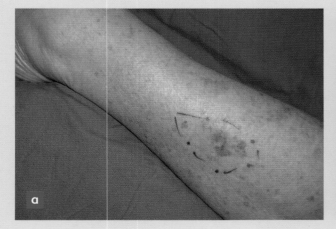

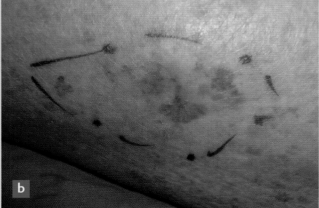

(a) Lesion of lateral left calf over the peroneal compartment.

(b) Close-up of lesion with surgical margins marked out.

FIGURE 8.1

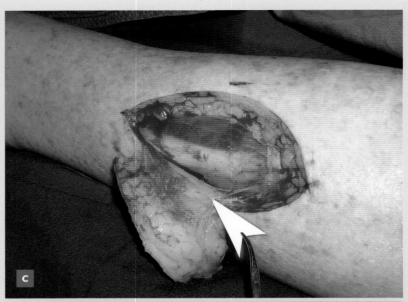

(c) Following the excision of skin, subcutaneous fat and deep fascia.

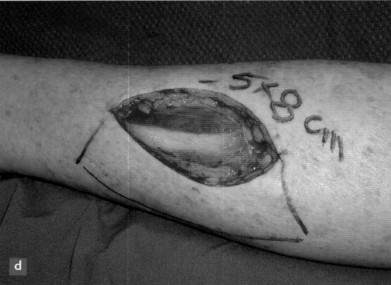

(d) The defect is 8 × 5 cm. A keystone flap is designed based on the posterolateral aspect of the calf.

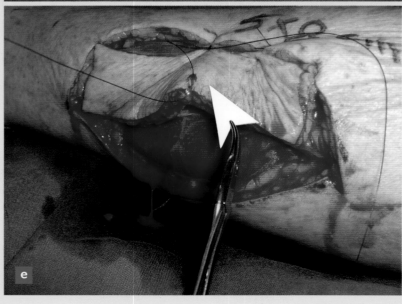

(e) Division of the deep fascia laterally permits improved flap movement. The substance of the calf musculature minimises dead space. The *red dot sign* (arrow) demonstrates the immediate vascular augmentation concept (IVAC) displayed with the keystone flap.

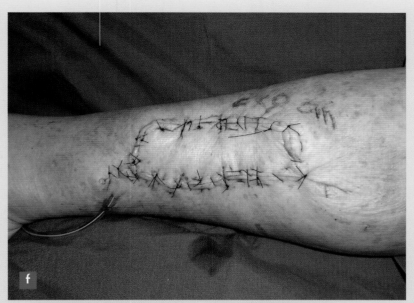

(f) On wound closure, the tension on the flap is distributed evenly, resulting in good cutaneous vascularity.

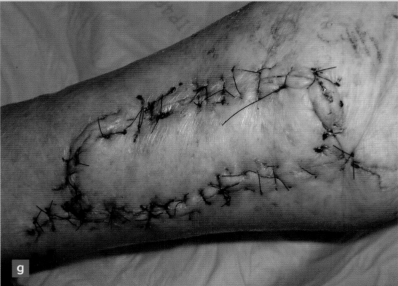

(g) Appearance 7 days following closure; pain-free.

(h) Appearance at 3 months.

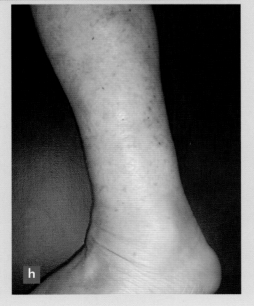

See video for Figure 8.1

TLC: Conjoint flap vascularity

Time (operation/cost)
45 minutes
Life quality (and aesthetics)
Good with early mobilisation and acceptable aesthetics
Complications
Nil

FIGURE 8.2

FIGURE 8.2 Recurrent melanoma of the calf following initial management with groin dissection and radiotherapy 1 year earlier in a 63-year-old female in whom excision of the recurrence and grafting resulted in lymphocele and a non-healing ulcer for 9 months

(Reproduced with permission from Behan FC, Lo CH 2009 Principles and misconceptions regarding the keystone island flap. Ann Surg Oncol 16(6):1722–3.)

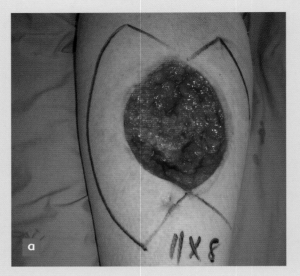

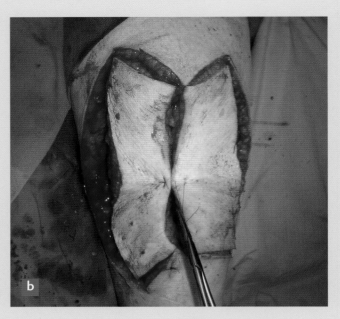

(a) The size of the re-excision defect is 11 × 8 cm and bilateral keystone flaps have been designed (more recently this type of closure has been adapted to a Yin Yang variant with greater success).

(b) Closure with a type III keystone flap (double opposing keystone) for direct closure.

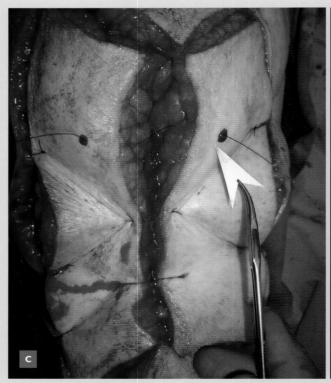

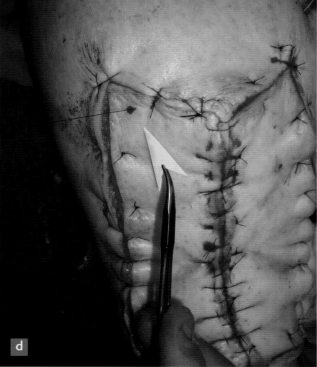

(c) Vascular dynamics showing *red dot signs* on both flaps indicating IVAC. The white lines of dermal tension are temporary and resolve following wound closure with even tension.

(d) *Red dot sign* at the extreme point of the flap. We now commonly use the Yin Yang variation for large defects of the calf.

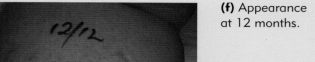

(e) On completion, closure has been achieved over a suction drain.

(f) Appearance at 12 months.

(g) Eventual result with significant reduction in peripheral oedema assisted by the use of compression stockings.

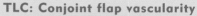

TLC: Conjoint flap vascularity

Time (operation/cost)
120 minutes

Life quality (and aesthetics)
Good, following healing, with no recurrence and no further need for compression garments, acceptable appearance

Complications
Slow healing with dressings for 8 weeks to fully heal in lymphoedematous leg

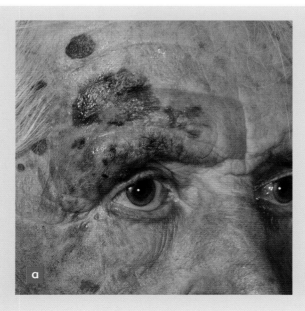

FIGURE 8.3 Hutchinson's melanotic freckle (HMF/lentigo maligna) of the right forehead in a 74-year-old farmer

(a) The lesion extends from the medial brow to the temple, from the mid forehead to the outer canthus of the right eye.

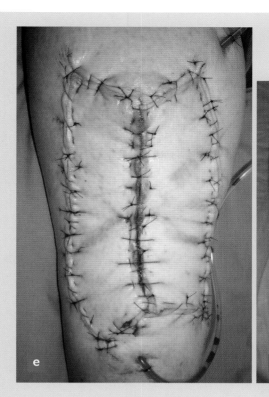

FIGURE 8.3

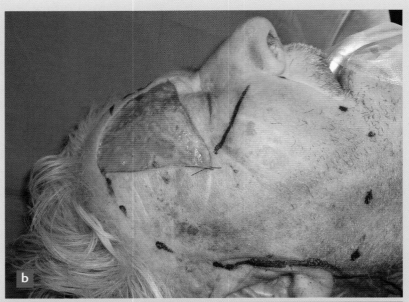

(b) DRAPE procedure—delayed reconstruction after pathology evaluation—leaves a defect of 7 × 7 cm.

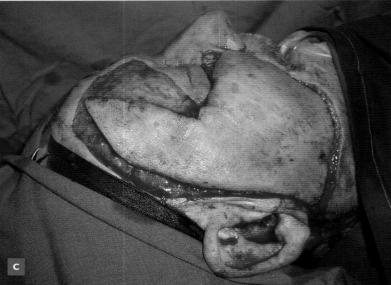

(c) Total cheek island flap (SMAS-based flap) based on the intact infraorbital neurovascular bundle and the facial vessels.

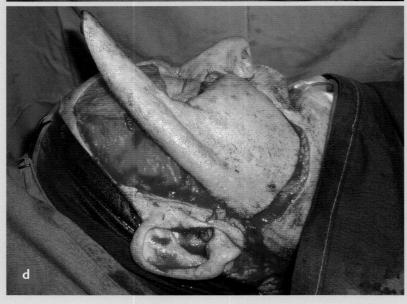

(d) Almost two-thirds of the flap is undermined to allow it to reach the medial brow.

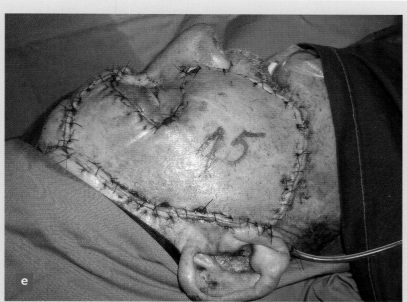

(e) Flap elevation and closure are complete within 45 minutes.

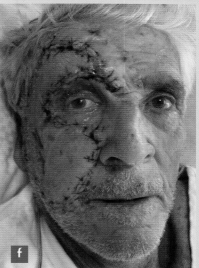

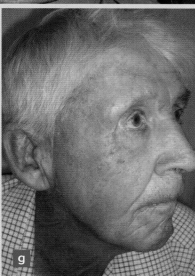

(f) Appearance at 2 days post operation.

(g) Appearance at 3 months.

See video for Figure 8.3

TLC: Conjoint flap vascularity

Time (operation/cost)
45 minutes
Life quality (and aesthetics)
Good with normal function and acceptable appearance
Complications
Nil

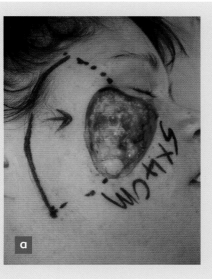

FIGURE 8.4 Recurrent desmoplastic melanoma of the right malar eminence in a 35-year-old female with concurrent thyroid cancer

(a) Re-excision of a desmoplastic melanoma of the right malar to produce a 5 × 4 cm defect after previous attempts undertaken elsewhere. A keystone flap based on the transverse facial vessels is planned.

FIGURE 8.4

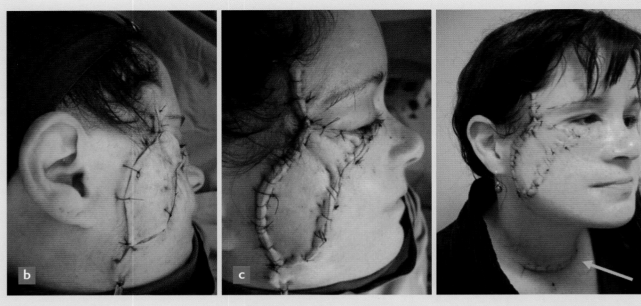

(b) Appearance following initial wound closure.

(c) Appearance at operation (left) and at 7 postoperative days (right).

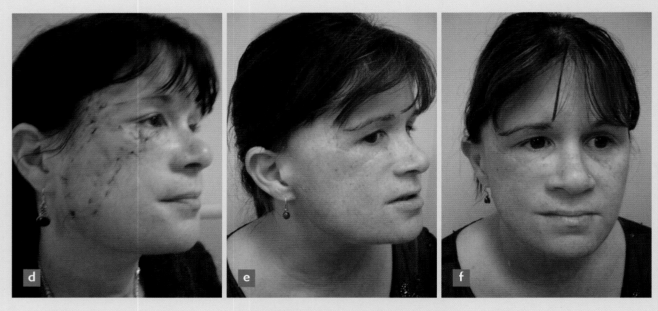

(d) Sequential removal of sutures by cutting the loops at 7 days, half the mattress sutures at 10 days and the tension sutures at 14 days (these may be revised downwards by the use of deep absorbable sutures).

(e) & **(f)** Improving aesthetics as the scar is settling.

(Reproduced with permission from Pelissier P, Gardet H, Pinsolle V, Santoul M, Behan FC 2007 The keystone design perforator island flap. Part II: clinical applications. J Plast Reconstr Aesthet Surg 60(8):889–91.)

TLC: Conjoint flap vascularity

Time (operation/cost)
60 minutes
Life quality (and aesthetics)
Good with normal function and acceptable appearance
Complications
Nil

FIGURE 8.5 Wide local excision of a T1b melanoma from the dorsum of the right hand following complete excision of visible melanoma previously by a poorly oriented transverse (rather than longitudinal) design in a 45-year-old dairy farmer

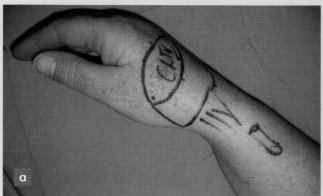

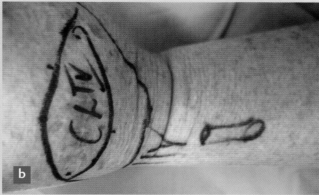

(a) Mark-out of the excision and proximal keystone flap based on the radial vessels.

(b) Additional neurovascular supply is provided by the superficial radial nerve (with its artery), which must not be damaged during blunt dissection.

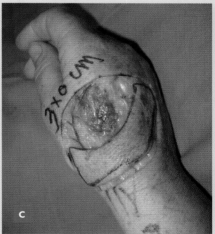

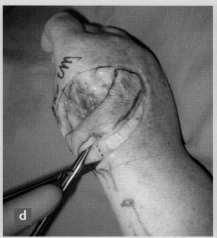

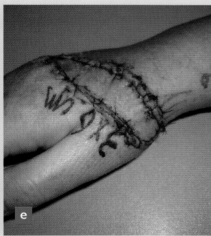

(c) The defect is 6 × 3 cm in size and unable to be closed primarily due to previous excision.

(d) Blunt dissection and stretch by teasing the tissues while maintaining the integrity of longitudinal structures.

(e) Closure with the wrist splinted in dorsoradial deviation.

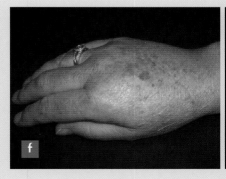

TLC: Conjoint flap vascularity	
Time (operation/cost)	
45 minutes	
Life quality (and aesthetics)	
Good with full mobilisation (2 weeks), acceptable appearance	
Complications	
Nil	

Postoperative appearance at 4 years (f) during normal resting position and (g) upon making a fist with a flexed wrist.

FIGURE 8.5

FIGURE 8.6

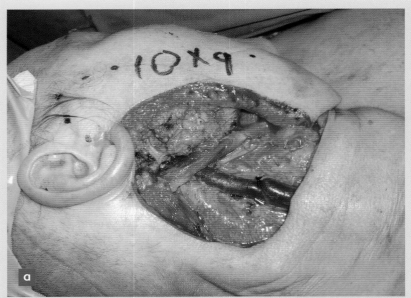

FIGURE 8.6 **Keystone flap closure of nodal metastases of the neck with cutaneous involvement. Previous 5.2 mm thick superficial spreading melanoma of the right preauricular region. Two months later, nodal recurrence appears clinically with cutaneous attachment**

(a) The mass in the neck was 8 × 6 cm in size, producing a 10 × 9 cm surgical skin defect.

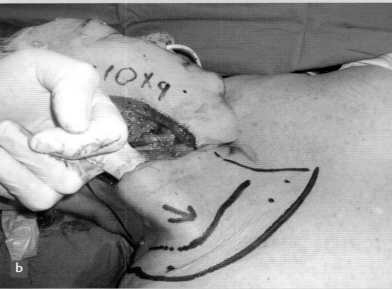

(b) Nodal clearance of levels II–IV in the neck with the degree of undermining of the neck indicated by the line below the flap edge. A keystone flap is designed to beyond the undermined region, designated by the left middle finger.

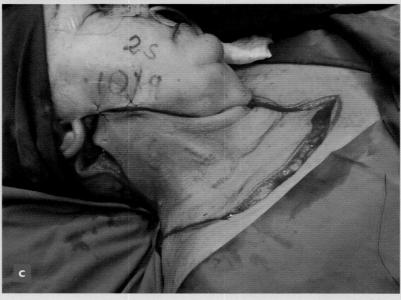

(c) The keystone flap used here is a design variant to run along the line of the clavicle. The ratio (undermined to non-undermined tissue) is 1:1 within the flap and the IVAC principle is evident with a pink flare within the whole flap following islanding.

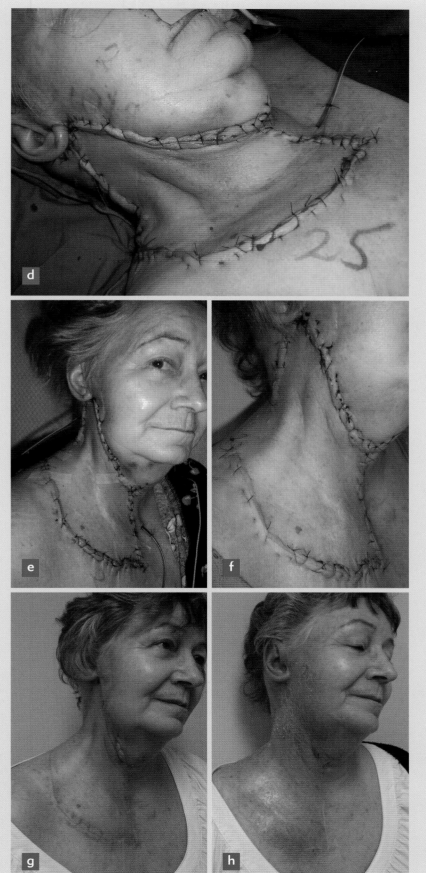

(d) Good vascularity to the tip of the flap despite undermining.

(e) Appearance at 3 days, with the patient experiencing some pain.

(f) Appearance at 13 days following cutting of the continuous loops of suture.

(g) Appearance at 3 weeks.

(h) Appearance on completion of radiotherapy in a timely manner.

See video for Figure 8.6

TLC: Conjoint flap vascularity

Time (operation/cost)
40 minutes
Life quality (and aesthetics)
Good and acceptable appearance
Complications
Nil

FIGURE 8.7

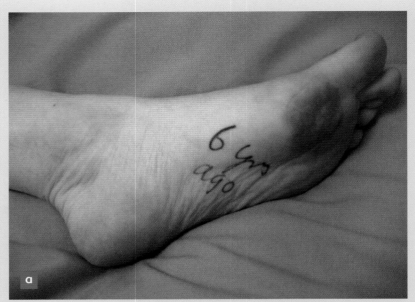

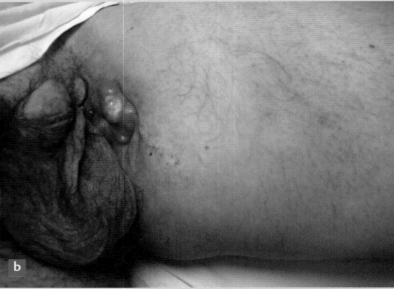

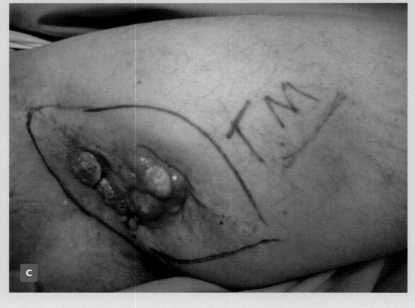

FIGURE 8.7 Quadriceps keystone flap closure of advanced metastatic spread of acral lentiginous melanoma of the left foot in a 45-year-old male with previous groin irradiation

(a) Acral lentiginous melanoma near the head of the first metatarsal in 1998.

(b) & **(c)** Cutaneous and nodal recurrence despite radiotherapy to treat the groin after 6 years (2004). The surgical defect is marked out as 15 × 10 cm in this irradiated field.

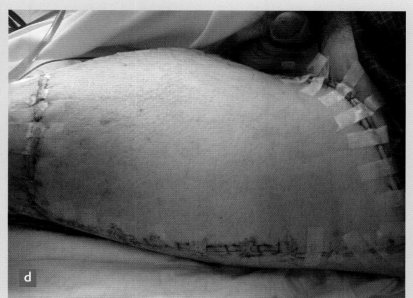

(d) A quadriceps keystone flap is used to close the defect of the left groin following full nodal clearance. The flap design must involve division of the iliotibial tract from the area of the greater trochanter to the suprapatellar region. Medially, the keystone flap design goes from the groin to the suprapatellar region. The transverse incisions create an island flap to establish improved vascularity (IVAC). With the division of the fascia supported by quadriceps perforators, the defect is easily closed with an upward and medial gliding movement.

(e) & **(f)** The closure of the groin wound at the point of suture removal. Due to the previous radiotherapy, final suture removal was delayed until 4 weeks.

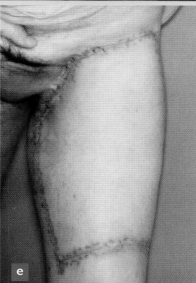

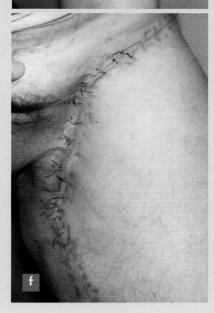

TLC: Conjoint flap vascularity

Time (operation/cost)
120 minutes
Life quality (and aesthetics)
Good with normal function and acceptable appearance
Complications
Nil

FIGURE 8.8

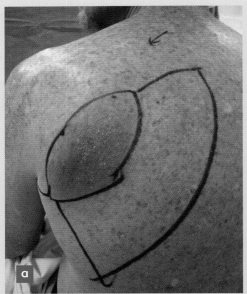

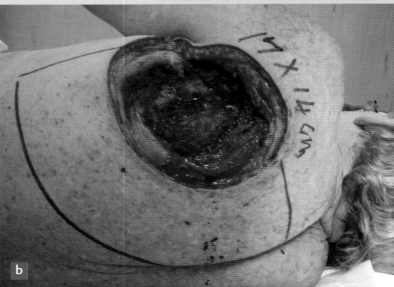

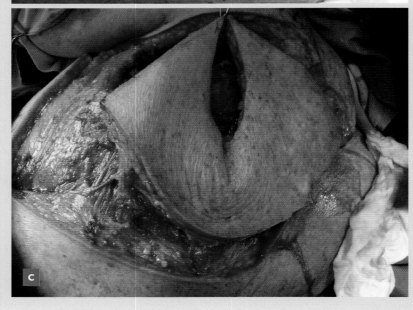

FIGURE 8.8 Use of the omega (Ω) variant of the keystone flap for closure of a large spindle cell tumour of the back in a 65-year-old male

(a) A melanoma/spindle cell tumour of the skin of the left scapula on biopsy with clinical evidence of left axillary lymph nodes.

(b) A 17 × 14 cm surgical defect is produced by tumour excision down to the infraspinatous muscles, with an axillary clearance in continuity. The design of the keystone flap indicates that the medial and lateral aspects of the flap can be undermined to facilitate defect closure following axillary clearance.

(c) The omega (Ω) variant is formed by transposing the ends of the flap towards each other based upon intercostal (T3–T6) perforators in the medial half of the flap.

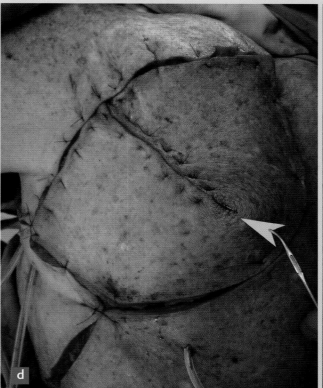

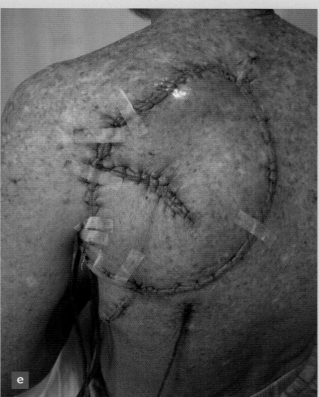

(d) Appearance following wound closure with even tension.

(e) Wound closure is complete over a suction drain (with a second drain for the axillary clearance). Note that vascular flare (IVAC) is present.

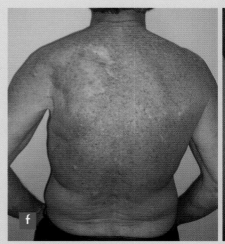

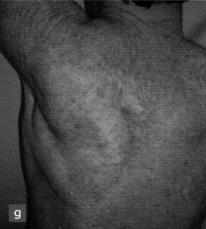

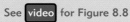

(f)–(h) Appearance at 2 years postoperatively with unrestricted movement of the left shoulder.

See video for Figure 8.8

TLC: Conjoint flap vascularity

Time (operation/cost)
120 minutes

Life quality (and aesthetics)
Good with patient walking in Himalayas by 4 weeks

Complications
Seroma, as a complication of the axillary dissection, was managed conservatively without sequelae

REVISIONAL SURGERY

The two most common reasons that revisional surgery may be necessary in keystone flap reconstruction of melanoma defects are when insufficient surgical margins have been taken or when surgical dog ears persist.

As discussed above, the need for wider excision can be reasonably common when immediate reconstruction is undertaken. This is particularly the case when a previous incisional biopsy has suggested that the lesion is less than 1 mm in thickness and without any additional adverse features (e.g. ulceration and >1 mitosis/mm^2) (ACN 2008), only to be identified as a thicker melanoma (e.g. >2 mm) subsequently. Here the margin may need revision to add an additional centimetre, depending on the radial margins of histopathological clearance. The use of DRAPE minimises this as an outcome in keystone flap reconstruction of melanoma defects. Where further excision is necessary, the simple geometry of the flap permits relatively easy planning for re-excision.

The revision of dog ears may be necessary in keystone flap surgery. The V–Y points of closure are sites that are prone to the development of dog ears. Any dog ears, even on the flap itself, can usually be excised at the time of surgery due to the robust blood supply to all regions of the dermis and skin, rather than any reliance on the dermal blood supply alone. For this reason, the need for dog-ear revision is less common with this approach than with other forms of flap reconstruction. Where revision is necessary, it is ideal to allow the patient to undergo any adjuvant therapies that may be required and, in the ideal scenario, allow maximal spontaneous resolution of the excess skin with time (6–12 months). When present on convex surfaces, dog ears improve readily, with the degree of resolution depending on the natural elasticity of the skin. Similar contour defects within concave areas are unlikely to resolve and will require early excision. The reliable healing and robust blood supply of these flaps minimises the chance that revisional surgery will be necessary and limits surgical misadventure to the flap should revisional surgery be necessary.

SUMMARY

Local control of invasive melanoma necessitates excision of the lesion plus an additional 2–4 cm of clinically uninvolved skin as a circumferential (1–2 cm) margin. This can make direct closure problematic, yet results in wounds that can be closed if a little more tissue could be imported. This size of defect is usually well-suited to locoregional flap reconstruction, but immediate reconstruction with complex local flaps can be problematic if incomplete excision or insufficient excision margins are present following excision. The keystone flap has relatively simple geometry, with readily identifiable reference points to indicate what area should be re-excised if insufficient margins occur. Where uncertainty is expected, the use of the DRAPE procedure with secondary keystone flap reconstruction is an effective solution, and keystone flaps can also be used to manage closure of metastatic disease, such as nodal metastasis with overlying skin involvement. As always, the surgery is relatively fast, with minimal morbidity for the patient, the wounds heal well and most patients experience good postoperative quality of life. As a result, the use of keystone island flaps for melanoma reconstruction (with variants) has increased markedly in the past decade, with significant benefits for patients over other available techniques.

BIBLIOGRAPHY

Australian Cancer Network (ACN) 2008 Clinical practice guidelines for the management of melanoma in Australia and New Zealand. National Health and Medical Research Council, Canberra.

Balch C M, Gershenwald J E, Soong S J, Thompson J F, Atkins M B, et al. 2009 Final version of 2009 AJCC melanoma staging and classification. J Clin Oncol 27(36):6199–206.

Behan F C, Lo C H, Findlay M 2010 Anatomical basis for the keystone island flap in the upper thigh. Plast Reconstr Surg 125(1):421–3.

Goldstein A M, Tucker M A 2001 Genetic epidemiology of cutaneous melanoma: a global perspective. Arch Dermatol 137(11):1493–6.

International Agency for Research on Cancer (IARC) 2008 GLOBOCAN 2008. Cancer incidence and mortality worldwide: IARC CancerBase no. 10. IARC, Lyon, http://globocan.iarc.fr/.

Morton D L, Cochran A J, Thompson J F, Elashoff R, Essner R, et al. 2005 Sentinel node biopsy for early-stage melanoma: accuracy and morbidity in MSLT-I, an international multicenter trial. Ann Surg 242(3):302–11; discussion 311–13.

Petersson F, Diwan A H, Ivan D, Gershenwald J E, Johnson M M, Harrell R, Prieto V G 2009 Immunohistochemical detection of lymphovascular invasion with D2-40 in melanoma correlates with sentinel lymph node status, metastasis and survival. J Cutan Pathol 36(11):1157–63.

Saint-Cyr M, Schaverien M, Wong C, Nagarkar P, Arbique G, Brown S, Rohrich R J 2009 The extended anterolateral thigh flap: anatomical basis and clinical experience. Plast Reconstr Surg 123(4):1245–55.

Thomas J M 2009 Concerns relating to the conduct and statistical analysis of the Multicenter Selective Lymphadenectomy Trial (MSLT-1) in patients with melanoma. J Plast Reconstr Aesthet Surg 62(4):442–6.

Whiteman D C, Whiteman C A, Green A C 2001 Childhood sun exposure as a risk factor for melanoma: a systematic review of epidemiologic studies. Cancer Causes Control 12(1):69–82.

Chapter 9
Radiotherapy

Insight, plus hindsight equals foresight.
Russell Murphy

The use of the keystone island flap in irradiated tissue, with its augmented cutaneous perfusion, can address this problem successfully.

INTRODUCTION

Radiotherapy plays an important part in the multidisciplinary approach to the management of cancers, particularly those in the head and neck, and skin (Ariyan 2006). It is imperative for the reconstructive surgeon to understand radiation injury and how it applies to reconstruction in order to optimise patient outcomes. Radiotherapy is the therapeutic use of ionising radiation for the control of rapidly dividing cells, such as those responsible for cancer. It is used with both curative and palliative intent, depending on the clinical situation and nature of the disease (e.g. tumour–node–metastases [TNM] staging, see Chapter 8). Cure has variable definitions, but it is most commonly expressed as remission or disease-free survival; where it fails to achieve cure, such treatment may increase life expectancy. Where cure is unachievable, radiotherapy can be employed palliatively in an attempt to improve quality of life for the patient's remaining time.

RADIOTHERAPY EFFECTS

Radiotherapy achieves these outcomes by combining direct effects on the tumour cells and indirect effects on the surrounding tissues, such as blood vessels, depending on their size and proximity to the treatment field. Ionising radiation causes covalent cross-linking of DNA nucleotides, affecting protein synthesis and cell replication. In normal cells, mismatch repair proteins delay division of cells until the DNA damage has been repaired; however, in rapidly dividing cells, there may be existing abnormalities of mismatch repair or cell cycle regulation and cell death can result. Cell death may be mitotic (death occurs when they undergo division) or during interphase (e.g. lymphocytes are destroyed

without cell division) (Baker & Krochak 1989, Stone et al. 2003). It may also accelerate apoptosis* (e.g. serous cells in the salivary gland) (Kerr et al. 1994, Stone et al. 2003). These cellular effects are applied to all cells receiving radiotherapy, but abnormal cells and those that are rapidly dividing show the greatest sensitivity (Hellman 1993, Mettler 1995, Rupnick et al. 2002).

Radiotherapy can have a major impact on tissues and a thorough understanding of its effects is essential to developing a safe approach to reconstruction in patients where radiotherapy is involved. The adverse effects of radiation and its clinical manifestations may be classified into early, consequential (chronic effects of acute toxicity) or late phases (Stone et al. 2003).

Acute radiotherapy effects

Acute changes are often described as radiation burns or dermatitis. This occurs during or immediately after the course of radiotherapy and predominantly affects proliferating tissues, such as the mucosa or skin (Mathes & Alexander 1996, Stone et al. 2003). Erythema may appear within the first hours of irradiation, caused by vessel damage or transient capillary dilatation secondary to vasoactive amines (Mathes & Alexander 1996, Brush et al. 2007). The basal cells of the epidermis that are responsible for producing the 10–20 layers of keratinising epithelial cells of the cornified layer of the skin may be lost (Brush et al. 2007). This dry desquamation may lead to moist desquamation or ulceration. Inflammation, warmth, tenderness, hypersensitivity or mucositis may lead to loss of appetite or difficulty eating (Mathes & Alexander 1996, Stone et al. 2003). These acute effects

---

* **Professor John Kerr, the discoverer of the phenomenon of apoptosis, tutored both F C Behan and M W Findlay in the early part of their surgical development at the Royal Brisbane Hospital in Queensland.**

are usually managed successfully with conservative measures, but can wreak havoc on inadequately healed wounds. Consequently, rapid healing of the surgical wound is vital so that radiotherapy can commence promptly at an oncologically appropriate stage.

Consequential effects of radiotherapy (chronic effects of acute toxicity)

There are a number of consequential effects of radiotherapy. Tissue oedema may be seen within hours or weeks following therapy (Mathes & Alexander 1996), reflecting injury to the vascular bed. Radiation causes degenerative change in the basement membrane and increased vascular permeability, resulting in transudation of plasma components into the extravascular space, compression of capillaries and lymphatic vessels, and impaired extracellular circulation (Baker & Krochak 1989, Tibbs 1997). The basement membrane itself thickens after about 30 days, increasing the resistance to the diffusion of oxygen and metabolites, further contributing to nutritional depletion (Baker & Krochak 1989). Smaller diameter vessels are more sensitive than larger vessels, with loss of capillaries and veins or venules (diameter less than 10 microns) before the destruction of larger ones (Baker & Krochak 1989). Progressive vessel loss occurs due to stasis, occlusion and reduced neovascularisation (Mathes & Alexander 1996). Any proliferations of new endothelial cells are abnormal. New capillaries are irregular in diameter and shape with a narrowed lumen, contributing to increased thrombosis and fibrous tissue replacement (Baker & Krochak 1989). Coexisting diabetes mellitus (microangiopathy) and/or hypertension (hyaline change) may increase the severity of these sequelae.

Irradiation can permanently damage fibroblasts (Tibbs 1997). Impaired fibroblast proliferation, function and collagen production/maturation may produce insufficient collagen production for normal wound healing.

Late effects of radiotherapy

Late changes of radiation injury usually begin 4–6 months after treatment (but may occur at any time) (Baker & Krochak 1989). Typical changes occur in tissues with slower cell turnover (e.g. muscle and fat), with atrophy of these tissues (Stone et al. 2003). These atrophic changes are probably a combination of direct cellular effects and an effect on the vascular volume within the tissue (with secondary effects on local reconstruction and healing). The skin becomes dry, with alopecia due to destruction of hair follicles and sweat glands (Mathes & Alexander 1996). Alopecia and dry skin are useful indicators of the extent of the radiotherapy field in the planning of flaps. The dermis becomes thinner with atrophy, and diagnostic telangiectasias of uncertain pathogenesis may arise. Impaired venous drainage and stasis, capillary damage resulting in dilatation

of other capillaries, and arteriovenous shunting and failure of regrowth of damaged vasculature are all proposed mechanisms (Brush et al. 2007). Increased enzymatic activity or destruction of melanocytes leads to pigmentation changes (Mettler 1995, Tibbs 1997). Small vessel changes include eccentric myointimal proliferation in small arteries and arterioles, capillary thrombosis and wall necrosis leading to progressive obliteration (endarteritis obliterans) (Teloh 1950). Increased vascular permeability, accumulation of extracellular fluid, collagen formation, progressive and irreversible tissue fibrosis and lymphoedema all contribute to a poor tissue environment. Reduced blood flow and decreased oxygen diffusion lower tissue oxygenation, resulting in poorer wound healing. As a consequence, the risk of ulceration and infection is increased (Tibbs 1997, Brush et al. 2007).

Other tissues are damaged, particularly in the head and neck. Irradiated bone (especially the mandible) is at significant risk of osteoradionecrosis, and radiotherapy damage to salivary glands (particularly the parotid) produces swelling, tenderness and xerostomia. Decreased and thickened oral secretions cause difficulties with eating, speech and wearing of dentures and increased dental caries (a possible contributing factor in osteoradionecrosis) (Stone et al. 2003). Irradiation is also associated with malignant degeneration of the skin, thyroid gland, breast and gastrointestinal tract, resulting in tumours and leukaemia (usually after a lag time of almost a decade) (Mathes & Alexander 1996, Stone et al. 2003).

The volume of some tissues (such as fat) is co-regulated with the volume of their blood vessels, growing or downsizing in parallel with each other (Rupnick et al. 2002, Dallabrida et al. 2003). In contrast, tumour cells often display the capacity to escape the normal cell cycle regulation of other cells and utilise mechanisms to increase their blood supply through tumour-related angiogenesis and vasculogenic mimicry (Hendrix et al. 2003). Despite these abilities, tumour cells are still dependent on blood vessels for their survival and growth. Radiotherapy causes endarteritis obliterans (of vessels), as well as limiting local angiogenic potential. This can have significant therapeutic benefit in cancer by minimising tumour blood flow and the potential for tumour angiogenesis and vasculogenic mimicry. The results can be the destruction of their existing blood supply, cessation of new blood vessel formation, tumour necrosis and a halt on further tumour growth (Hellman 1993).

PRESENTATIONS INVOLVING RECONSTRUCTION AND RADIOTHERAPY

Three different scenarios are possible where radiotherapy and reconstruction interact. The first is where the patient has never had radiotherapy but will receive radiotherapy as an adjuvant treatment in the postoperative setting to maximise oncological clearance. In this setting, any prolonged delay in the commencement of radiotherapy can affect disease control (Studer et al. 2006). Therefore, it is important that reconstructive approaches promote rapid healing in a reliable manner. As discussed above, radiotherapy can cause burns to the reconstructed skin, with ulceration. For this reason, skin grafts usually respond poorly to radiotherapy and alternative forms of reconstruction are preferable rather than risking exposure of the underlying structures. The robust circulation of the keystone island flap, along with its rapid healing, make it an ideal form of reconstruction where radiotherapy is anticipated in the postoperative setting. If skin grafts are used for the donor defect in keystone island flaps, these are usually away from the immediate field of radiation and do not usually cover any vital structures. Many of the keystone flap reconstructive cases for oncological defects presented in previous chapters (e.g. Chapters 4 and 8) are examples of the use of the keystone island flap to provide reconstruction with reliable healing, minimal morbidity and timely commencement of adjuvant radiotherapy. As a result, the clinical cases presented in this chapter will focus on flap elevation in irradiated tissue beds (see below) where regional or free-tissue reconstruction would otherwise have been used.

Reconstruction in previously irradiated tissues

The second scenario where radiotherapy and reconstructions meet is where the patient develops radio-recurrent or new disease in a previously irradiated tissue bed. This usually indicates that the tumour involved is aggressive, since it is capable of growth despite previous radiotherapy to control tumour growth. In this case, any further surgery is undertaken in tissue that has reduced local blood flow, lower oxygenation, poorer wound healing and lower wound tensile strength/ increased risk of wound dehiscence (Baker & Krochak 1989, Tibbs 1997). Traditionally, radiotherapy has been a contraindication to the use of locoregional flap reconstruction. The importation of fresh, non-irradiated tissue in the form of regional or free-tissue transfers represents the gold standard in fasciocutaneous reconstruction of these defects. Our experience with use of the keystone island flap in irradiated tissue brings into question the suitability of this standard. Both of these forms of reconstruction are not always achievable without significant additional morbidity, especially in the elderly. The pedicled pectoralis major flap has been a reliable workhorse in head and neck reconstruction (Mathes & Alexander 1996). However, as discussed in Chapter 4, the muscle is bulky, requiring time to atrophy, its arc of rotation can be difficult and its reach is limited to the level of the zygomatic arch. Free-tissue

transfer imports well-vascularised, non-irradiated tissue for coverage. However, the recipient vessels can be friable and difficult to dissect due to the loss of tissue planes and fibrosis, increasing the potential morbidity of an already complex procedure. Patients with radio-recurrent disease have aggressive disease by definition. Therefore, where possible, the reconstructive surgeon should try to limit the morbidity of any form of reconstruction used. The keystone island flap is well-suited to meeting this need.

When considering reconstruction using local tissues, an assessment of the degree of radiotherapy-related and comorbidity-related tissue compromise is worthwhile. For example, if the patient suffers from comorbidities such as hypertension or diabetes mellitus, these can adversely add to the impairment induced by radiotherapy (Baker & Krochak 1989). Quantification of the radiation dose already applied has two uses. It permits an assessment of the likely severity of radiotherapy changes and, second, it will determine whether any additional radiotherapy is possible. Relevant treatment-related factors include the type of radiation, total radiation dose, dose per fraction, volume of irradiated tissue, the time interval between treatments and protraction of treatments (Sandel & Davison 2007). Some chemotherapeutic agents, including actinomycin D, bleomycin and methotrexate, may exacerbate radiation injury (Mathes & Alexander 1996). The keystone island flap has demonstrated reliable vascularity and increased skin erythema following islanding in normal skin (immediate vascular augmentation concept, IVAC). This provides additional protection against necrosis relative to non-islanded flaps for local defect reconstruction. As a result, in our centre the keystone island flap has been applied successfully for the reconstruction of the majority of fasciocutaneous defects in previously irradiated fields.

As with any surgery, in irradiated tissue the technique is adapted to suit the additional needs that irradiation places on the tissues. For example, general considerations in irradiated fields include careful tissue handling, judicious use of systemic antibiotic therapy perioperatively, and separation of surgery and radiotherapy by a period of at least 3–4 weeks (Tibbs 1997). In addition to these considerations, some specific adaptations are useful when using keystone island flaps for the reconstruction of irradiated defects.

First, any keystone island flap in irradiated tissue is designed to be larger than might otherwise be necessary in other tissues so that non-physiological tension is minimised. Strategic use of haemostatic clips (rather than diathermy) during flap elevation seeks to achieve a balance between minimising blood loss and additional damage to the local vasculature. Use of suction drainage, where appropriate, minimises additional complications. Designs that incorporate a conjoint blood supply (perforator/direct vessel and neurovascular supplies) can improve the reliability of the flaps. Suture removal is delayed by an additional 1–2 weeks relative to the normal postoperative schedule (up to 4 weeks) to avoid wound dehiscence from radiotherapy-induced delayed healing and tensile wound strength. As a rule of thumb, when marked bleeding occurs following removal of a non-buried suture, further suture removal is delayed for an additional 1–2 weeks.

The standard use of the keystone island flap is relatively safe in irradiated fields but the normal vascular changes seen upon islanding may be significantly blunted by the previous radiotherapy, causing concern. Utilising these additional principles of greater flap size, strategic haemostasis and delayed suture removal increases the buffer between a successful reconstruction and a problematic postoperative course. Timely healing

and lower complication rates have been our experience with the use of keystone island flaps in previously irradiated tissue (Behan et al. 2006).

Figure 9.1 demonstrates the safe use of a standard keystone island flap for closure of a melanoma defect in the cheek where the upper limit of the irradiated field for a previous cancer (laryngeal cancer) extended to the level of the angle of the mandible. Figure 9.2 goes further, by demonstrating the use of two keystone island flaps in an irradiated field, with one used principally for tissue salvage (of an ear remnant) by islanding (IVAC). Figure 9.3 shows what can happen if suture removal is not delayed in the setting of radiotherapy, and Figures 9.4 and 9.5 (with salvage) demonstrate examples of where all these principles have been applied successfully for keystone island flap reconstruction in irradiated fields.

FIGURE 9.1

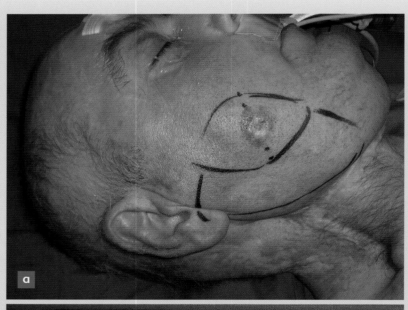

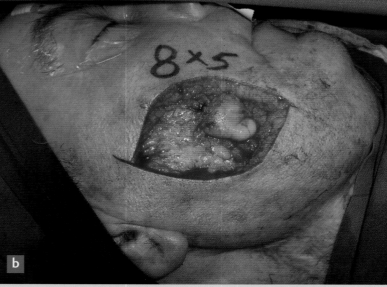

FIGURE 9.1 Male with previous history of laryngeal cancer treated with radiotherapy and a radionecrotic ulcer covered with a previous pectoralis major flap presents with a new melanoma of the right cheek

(a) Invasive melanoma centrally in a field of in-situ melanoma is planned for an excision of 2 cm from the invasive disease and 1 cm from the in-situ disease.

(b) Excision creates an 8 × 5 cm defect of the right cheek that cannot be closed primarily.

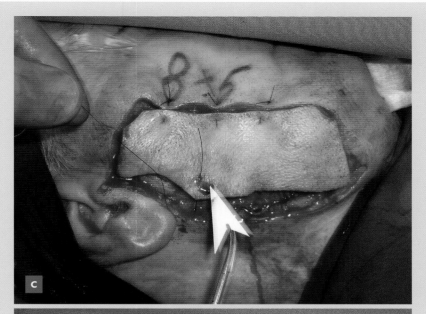

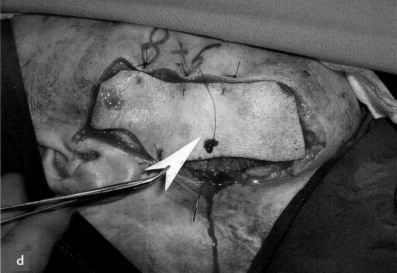

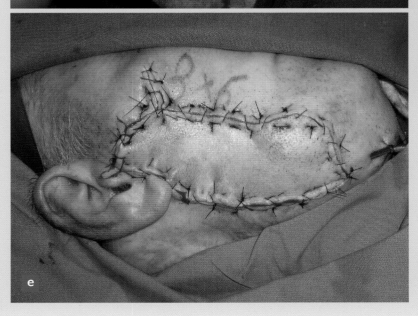

(c) A posteriorly based keystone flap is elevated (part of the flap is within an irradiated field), based on facial and superficial temporal artery perforators. Despite having similar transverse dimensions to the defect size, the flap is markedly paler than most keystone flaps following islanding, especially in the lower irradiated region of the flap.

(d) A cyanotic *red dot sign* (arrow) is of concern initially, but the flap colour improves on completion of the procedure.

(e) Flap colour never improves to normal levels for keystone flaps (vascular flare of quaternary response).

(f) Despite this concern, the flap healed without incident and acceptable aesthetics at 2 months post operation.

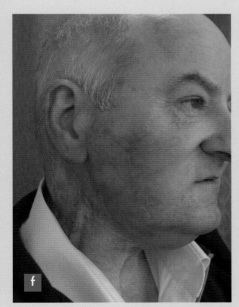

TLC: Conjoint flap vascularity

Time (operation/cost)
50 minutes
Life quality (and aesthetics)
Good with normal acceptable appearance
Complications
Nil

FIGURE 9.2

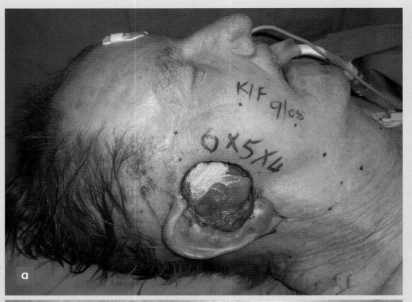

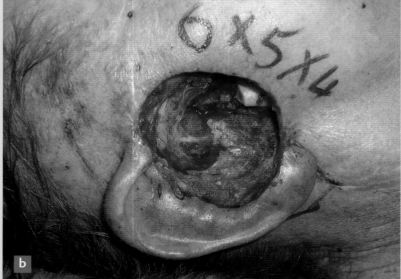

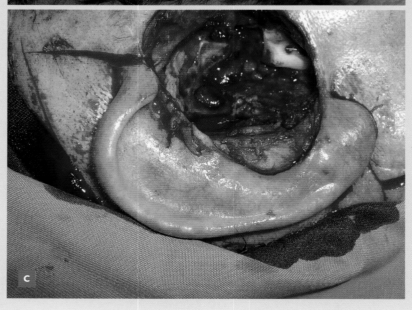

FIGURE 9.2 **Radio-recurrent squamous cell carcinoma (SCC) of the parotid with cutaneous involvement in this elderly man demonstrates the use of IVAC to provide salvage of poorly vascularised tissues (the remaining part of the ear) by islanding, even in an irradiated bed**

(a) Following excision of the SCC, a 6 × 5 cm defect (4 cm deep) is produced along with decreased vascularity to the ear due to a small cutaneous attachment posteriorly. Note the scar on his cheek of his previous SMAS-based keystone flap for initial primary SCC 1 year earlier.

(b) Following haemostasis of the deep wound with exposed bone after bony resection to complete oncological clearance, the vascularity of the ear is progressively worsening with obvious venous insufficiency. At this point, the respective surgeon advocated for amputation of the ear. However, it was salvaged by islanding within a post-auricular keystone flap to improve its vascularity and viability.

(c) Following incorporation of the devitalised ear remnant into a posterior keystone island flap, the flap rapidly undergoes improved vascularity with loss of venous congestion. A salvage manoeuvre to revitalise suspiciously cyanotic tissue.

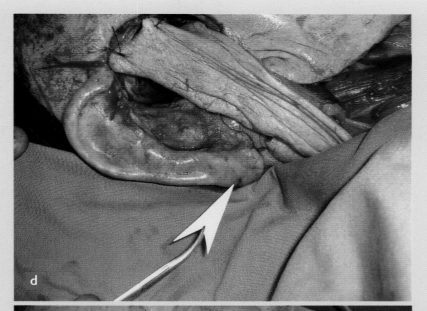

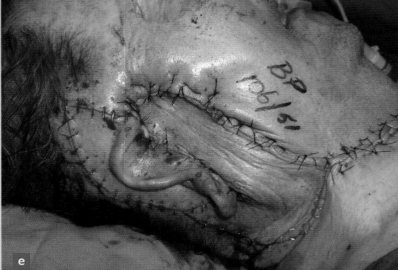

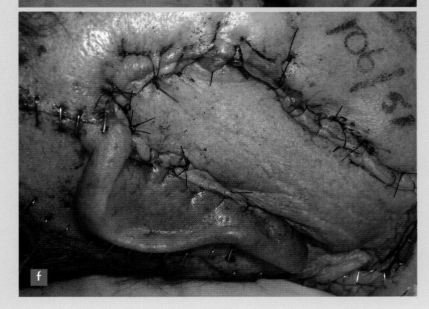

(d) A cervicosubmental island (CSI) flap is elevated in the neck and transposed into the defect. Note the bleeding from the lobule of the ear.

(e) Upon wound closure, the flap and the ear are viable. Additional procedures to improve the positioning of the ear are delayed so as to avoid any return of vascular compromise to the ear.

(f) Two days post operation, both the flap and the ear are nicely perfused.

(g) Appearance at 6 months with full survival of the ear remnant and flap. The patient was happy with the shape and position of the ear and did not want any subsequent correction.

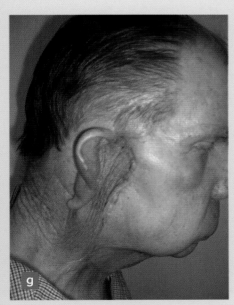

TLC: Conjoint flap vascularity

Time (operation/cost)
50 minutes
Life quality (and aesthetics)
Good with normal function and acceptable aesthetics
Complications
Nil

FIGURE 9.3

FIGURE 9.3 A 60-year-old female with previous SCC (T2) of the tongue treated with surgical excision and postoperative radiotherapy (60 Gy) to the operative field and neck

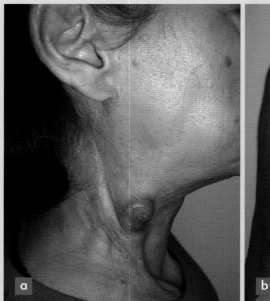

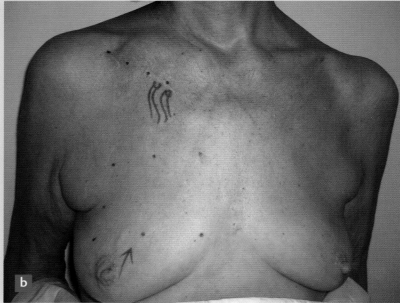

(a) Radio-recurrent disease developed in the neck.

(b) Previous surgery to the right clavicle as a child, 50 years earlier, was a potential contraindication to the use of the pectoralis major flap (no preoperative vascular imaging undertaken).

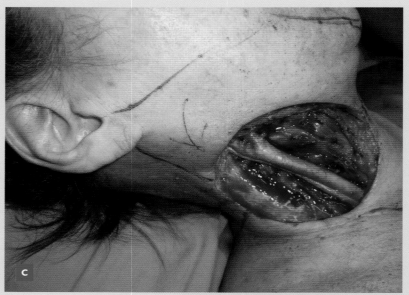

(c) An 8 × 8 cm defect is produced following surgical excision of the tumour with local nodes and exposure of the internal jugular vein.

(d) The pathology specimen.

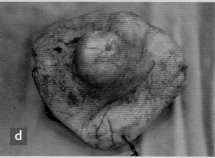

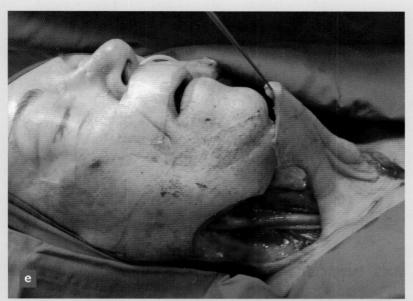

(e) A suprasternal keystone flap is raised with transposition of the skin (with platysma) from the contralateral (left) submandibular region, with a turnover to reach the right angle of the jaw to assist coverage of the major vessels. A second flap was not necessary at this time and direct closure of the donor site was undertaken.

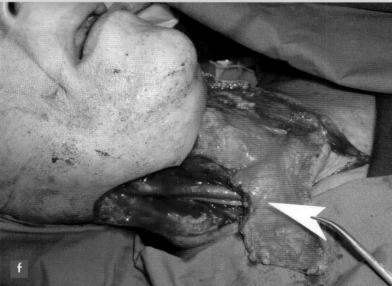

(f) The neurovascular structures from the supraclavicular nerves (with associated vessels), along with local perforators (arrow).

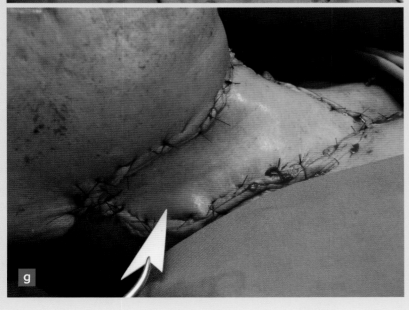

(g) IVAC on closure, with marked erythema of the flap.

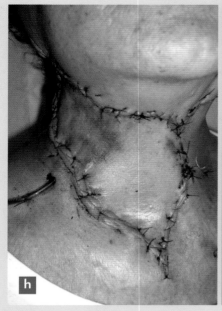

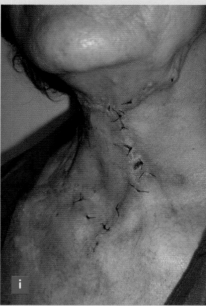

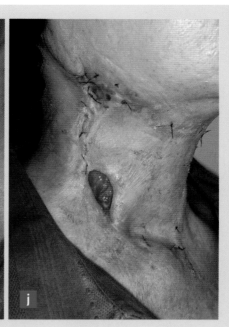

(h) Appearance on the first postoperative day, demonstrating some bruising but, otherwise, a well-vascularised flap and good neck mobility.

(i) Appearance 2 weeks post operation.

(j) Premature removal of sutures in an irradiated field at 2 weeks resulted in wound dehiscence posteriorly and superiorly.

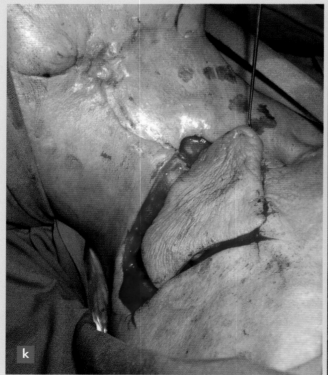

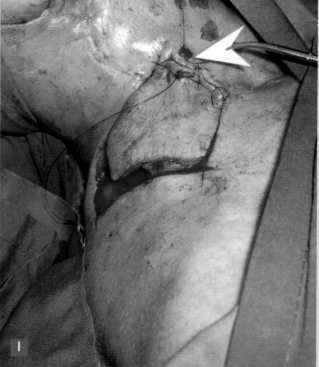

(k) A smaller supraclavicular keystone flap is elevated based upon perforators of the transverse cervical/superficial cervical vessels for closure of the lower dehiscence.

(l) *Red dot signs* are evident on both sides of the suture line here because both are islanded keystone flaps.

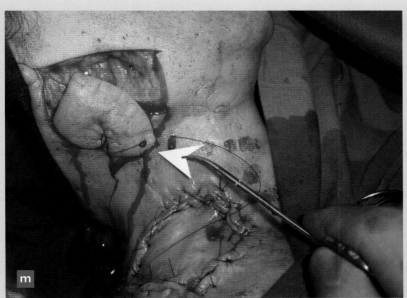

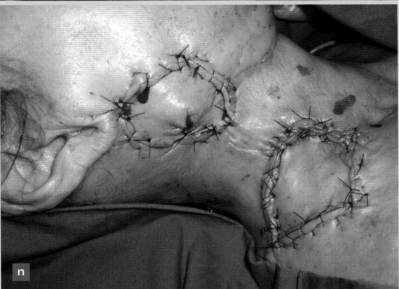

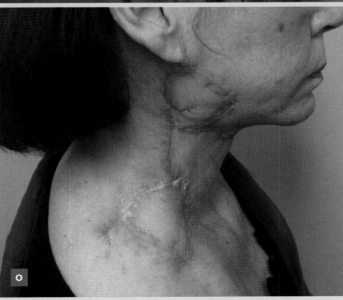

(m) A second keystone flap is elevated over the angle of the jaw and transposed as an omega (Ω) variant to cover the upper dehiscence. Again, *red dot signs* are evident from both flaps.

(n) The donor sites for both flaps are closed primarily and reliable vascularity is noted in both flaps despite reoperation and previous radiotherapy.

(o) Postoperative appearance at 6 weeks when erythema of the suture lines is most marked. No further issues with wound healing were experienced and appropriate scar management was undertaken.

See 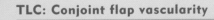 for Figure 9.3

TLC: Conjoint flap vascularity

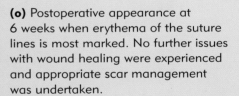

Time (operation/cost)
90/15/60 minutes—three operations (first keystone flap, resuturing, second keystone flap)

Life quality (and aesthetics)
Good following eventual healing and acceptable function

Complications
1. Wound dehiscence following premature removal of sutures by inexperienced clinician
2. Resuturing unsuccessful
3. Second keystone flap for carotid coverage—no complications

FIGURE 9.4

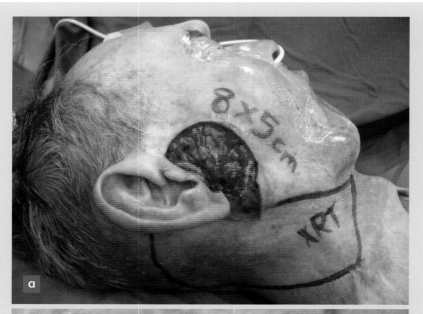

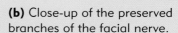

FIGURE 9.4 A 78-year-old male with metastatic SCC of the parotid (the Australian disease), having previously had a free deep circumflex iliac artery bone flap reconstruction of his right hemi-mandible following invasive SCC of his lower lip that invaded the mental (and inferior alveolar) nerves, followed by radiotherapy

(a) Following excision of the SCC and superficial parotidectomy, an 8 × 5 cm skin defect is created.

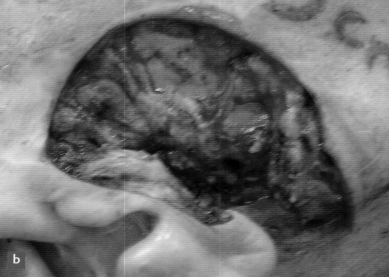

(b) Close-up of the preserved branches of the facial nerve.

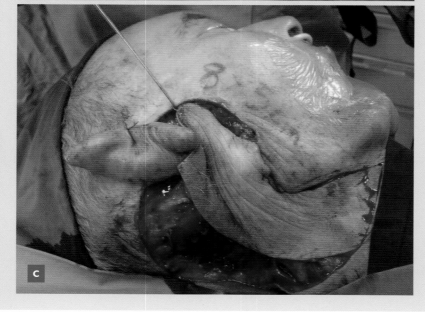

(c) A posterior CSI flap is transposed into the defect, having been planned to be a little larger than would normally be used to ensure only physiological wound tension upon closure.

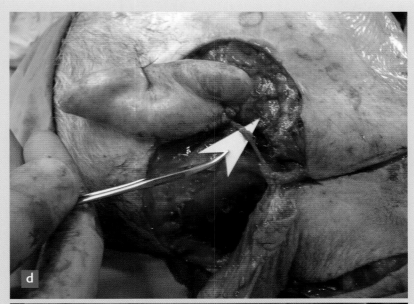

(d) The arrow demonstrates a branch of the great auricular nerve (part of the C2–C3 dermatome) exiting the superior border of the flap, confirming the neurovascular support for the flap, along with the likely perforator support from external carotid branches medially (conjoint supply).

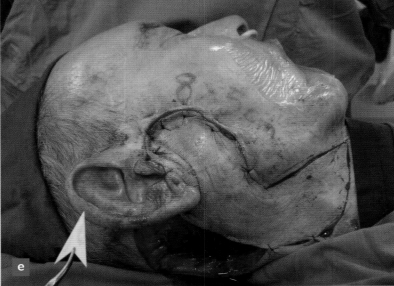

(e) Following initial closure where a vascular flare would normally be evident, the blood supply to the flap looks normal (rather than hyperaemic), indicating good blood supply despite previous radiotherapy. Note the small folds of the flap as it curves around the ear base.

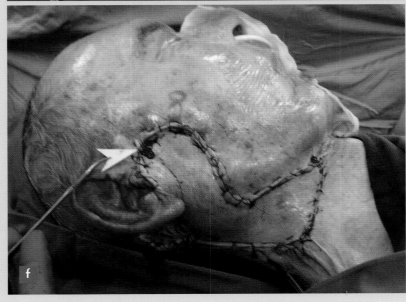

(f) A *red dot sign* at the apex of the flap, demonstrating good arterial supply despite the paler appearance of the posterior neck skin within the field of post-radiotherapy telangiectasia surrounding the flap. A small, fenestrated full-thickness skin graft has been used to assist closure of the donor site.

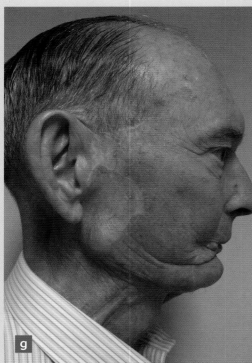

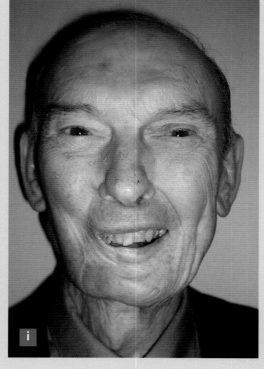

(g) The healed wound, with the patient adamant that he had not felt any significant pain during his postoperative recovery.

(h) Posterior view of his healed wounds.

(i) Recovery of most facial nerve function.

(Reproduced with permission from Behan F, Sizeland A, Gilmour F, Hui A, Seel M, Lo CH 2010 Use of the keystone island flap for advanced head and neck cancer in the elderly—a principle of amelioriation. J Plast Reconstr Aesthet Surg 63(5):739–45.)

TLC: Conjoint flap vascularity

Time (operation/cost)
90 minutes

Life quality (and aesthetics)
Good—this doctor reports he was totally pain-free and still working at 78 years of age, acceptable aesthetics

Complications
Nil

FIGURE 9.5 **A 78-year-old female with SCC of the left tonsil treated with radiotherapy to the primary site and neck in 2006. In 2009, she developed cutaneous recurrence over the mastoid**

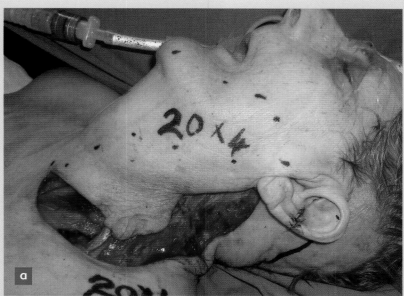

(a) Excision of the radio-recurrent lesion and neck clearance created a defect 20 × 4 cm in an irradiated field. Note the early vascular changes in the undermined anterior neck flap.

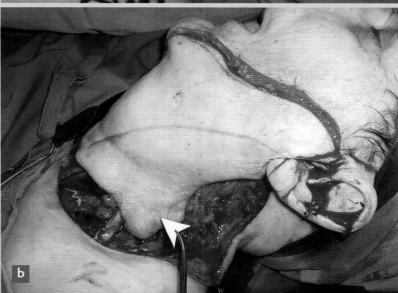

(b) Use of IVAC to improve functional perfusion to the undermined anterior neck skin. The line over the flap indicates the level of undermining. Superomedial to this, the flap is attached to the underlying tissues and, here, facial artery perforators are supplying the flap. Pre- and post-platysma plexuses provide supply to the tip of the flap.

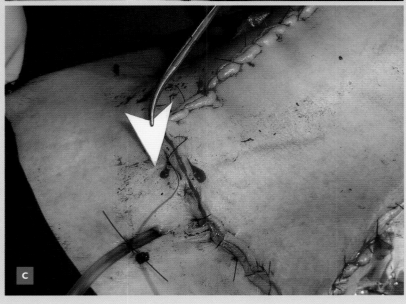

(c) A *red dot sign* is larger on the flap side than on the non-flap side.

FIGURE 9.5

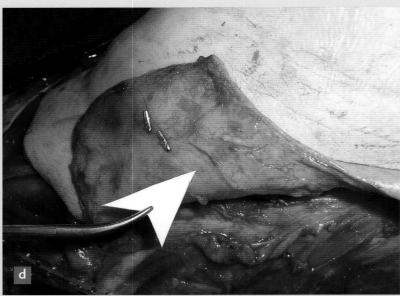

(d) Haemostasis on the deep surface of the neck flap is achieved with surgical clips.

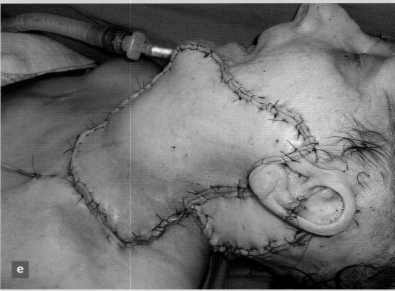

(e) On closure, there is good vascular perfusion throughout the flap.

(f) Day 5 following surgery with a reliable, pain-free recovery and good neck mobility.

See video for Figure 9.5

TLC: Conjoint flap vascularity

Time (operation/cost)
90 minutes
Life quality (and aesthetics)
Good, acceptable aesthetics
Complications
Nil

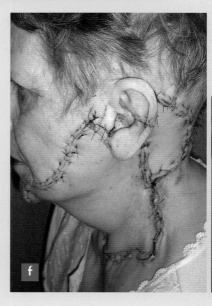

(g) Appearance after staged removal of sutures—the interrupted mattress sutures are left for 4 weeks in this irradiated field.

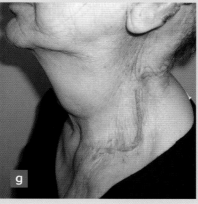

Reconstruction of radionecrosis

The final scenario where reconstruction and radiotherapy collide is in the management of long-term radiotherapy complications, such as radionecrosis. The development of non-healing ulcers, usually occurring quite some time after the course of radiotherapy, is an all too common diagnostic and management problem for the reconstructive surgeon working in multidisciplinary centres. These ulcers usually occur in the elderly, often in patients with multiple comorbidities that may contribute to the problem and limit the reconstructive options. Appropriate management of these patients necessitates thorough preoperative work-up with optimisation of the comorbidities prior to consideration of any surgical procedure. Exclusion of tumour recurrence, radiotherapy-related malignant degeneration or incidental new tumour formation is essential. Hyperbaric oxygen therapy (HBOT) can be a useful adjunct to assist healing of non-malignant late radiotherapy ulceration, with multiple studies, including an appropriately performed meta-analysis (Bennett et al. 2005), finding a benefit from its use. However, where the defect size is large or involves the exposure of important structures (e.g. bone, tendon),

surgical reconstruction may hasten the time to healing and minimise contracture formation. Surgery in this situation must be staged, incorporating the use of tissue biopsies in the first instance (to exclude malignancy), followed by subsequent reconstruction where there is no evidence of tumour. Punch biopsies or incisional biopsies are useful if they are positive for malignancy, but will fail to exclude malignancy with a negative result. Therefore, excisional ulcer debridement with the specimen sent for histopathology is the mainstay of our initial approach to this problem (delayed reconstruction after pathology evaluation [DRAPE] procedure). After excision, the wound is dressed and elevation of the wound undertaken for the few days necessary for the histopathology result. This elevation minimises local tissue oedema, thereby minimising its impact on local microvascular tissue perfusion, and limits further tissue necrosis related to the surgery. A reconstructive plan can then be made once the histopathology is clear. Keystone flap reconstruction can be undertaken in this setting using similar principles to those used for radio-recurrent disease. Figure 9.6 demonstrates the use of keystone island flap closure for both radionecrotic ulceration and radio-recurrent disease.

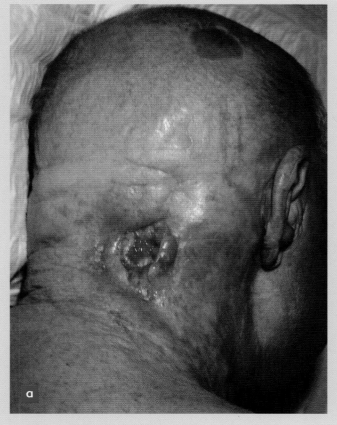

FIGURE 9.6 A 75-year-old male with a recurrent SCC of the right occipital region despite radiotherapy, 6 months after treatment of the original lesion in the right parietal region.

FIGURE 9.6

(a) The appearance of the primary site and the secondary lesion in the occiput.

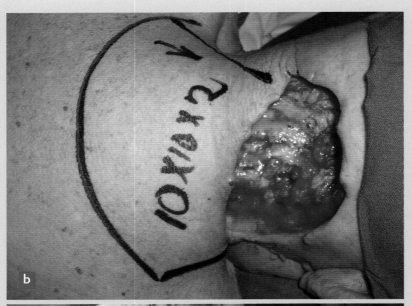

(b) The surgical defect, following excision down to the cervical spine, measuring 10 × 10 × 2 cm.

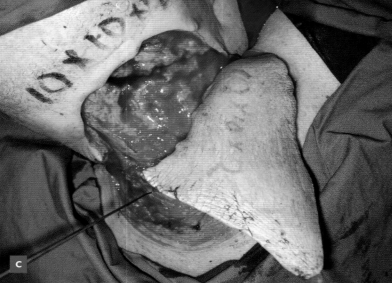

(c) The keystone flap raised on the left paraspinal perforators, facilitating an arc of rotation to close the surgical defect with moderate tension.

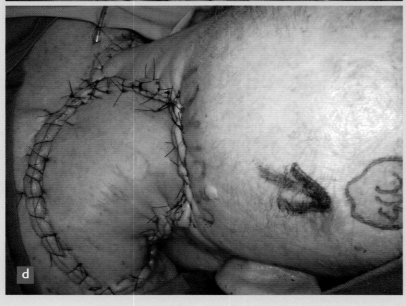

(d) The operation on completion (80 minutes). Note the increasing vascularity present, called the hyperaemic phase.

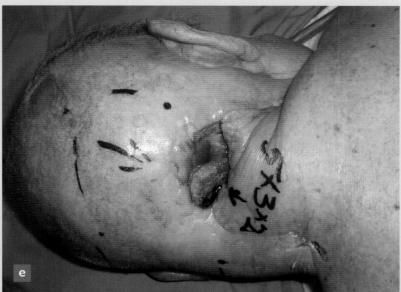

(e) Complication of wound breakdown at 4 weeks in the irradiated field with undue flexion of the neck contributing to this setback.

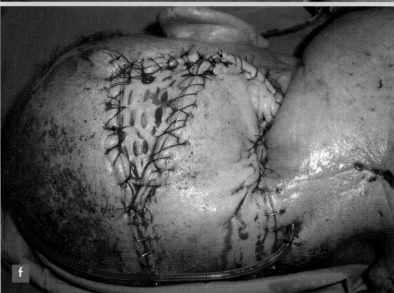

(f) Left occipital island flap, keystone in design, to close the hole, with a secondary scalp defect covered with a fenestrated full-thickness graft.

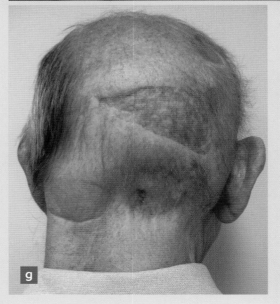

(g) The healed wound after some months of dressings, the patient refusing further surgery.

(Reproduced with permission from Behan F, Sizeland A, Gilmour F, Hui A, Seel M, Lo CH 2010 Use of the keystone island flap for advanced head and neck cancer in the elderly—a principle of amelioriation. J Plast Reconstr Aesthet Surg 63(5):739–45.)

TLC: Conjoint flap vascularity

Time (operation/cost)

80 minutes for first operation; 80 minutes for second procedure

Life quality (and aesthetics)

Good with normal function following eventual healing— 3 months (patient declined further surgery), acceptable aesthetics

Complications

Wound breakdown on marked neck flexion requiring revision

SUMMARY

The classical teaching of avoiding local flap reconstruction in irradiated tissue has been challenged by the development of the keystone island flap (and its variants). It appears to be reliable and safe for use in the reconstruction of defects within irradiated tissue beds. Its excellent cutaneous perfusion and reliable healing offset many of the problematic issues associated with flaps and healing within irradiated tissues, while it provides fasciocutaneous reconstruction with minimal morbidity in a patient population that tends to be elderly and infirm. Consideration should be given to its use as an alternative to microsurgical reconstruction in some situations, with additional precautions as discussed in this chapter. Ideally, the reconstructive surgeon should have both options available—'both barrels loaded' (Behan et al. 2006).

BIBLIOGRAPHY

Ariyan S 2006 Management of regional metastatic disease of the head and neck: diagnosis and treatment. In: S J Mathes & V R Hentz, eds. Plastic surgery, 2nd edn. WB Saunders, Philadelphia, 465–74.

Baker D G, Krochak R J 1989 The response of the microvascular system to radiation: a review. Cancer Invest 7(3):287–94.

Behan F, Sizeland A, Porcedu S, Somia N, Wilson J (2006). Keystone island flap: an alternative reconstructive option to free flaps in irradiated tissue. Aust N Z J Surg 76(5):407–13.

Bennett M H, Feldmeier J, Hampson N, Smee R, Milross C 2005 Hyperbaric oxygen therapy for late radiation tissue injury. Cochrane Database Syst Rev 20(3):CD005005.

Brush J, Lipnick S L, Phillips T, Sitko J, McDonald J T, McBride W H 2007 Molecular mechanisms of late normal tissue injury. Semin Radiat Oncol 17(2):121–30.

Dallabrida S M, Zurakowski D, Shih S C, Smith L E, Folkman J, Moulton K S, Rupnick M A 2003 Adipose tissue growth and regression are regulated by angiopoietin-1. Biochem Biophys Res Commun 311(3):563–71.

Hellman S 1993 Principles of radiation therapy. In: V T DeVita Jr, S Hellman, S A Rosenberg, eds. Cancer: principles and practice of oncology. Lippincott, Philadelphia: pp 248–75.

Hendrix M J, Seftor E A, Hess A R, Seftor R E 2003 Vasculogenic mimicry and tumour-cell plasticity: lessons from melanoma. Nat Rev Cancer 3(6):411–21.

Kerr J F, Winterford C M, Harmon B V 1994 Apoptosis. Its significance in cancer and cancer therapy. Cancer 73(8):2013–26.

Mathes S J, Alexander J 1996 Radiation injury. Surg Oncol Clin N Am 5(4):809–24.

Mettler F U 1995 Medical effects of ionising radiation. WB Saunders, Philadelphia.

Rupnick M A, Panigrahy D, Zhang C Y, Dallabrida S M, Lowell B B, Langer R, Folkman M J 2002 Adipose tissue mass can be regulated through the vasculature. Proc Natl Acad Sci U S A 99(16):10730–5.

Sandel H D, Davison S P 2007 Microsurgical reconstruction for radiation necrosis: an evolving disease. J Reconstr Microsurg 23(4):225–30.

Stone H B, Coleman C N, Anscher M S, McBride W H 2003 Effects of radiation on normal tissue: consequences and mechanisms. Lancet Oncol 4(9):529–36.

Studer G, Furrer K, Davis B J, Stoeckli S S, Zwahlen R A, Leutolf U M, Glanzmann C 2006 Postoperative IMRT in head and neck cancer. Radiat Oncol 1:40.

Teloh H 1950 Histopathology of radiated tissue. Surg Gynecol Obstet 90:335.

Tibbs M K 1997 Wound healing following radiation therapy: a review. Radiother Oncol 42(2):99–106.

Chapter 10
Trauma

We give advice, but we cannot give the wisdom to profit by it.
La Rouchefoucauld

The keystone flap is emerging as a useful reconstructive tool for specific traumatic defects due to its robust vascularity, minimal morbidity, relatively pain-free recovery, early return of function and acceptable aesthetics.

INTRODUCTION

Trauma can occur in an instant. Rarely should reconstruction of traumatic defects be undertaken in such a time frame. A considered, methodical approach can improve patient safety, optimise outcomes and avoid more complex forms of reconstruction. Thorough assessment of patient factors (e.g. age, site, comorbidities), the defect complexity and the available donor tissues (locoregional and distant) can highlight reconstructive options that might otherwise have been overlooked. For example, locoregional reconstruction is a simple, minimally intrusive, low expense (i.e. from the point of view of the patient, surgeon and hospital) reconstructive option suitable for many defects that might otherwise receive more complex approaches in some centres. The reasons for choosing a more complex form of reconstruction need to be explicit and in keeping with optimising quality of life for the patient.

Trauma presentations represent a spectrum from relatively simple, isolated injuries (e.g. pretibial lacerations from mechanical falls in the elderly) through to complex, life-threatening multi-traumas (e.g. high-speed motor vehicle accidents). As trauma complexity increases, so too does the need for a systematic approach to the trauma patient. The principles of Emergency Management of Severe Trauma/Advanced Trauma Life Support (EMST/ATLS) following primary, secondary and tertiary surveys is pivotal to ensuring life- and limb-threatening injuries are identified and managed in an appropriate and timely manner. In severe trauma, a multidisciplinary approach is essential, involving specialists in emergency medicine, intensive care, general surgery, orthopaedic surgery, neurosurgery and plastic surgery. Based on the assessments of these teams, a prioritised management plan can be devised

that focuses on the most life- or limb-threatening issues for the patient. This approach not only maximises patient survival and well-being, it also permits an appreciation of the likely long-term outcomes for the patient. This is an important consideration in the planning of any reconstruction, where the morbidity of any reconstructive procedure must be weighed carefully against the presumed benefit to the patient. Free-tissue transfer can provide revascularisation (via flow-through flaps), numerous tissue types (including vascularised bone, functional or denervated muscle, skin and fat) and flap dimensions to reconstruct most traumatic defects. The perennial problems associated with free-tissue transfer, including operative and donor site morbidity (Parrett et al. 2006), questionable aesthetics from the use of non-matched distant tissue (non-like for like) (Posch et al. 2007) and the need for additional surgery and cost, have been well-documented. The combination of these problems and the recent availability of temporising measures (e.g. vacuum-assisted closure) has seen an increase in the use of other reconstructive options, including locoregional reconstruction, over the past decade (Parrett et al. 2006). Less morbid reconstructive options may provide adequate soft tissue coverage without many of the problems associated with free-flap reconstruction, thereby improving quality of life.

THE NATURE AND SEVERITY OF TRAUMA

Trauma encompasses many diverse forms of injury—whether blunt, sharp, burns, high- or low-velocity injuries (or a combination of all of these), the aetiological factors are wide-ranging. For our purposes, when deciding upon the reconstructive options, our rationale takes into consideration four pathways/axes. The first axis is isolated trauma versus multi-trauma, the second is low-energy versus high-energy injuries, the third is simple mechanism versus complex mechanism injuries and the fourth is acute versus chronic trauma manifestations. The purpose of these considerations is to determine to what degree the surrounding tissues can be relied upon as a source of donor tissue for reconstruction.

Isolated trauma versus multi-trauma

The same defect can occur either in isolation from any other injury, or as part of a constellation of tissue insults to the patient in the form of multi-trauma. Isolated trauma is well-suited to consideration of keystone flap reconstruction depending on the nature of the defect and available tissues (see Fig 10.1). However, multi-trauma encompasses more than just the potential for multiple injuries. It indicates that the severity of the injury to the patient is of sufficient magnitude that the patient may mount a systemic reaction to the injury. For example, a systemic inflammatory response syndrome (SIRS) can result, along with the potential for organ dysfunction and failure (Bone et al. 1992). These patients are, therefore, more complex in nature and require the multidisciplinary approach introduced above, including a potential intensive care admission. Strong consideration must be given to their general status at the time of any reconstruction, and reconstructive decision-making will be strongly influenced by competing (sometimes conflicting) interests. Keystone flap reconstruction can be considered in these patients and can contribute to minimising systemic injury, but the severity of the injuries (especially in devascularisation) often necessitates more complex reconstructive options.

Low-energy versus high-energy trauma

Low-energy injuries are those in which the total kinetic energy involved in the trauma is relatively low. For example, mechanical falls from standing or sitting heights can lead to injuries with soft tissue defects. These defects do not demonstrate extensive areas of damaged, devitalised tissue, and endothelial dysfunction of vessels within the local tissues is minimal. Low-energy trauma is, therefore, very well-suited to keystone flap reconstruction (see Fig 7.16). High-energy trauma (e.g. motor vehicle accidents at >80 km/h or falls from multiple storeys) often results in significant devascularisation of tissue, periosteal stripping and even segmental loss (see Fig 10.2). In these injuries, assessment of the initial injury may mean that the injury looks similar to lower velocity injuries, but the degree of injury to the surrounding tissues is much greater, including discrete vascular injury or significant regions of endothelial dysfunction. For this reason, the use of local tissues for reconstruction of high-energy trauma should be undertaken with caution. A delay in reconstruction is often advisable

to promote healing within the surrounding tissues, as found by Behan and colleagues (1994) during the early use of fasciocutaneous island flaps (a forerunner of the keystone island flap) for traumatic defects.

Simple versus complex mechanisms

A complex mechanism of trauma is where two or more injurious agents are involved, such as blunt trauma and burns (e.g. a patient sustaining lower limb trauma jumping out of a burning building or central tissue loss from a fall from a motorcycle with surrounding friction burns from contact with the road at speed). In complex trauma, the use of locoregional flaps may be inappropriate where there is injury to surrounding potential donor sites. Even if the tissues around the blunt trauma are not burned, wound healing and immune function may be impaired in severe complex trauma (e.g. major burns), so the timing of keystone flap reconstruction (though not precluded) should be considered carefully.

Acute versus chronic trauma

Trauma often results in a central zone of tissue destruction (with possible tissue necrosis) at the site of injury. The surrounding tissue is subject to initial oedema and lowered oxygen tension following this insult, which places additional tissue at risk of necrosis and poor wound healing. Flap elevation within the injured zone during this precarious time can result in flap loss (complete or partial), delayed wound healing and increased tissue loss (although the immediate vascular augmentation concept [IVAC] and keystone island flap salvage may assist in specific situations; see Chapter 3). Vacuum-assisted dressings can be used successfully to temporise wounds while the zone of injury undergoes healing. This period also permits appropriate debridement and serial wash-outs of the wound to ensure a clean bed for flap coverage. After appropriate tissue recovery, keystone flap reconstruction of soft tissue defects can then be undertaken safely. Keystone flap reconstruction in cases of acute (immediate) trauma can be problematic but its use in subacute injuries (after a period of 3–7 days) is an optimal time of application and can result in predictable outcomes with good flap preservation and timely healing. This is comparable to the staged early closures (within the first 3–5 days) reported with other flaps in the literature that demonstrate lower infection rates and improved outcomes, but may provide lower morbidity (Byrd et al. 1981, Godina 1986, Lo et al. 2007).

Chronic injuries (see Fig 10.4) have a more stable wound bed but may demonstrate long-term sequelae that can affect healing and surgical reconstruction (e.g. as shown in Fig 8.2). For example, previous vascular or lymphatic injury may result in poor tissue quality, lymphoedema and the loss of some sites for flap elevation. The blood supply of the keystone flap is generally reliable and it may solve many chronic traumatic injuries, but where there are significant traumatic sequelae, the importation of undamaged, healthy vascularised soft tissue coverage warrants consideration.

Chronic wounds have two additional considerations not generally present in more acute injuries. The exclusion of malignant ulceration in the form of a Marjolin's ulcer (squamous cell carcinoma as a result of inflammation at the site of a chronic wound) is essential in all chronic non-healing wounds. Failure to do so will result in flap reconstruction over a mitotic lesion with reconstructive failure and potential contamination of the operative field by tumour. Keystone flap loss or poor flap wound healing are sufficiently unusual that they can represent a clinical indicator of undiagnosed malignancy (recurrent or de novo). For example, extensive metastatic melanoma was identified shortly after wound dehiscence of a keystone flap for reconstruction of a melanoma-wide local excision of the back. In the vast majority of cases, tissue biopsies of non-healing or chronic ulcers should be undertaken prior to reconstruction.

The other significant issue to address in chronic injury is vascular compromise (either arterial/venous or both). The correction of chronic arterial occlusion may resolve non-healing ulcers without the need for surgery, as well as avoid the creation of a larger defect by surgery in a poorly perfused region.

In addition to biopsies and vascular investigations, other information may be garnered by medical imaging, including computerised tomographic (CT) scans looking at bony injury, plain X-rays and magnetic resonance imaging (MRI) for osteomyelitis, and Doppler ultrasound/CT angiography to examine the local vasculature. There is little excuse for a poorly considered, under-investigated and hasty reconstruction of the chronic soft tissue defect.

SPECIFIC SITES

Chapters 4–7 have described the various regions of the body and highlighted their specific needs during reconstruction. In traumatic defects, some specific body regions, such as the lower leg and the hand, are worthy of special mention due to the additional demands placed upon the reconstructive surgeon in these areas.

Lower third of leg
Few areas of the body are as challenging in terms of reconstruction as the lower one-third of the leg. Trauma to this region is common, with falls and motor vehicle accidents representing two of the most common causes. This region displays minimal soft tissue laxity, and soft tissue defects in this area can expose bone, joint, multiple vessels and tendons that will require definitive coverage. With the exception

of the foot, it is the most dependent region in the body and can suffer from chronic problems, such as venous or arterial insufficiency, lymphoedema and neuropathies. Any reconstructive options should have reliable vascularity, especially for its venous drainage, and promote early mobilisation and rapid return of daily activities of living/quality of life. As a result of these features, soft tissue reconstruction in this region is problematic and often few options may seem available except free-tissue transfer. The keystone island flap (and its design variants) can provide reliable soft tissue coverage of these defects where appropriate patient and defect selection is undertaken. Closure of the defect with only physiological tension may necessitate the use of a small skin graft to the donor site, but this can usually be undertaken without significant additional risk or morbidity (as shown in Figs 10.1 and 10.3).

Hand trauma
The hand is densely constructed of important nerves, vessels, tendons, bones and joints, with overlying soft tissues arranged to provide appropriate glide planes for these structures to permit the complex hand movements required for the activities of daily living. Each of the subregions of the hand displays site specialisation to permit the various functions of the hand. Few sites outside the hand can recreate the features and characteristics of native hand tissues, and 'like with like' reconstruction should be considered the gold standard. As described in Chapter 5, there are numerous suitable vascular perforators throughout the hand for use in locoregional flap reconstruction. The inherent focal elasticity of regions of the hand can be utilised to provide tissue for reconstruction of even modest-sized defects. Trauma to the hand is treated in a similar manner to the lower limb, focusing on appropriate patient assessment and management as a whole, bony stabilisation and timely vascularised soft tissue coverage of surgically prepared wounds that emphasises return to function as early as possible. Figures 10.5 and 10.6 demonstrate two cases where these principles have been applied for soft tissue reconstruction following trauma to the upper limb.

MANAGEMENT OF THE PRIMARY DEFECT

Assuming that an appropriate assessment of the patient and the injury(ies) is undertaken, management of the primary defect involves the surgical debridement of the wound with removal of all devitalised tissue followed by appropriate wash-out. Tissue biopsies may be taken at this time if needed. Temporary or definitive bony fixation will assist wound closure and minimise ongoing tissue damage. As described above, where injury is significant or the surrounding potential donor sites are within the zone of injury, a delay in reconstruction by the use of dressings and elevation is prudent to ensure an adequately stable and clean wound bed for subsequent flap coverage. Vascular imaging is not used as a rule but can be useful in specific instances where pre-existing vascular compromise or local vascular injury is suspected. Where reconstruction is to be undertaken as part of a team, sound communication during this process is vital to surgical success.

Identification of the type of defect and nature of reconstruction then directs the type of flap used. Where the defect is of fasciocutaneous tissue only, locoregional reconstruction with the keystone island flap (or its design variants) is a reliable approach when the geometry of the defect is relatively straightforward. In cavitating injuries or those with significant dead space, muscle-based flaps (pedicled or free) often provide better dead space obliteration with improved outcomes relative to keystone or other fasciocutaneous flap reconstructions (including free flaps, such as the anterolateral thigh flap) (Engel et al. 2011).

Keystone flap reconstruction, with or without skin grafting of the secondary defect, is a simple and reliable reconstructive tool for the management of trauma, even in difficult areas such as the lower third of the leg. Figure 10.1 demonstrates an example of its use in acute trauma in this region. Where a skin graft is used for the secondary defect, this compares favourably with alternative forms of reconstruction, such as free-tissue transfer, where split-thickness skin may be used directly on muscle flaps with poor cosmetic and functional results, or with skin grafting to the donor site in some free fasciocutaneous flaps. Keystone flap reconstruction provides a shorter, less morbid operation that limits surgical morbidity to the affected area alone, while demonstrating reliable healing and acceptable aesthetics. It is an excellent reconstructive choice for many defects, especially where specific indications for free-tissue transfer (e.g. provision of vascularised bone, functional or denervated muscle transfer, revascularisation, or defects with insufficient local donor tissue availability) are not met.

FIGURE 10.1

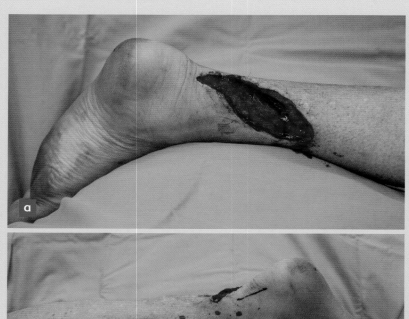

FIGURE 10.1 A 39-year-old man presents with a circular saw injury to his left posteromedial calf involving transection of the Achilles tendon and significant soft tissue loss (4 × 13 cm soft tissue defect)

(a) Following excisional wound debridement and pulsed lavage, the Achilles tendon is ready for reconstruction.

(b) Doppler ultrasound is used to identify peroneal artery perforators as the basis for a laterally based flap due to the proximity of the defect to the tibia medially and the oblique angle of the wound. The lowest perforator is sought so that the flap may be narrowed to limit exposure over the fibula at the flap donor site.

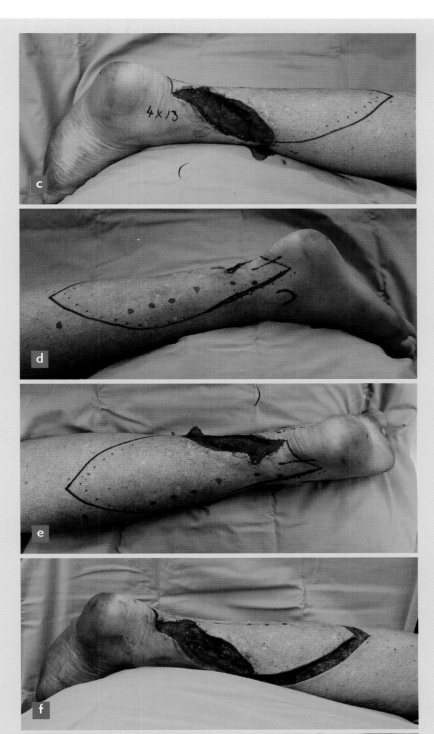

(c) & **(d)** A peroneal perforator keystone island flap is designed to incorporate the posterior aspect of the calf.

(e) The flap incorporates numerous perforators and would permit the narrowed area of the lower part of the flap without compromise. This would not be as certain without identification of nearby perforators in the keystone flap. Any number of flaps could be elevated on the identified perforators.

(f) & **(g)** The Achilles tendon repair is complete and the flap islanding is undertaken circumferentially through the deep fascia, with preservation of longitudinal neurovascular structures, such as the short saphenous vein and sural nerve.

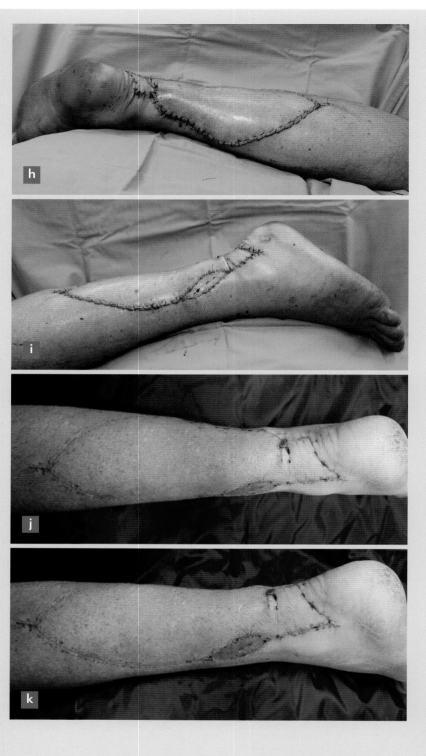

(h) The medial aspect of the wound is closed using 3/0 and 4/0 nylon.

(i) A small, full-thickness skin graft is applied laterally to avoid excessive tension.

(j) & **(k)** At 3 weeks, the wounds have healed, with the exception of a small granulated area that responded well to simple dressings within 1 week. The patient progressed to normal weight-bearing, walking and activities as directed by his Achilles tendon repair, with acceptable aesthetics and function.

TLC: Conjoint flap vascularity

Time (operation/cost)	
90 minutes	
Life quality (and aesthetics)	
Good with normal function and acceptable aesthetics not limiting recovery of Achilles tendon repair	
Complications	
Single site of granulation healed after 4 weeks	

CLINICAL CASES

The usefulness of the keystone island flap as a reconstructive tool for a variety of traumatic defects is demonstrated in the following clinical cases shown in Figures 10.2 to 10.7.

FIGURE 10.2

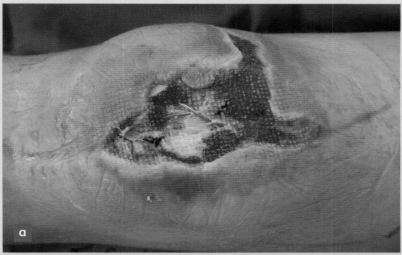

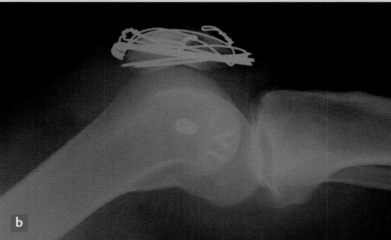

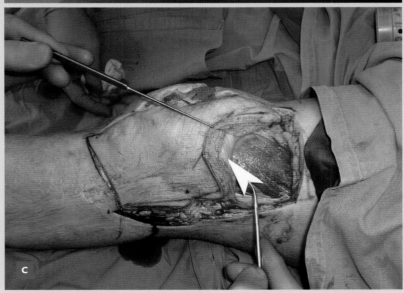

FIGURE 10.2 A referral was made to our tertiary hospital from an outside health centre of a truck driver managed by a local orthopaedic unit following a truck accident

(a) Appearance at 4–5 weeks following orthopaedic fixation of his patellar fracture. Exposed metal and bone are evident, with slough along the wound margins.

(b) Plain X-ray demonstrates a copious volume of metal wiring for fixation of the patella, yet good articular alignment.

(c) Following wound debridement, an inferiorly based keystone flap is raised medially with sharp incision through the skin followed by blunt dissection for flap elevation. The lower third is left attached to capture medial geniculate perforators along with neurovascular supply to the region. The flap is aligned along the L3 dermatome.

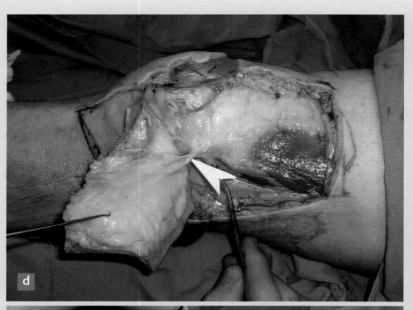

(d) The arrow indicates perforator support for the flap as it is raised during blunt dissection.

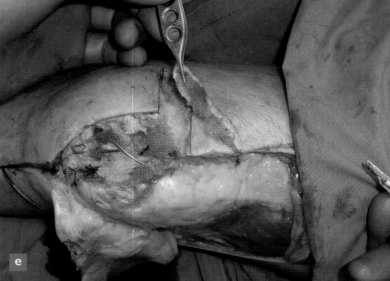

(e) With the flap in position, the debridement is completed to fit in with the flap alignment.

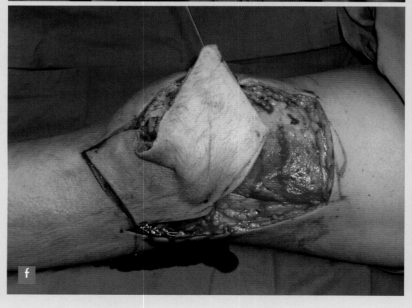

(f) With the tourniquet still applied, the *red dot sign* understandably demonstrates a cyanotic tinge.

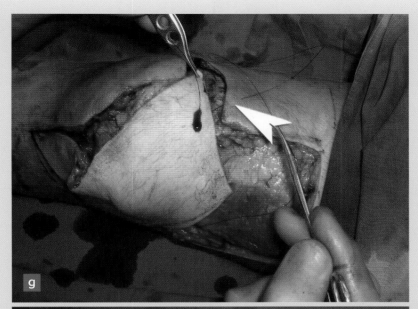

(g) Upon release of the tourniquet, a vascular flare gradually becomes evident. The white lines of tension in the subdermal plexus are temporary phenomena while the perfusional dynamics are supported by the underlying perforator system.

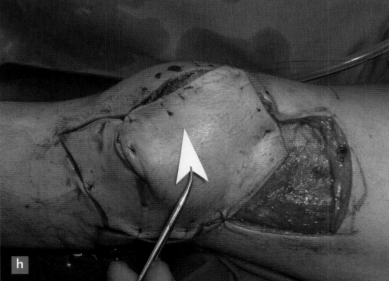

(h) & **(i)** The wound on closure with suction drainage and the arrow indicating another point of red dot reactive hyperaemia.

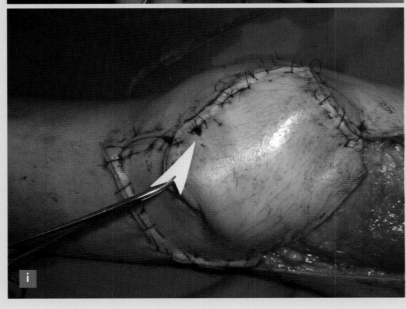

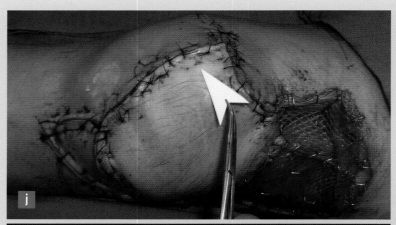

(j) A meshed split-thickness skin graft is applied for secondary defect closure. Additional V–Y advancement would normally be possible but caution was exercised to limit tension in the oedematous wound bed of the 4-week-old subacute wound.

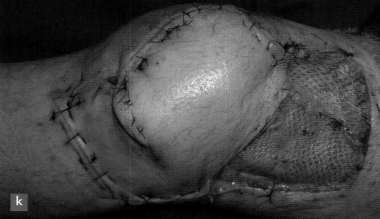

(k) Appearance at 7 days indicating good skin graft take and reliable flap healing. The patient refused long-term follow-up.

(l) The appearance at 3 weeks with a full range of movement.

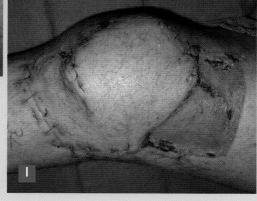

TLC: Conjoint flap vascularity

Time (operation/cost)
120 minutes

Life quality (and aesthetics)
Patient returned to driving his truck and refused further reviews as he had no further issues

Complications
Nil

See video for Figure 10.2

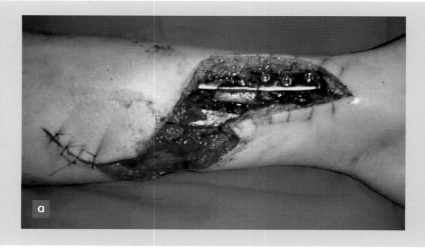

FIGURE 10.3

FIGURE 10.3 A 26-year-old male with compound tibial fracture managed with internal fixation and plating. Attempted closure by the orthopaedic unit was suboptimal, so temporising measures were instituted and plastic surgery referral made. Options of free-tissue transfer or locoregional fasciocutaneous flap reconstruction with a keystone flap variant were considered

(a) Wound appearance at referral following removal of tension sutures with exposed metal work, fracture and devitalised tissue margins.

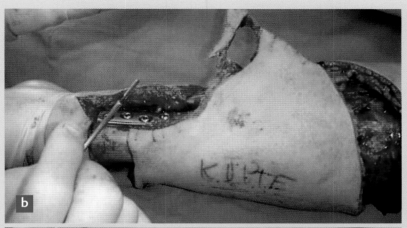

(b) A keystone flap was elevated based upon peroneal perforators and superficial peroneal branches for neurovascular support. Debridement of the flap edge once sufficient flap mobility is provided to enable wound closure under physiological tension.

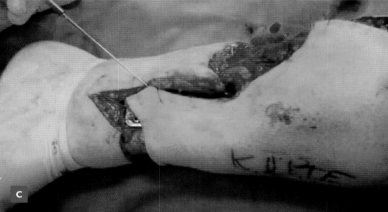

(c) Alignment with a skin hook to note appropriate apposition.

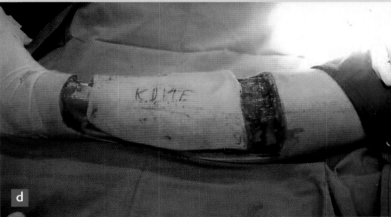

(d) The flap is completely islanded, with good supply from the underlying peroneal perforators.

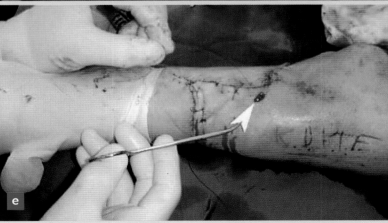

(e) *Red dot sign* confirming the hypervascularity (part of the quaternary response).

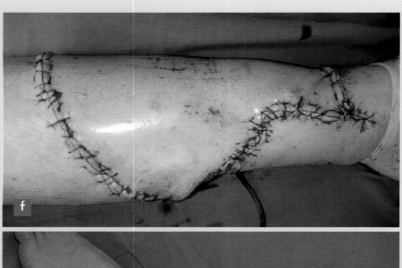

(f) On completion, the vascular flare demonstrates another part of the quaternary response, ensuring rapid healing. The patient's compliance postoperatively was problematic, with the patient self-discharging against medical advice for social reasons. The reliability of the flap withstood the issues with compliance despite this self-discharge within 24 hours.

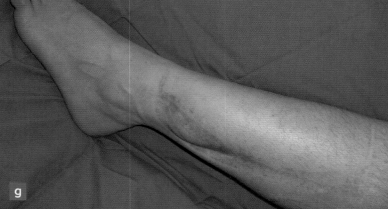

(g) Appearance 3 months postoperatively demonstrating good healing, including of the split-thickness skin graft above the lateral malleolus.

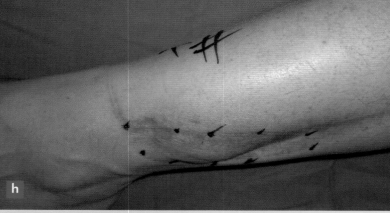

(h) The site of previous skin grafting is dotted out.

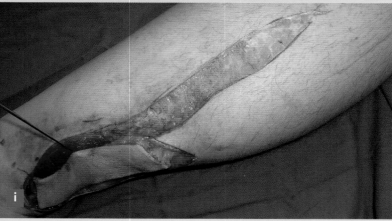

(i) At the request of the patient, a scar revision was undertaken. Following excision of the skin graft, a posteriorly based keystone flap is elevated and used to close the skin graft excision site directly.

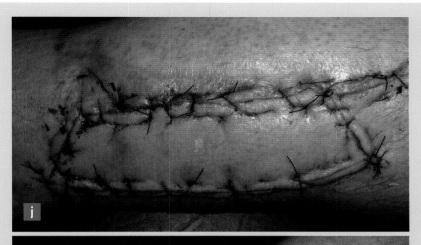

(j) The flap is inset and undergoes reliable healing, as seen in (k).

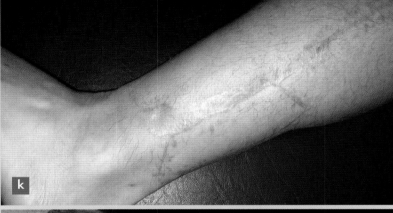

(l) The contralateral leg has a sizeable tattoo. The patient planned a tattoo for the operative leg once it was healed.

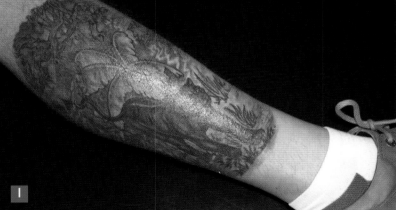

TLC: Conjoint flap vascularity

Time (operation/cost)	Life quality (and aesthetics)	Complications
80 minutes	Non-compliant—patient signed self out of hospital to take possession on settlement of his recently purchased house	Nil
40 minutes (scar revision and keystone flap)	Good with normal function and acceptable appearance	Nil, patient undertook tattooing over the site

FIGURE 10.4

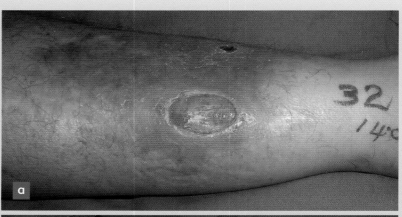

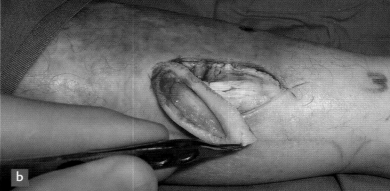

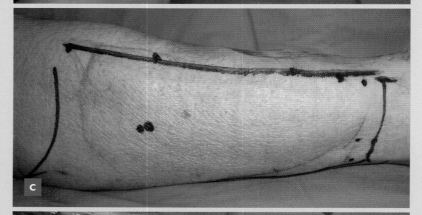

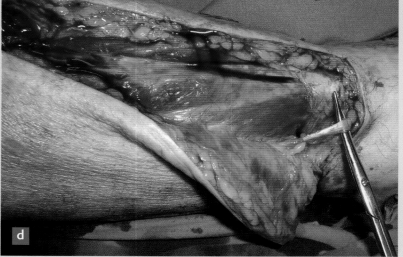

FIGURE 10.4 A 48-year-old male with a chronic non-healing ulcer over a compound tibial fracture from 32 years previously. Fourteen operations had failed to resolve the ulcer and unstable scar. Marked unilateral lymphoedema significantly limited activities of daily living/quality of life

(a) Chronic ulcer of anterior shin directly over the previously fractured tibia.

(b) Excisional debridement of the ulcer is undertaken, with thorough wash-out of the wound.

(c) A laterally based keystone flap is planned.

(d) The lower end of the keystone flap is elevated while maintaining important neurovascular structures.

(Reproduced with permission from Behan FC, Lo CH, Shayan R, Findlay M 2009 The keystone technique for resolution of chronic lower limb wound with lymphedema. J Plast Reconstr Aesthet Surg 62(5):701–2.)

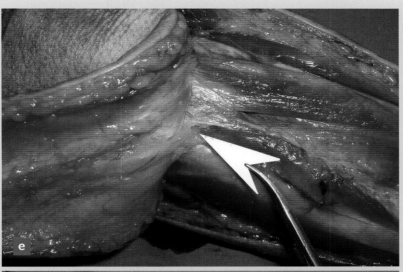

(e) Blunt dissection deep to the deep fascia is performed, with preservation of cutaneous perforators (arrow).

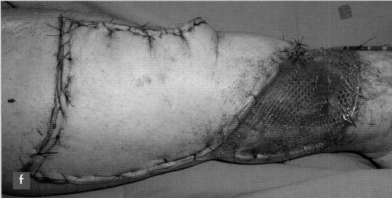

(f) Transposition of the distal end of the flap achieves wound closure, and split-thickness skin grafting is undertaken for the secondary defect.

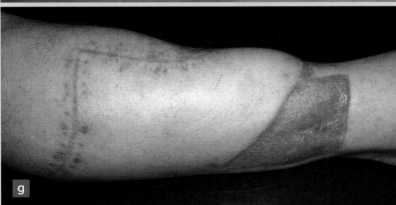

(g) & **(h)** Following uneventful wound healing, the lymphoedema resolved, with the patient able to stand and work all day without significant swelling and with resolution of peripheral oedema after 32 years. His quality of life improved dramatically by 1 year despite the addition of more scars.

See **video** for Figure 10.4

TLC: Conjoint flap vascularity

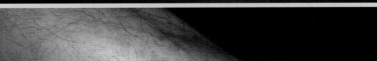

Time (operation/cost)
68 minutes
Life quality (and aesthetics)
Good, with loss of lymphoedema during normal work day (32-year history previously), and acceptable aesthetics
Complications
Nil

FIGURE 10.5

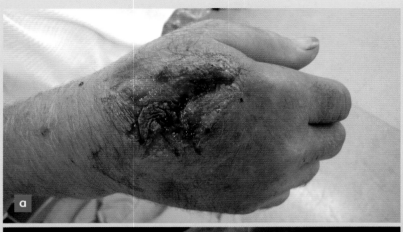

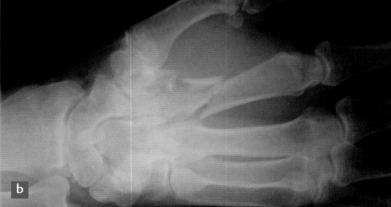

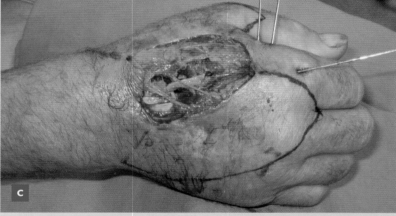

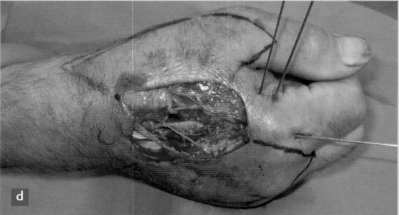

FIGURE 10.5 **A 78-year-old retired pilot received a compound fracture to his right (dominant) second metacarpal as a result of starting the propeller of an original World War II fighter plane by hand**

(a) The initial appearance does not demonstrate significant soft tissue loss, but the open fracture is hidden by the skin that has been pushed down within the fracture.

(b) X-ray demonstrates the comminuted nature of the fracture to the base of the second metacarpal.

(c) Following appropriate wound debridement, the fracture fragments are evident within the central aspect of the wound and the cutaneous defect is significantly larger. A single axial K-wire is used to maintain alignment and an additional two transverse wires are used to control the fragments. An ulnar-based keystone flap is devised to assist wound closure following pulsed lavage.

(d) An additional radially based keystone flap is devised, based upon the size of the defect and swelling within the tissues.

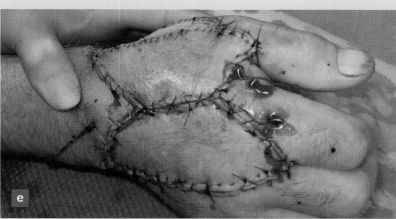

(e) A bilateral flap advancement (type IV) is undertaken over a small suction drain.

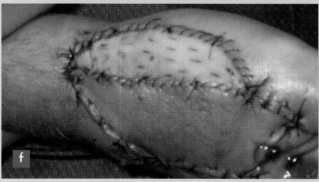

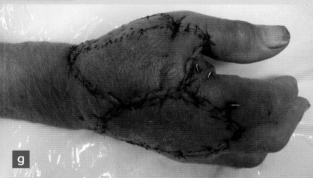

(f) Due to untoward tension, a small fenestrated full-thickness skin graft is applied to the radial flap's secondary defect over the thumb.

(g) Appearance at 9 days, showing good skin graft take and reliable healing of both keystone flaps. Protected range of motion exercises are begun for the thumb, little and ring fingers.

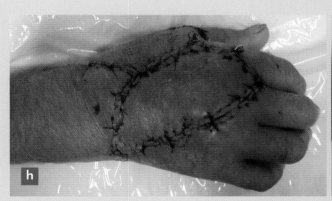

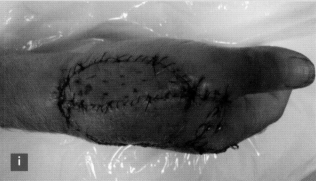

(h) Despite swelling, the V–Y points of the ulnar flap are progressing well.

(i) Excellent skin graft take is evident. Good mobility with no significant restriction in function compared with preinjury levels was evident at 6 months follow-up.

TLC: Conjoint flap vascularity

Time (operation/cost)
90 minutes
Life quality (and aesthetics)
Good with normal function and acceptable aesthetics
Complications
Nil

See video for Figure 10.5

FIGURE 10.6

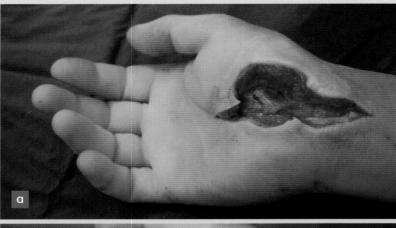

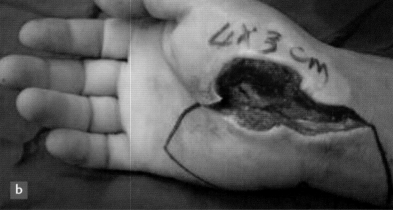

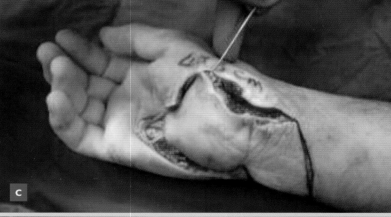

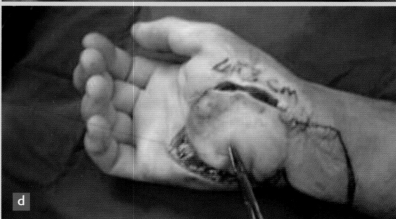

FIGURE 10.6 A 42-year-old, right-handed man who fell off his bicycle injured the palmar surface of his right hand, with full-thickness tissue loss

(a) Staged debridement of the injury resulted in exposure of the median nerve proximally and the transverse carpal ligament in the palm via a 4 × 3 cm defect. Immediate reconstruction was a necessity.

(b) A hypothenar keystone island flap based on a conjoint supply via perforators from the ulnar neurovascular bundle and the palmar cutaneous branch of the ulnar nerve, with division of the radial aspect of Guyon's canal to facilitate advancement into the defect.

(c) & **(d)** The inherent laxity of the hypothenar complex permitted direct closure of the defect.

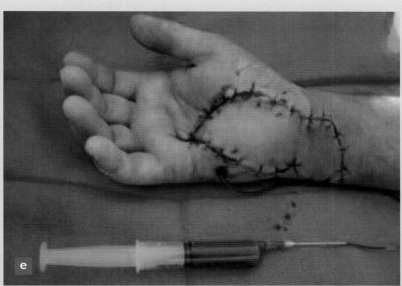

(e) Closure is undertaken over a small suction drain with the use of Luer-Lok syringe-based suction.

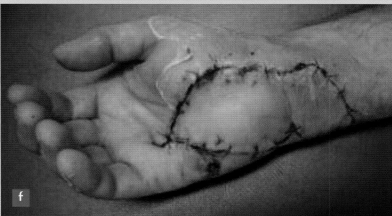

(f) Appearance at 7 days post operation with sound early healing and noticeable keratosis from rest in a splint.

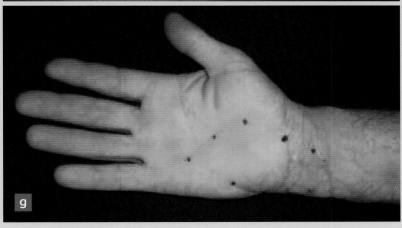

(g) Appearance at 6 weeks with good function and aesthetics.

TLC: Conjoint flap vascularity

Time (operation/cost)
45 minutes
Life quality (and aesthetics)
Good—back to riding his bike to collect his wine, acceptable appearance
Complications
Nil

FIGURE 10.7

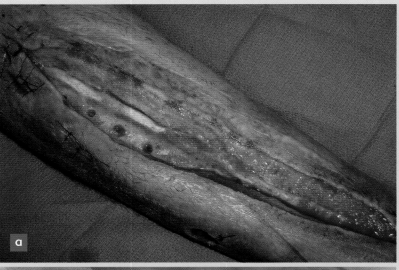

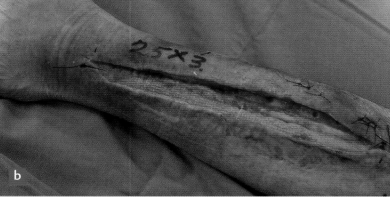

FIGURE 10.7 A 46-year-old male with previous open reduction, internal fixation and, following removal of the plate fixation, wound breakdown that occurred with exposure of the full length of the fibula. Free-flap reconstruction was considered but a local option was sought

(a) & **(b)** Defect size 25 × 3 cm with noticeable screw hole defects in the bone.

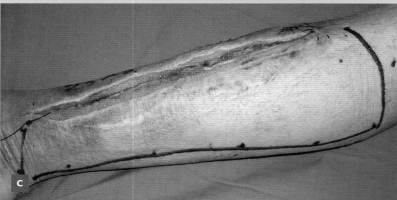

(c) A keystone flap over the posterolateral aspect of the leg is devised, based on peroneal musculocutaneous perforators, with previous trauma to the flap indicated by a healed split-thickness skin graft.

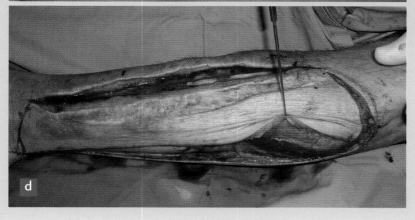

(d) The flap is elevated with division of the deep fascia.

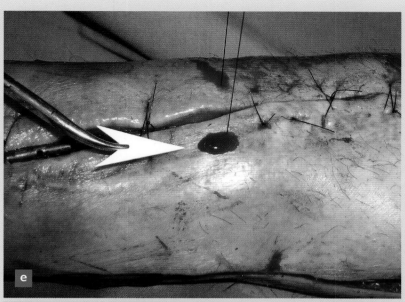

(e) The *red dot sign* indicated reliable vascularity (the quaternary response).

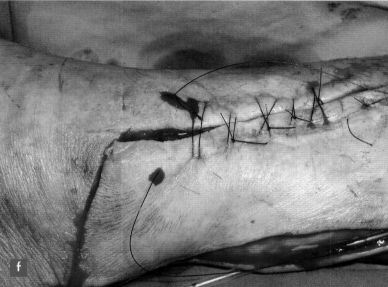

(f) A vascular flare is evident, including within the skin graft on the flap.

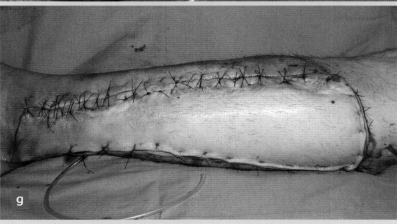

(g) Appearance once the flap is inset with even tension and subsequent good wound healing.

TLC: Conjoint flap vascularity

Time (operation/cost)
70 minutes
Life quality (and aesthetics)
Good with normal function and acceptable aesthetics
Complications
Nil

SUMMARY

Flap reconstruction in trauma should follow the principle of complex assessment followed by the use of the simplest, most appropriate solution. Thorough assessment of the trauma patient is essential for successful outcomes. In cases of severe trauma, there are often multiple competing problems. Free-tissue transfer is a complex form of reconstruction for traumatic defects, and is most suitable where revascularisation, composite tissue or large volume reconstructions are required. Careful consideration of all reconstructive options in the given patient (and setting) maximises the chances of correctly identifying the simplest form of reconstruction that will achieve the most appropriate outcome. The keystone flap provides reliable, robust vascularised soft tissue coverage that is suitable for many traumatic defects and has suitable aesthetics. It is most suited to isolated, simple low-velocity trauma in the subacute setting, but can be used very effectively in other presentations with consideration and care. A systematic approach to the trauma patient should correctly identify those patients with the most to benefit from such a reconstructive approach.

BIBLIOGRAPHY

Behan F C, Terrill P J, Ashton M W 1994 Fasciocutaneous island flaps for orthopaedic management in lower limb reconstruction using dermatomal precincts. Aust N Z J Surg 64(3):155–66.

Bone R C, Balk R A, Cerra F B, Dellinger R P, Fein A M, Knaus W A, Schein R M, Sibbald W J 1992 Definitions for sepsis and organ failure and guidelines for the use of innovative therapies in sepsis. The ACCP/SCCM Consensus Conference Committee. American College of Chest Physicians/Society of Critical Care Medicine. Chest 101(6):1644–55.

Byrd H S, Cierny G 3rd, Tebbetts J B 1981 The management of open tibial fractures with associated soft-tissue loss: external pin fixation with early flap coverage. Plast Reconstr Surg 68(1):73–82.

Engel H, Lin C H, Wei F C 2011 Role of microsurgery in lower extremity reconstruction. Plast Reconstr Surg 127 (Suppl 1):228S–238S.

Godina M 1986 Early microsurgical reconstruction of complex trauma of the extremities. Plast Reconstr Surg 78(3):285–92.

Lo C H, Leung M, Baillieu C, Chong E W, Cleland H 2007 Trauma centre experience: flap reconstruction of traumatic lower limb injuries. Aust N Z J Surg 77(8):690–4.

Parrett B M, Matros E, Pribaz J J, Orgill D P 2006 Lower extremity trauma: trends in the management of soft-tissue reconstruction of open tibia-fibula fractures. Plast Reconstr Surg 117(4):1315–22; discussion 1323–4.

Posch N A, Mureau M A, Dumans A G, Hofer S O 2007 Functional and aesthetic outcome and survival after double free flap reconstruction in advanced head and neck cancer patients. Plast Reconstr Surg 120(1):124–9.

Index

A

abdominal reconstruction 120–6
absorbable sutures 30, 116
    continuous 130
acral lentiginous melanoma of the foot 174–5
acute trauma 200–1
    see also trauma
Advanced Trauma Life Support (ATLS) 199
    see also trauma
aesthetics 9, 40, 47, 49, 55, 57, 70
afferent sensory neurons 16
    see also cutaneous vascular physiology
ageing population 3
American Joint Committee on Cancer (AJCC) guidelines for
    melanoma 161
anatomical layers of the face 57–8
anatomy *see* fasciocutaneous tissue anatomy; vascular
    anatomy
angiosome concept 5–7
angiotome concept 4–5
ankle reconstruction
    ankle vessels 142
    anterior ankle region arteries 141
    cutaneous vascular anatomy 141–2
    flap elevation 150–1
    sinus of lateral aspect of ankle 150–1
    see also lower limb reconstruction
antidromic vasodilation 20
architectural nomenclature 8
arterial perforators 12
    see also fasciocutaneous tissue anatomy
arterioles 16
    see also fasciocutaneous tissue anatomy
arteriovenous anastomoses (AVAs) 16
    see also fasciocutaneous tissue anatomy
atypical fibroxanthoma of vertex of scalp 88–9

B

back reconstruction 114–16
basal cell carcinoma (BCC)
    conchal bowl 69
    iliac fossa 121–3
    multiple 74–6
    nose, advanced 77–9
    of the back 41–3
    right malar eminence 40
BCC *see* basal cell carcinoma
Bezier curve flap 6, 8
biopsy for melanoma 161–2
biopsy-proven melanoma of calf 163–5
bipedicled flap 28
blood supply *see* vascular anatomy

breast reconstruction 116–19
bridge flap variant 35, 50–1, 70
buttock and perianal reconstruction 131–4

C

cadaveric studies 4, 6
calf reconstruction
    biopsy-proven melanoma 163–5
    chronic ulcer 18–19
    melanoma of posterior 148–9
    posteromedial calf injury, trauma 202–4
    recurrent melanoma 166–7
    see also lower limb reconstruction; lower limb
        reconstruction demonstrations
capillaries 16
    see also fasciocutaneous tissue anatomy; vascular anatomy
cervicosubmental (CSM) keystone island flap 31, 32, 35, 72,
    74, 77, 80
    clinical demonstrations 32–4, 56, 63, 73, 75, 84, 95–6,
        185
cheek and temple defects 77
    clinical demonstration 32–4
chest wall and breast reconstruction 116–19
chronic calf ulcer 18–19
chronic non-healing ulcer 212–13
chronic trauma 200–1
    see also trauma
classification
    fasciocutaneous flap 12
    keystone island flap 31–2
    vascular pattern 12–13
    vascular pattern of peripheral nerves 14
clinical demonstrations
    cervicosubmental (CSM) keystone island flap 32–4
    chronic calf ulcer 18–19
    grid pattern application 26
    melanoma involving the parotid 56
    metastatic melanoma 22–5
    multiple facial skin cancers 20–2
    neurovascular-based keystone island flap 15
    preserving neurovascular supply 73–4
    see also design variation demonstrations; head and
        neck demonstrations; lower limb reconstruction
        demonstrations; melanoma demonstrations; planning
        a keystone island flap; trauma demonstrations;
        trunk reconstruction demonstrations; upper limb
        reconstruction demonstrations
compound fracture to second metacarpal 214–15
compound tibial fracture 208–11
Cormack and Lamberty vascular pattern classification 12–13
cross-sectional anatomy of leg 141
CSM *see* cervicosubmental

cutaneous nerve territories 14
cutaneous vascular anatomy *see* vascular anatomy
cutaneous vascular perforators
    ankle 142
    anterior trunk 117
    arterial perforators 12
    buttock 131
    deep inferior epigastric perforator (DIEP) 5–6
    dermatomal axes–perforator zones 29–30
    dorsal trunk 115
    foot 142
    hand 102
    hypogastric flap 5
    internal pudendal artery 128
    lateral aspect of leg 140
    lateral trunk 116
    lower limb 137–8
    medial aspect of foot 142
    septocutaneous nature of perforators 100
cutaneous vascular physiology 16–17
    afferent sensory neurons 16
    autoregulation 17
    inflammatory response 16
    microcirculation 16
    neurovascularisation patterns 13–15
    sympathetic innervation 16
    see also fasciocutaneous tissue anatomy; vascular anatomy

D

deep fascia/panniculus carnosus remnants 34
    see also planning a keystone island flap
deep inferior epigastric perforator (DIEP) 5
de-epithelialisation 35
    see also planning a keystone island flap
delayed reconstruction after pathology evaluation (DRAPE)
       90, 161–2, 153, 168
delto pectoral flap 5
deltoid region 99–100
dermatomal axes–perforator zones 29–30
dermatomal roadmap 14
    see also fasciocutaneous tissue anatomy
design 17, 28
    cervicosubmental (CSM) flap 32–4, 56, 63, 65
    clinical demonstrations 20, 23, 46
    longitudinal 44
    preauricular region 48
    transverse orientation 38–9
    see also cervicosubmental (CSM) keystone island flap;
       omega variant; planning a keystone island flap; Yin
       Yang variant
design variation 34–5
    deep fascia/panniculus carnosus remnants 34
    de-epithelialisation 35
    flap movement into the defect 35
    flap subdivision 35
    islanding 35
    skin incision shape 35–6
design variation demonstrations
    basal cell carcinoma of right malar eminence 40
    basal cell carcinoma of the back 41–3
    bridge flap variant 50–1

    early type 1 keystone flap 38–9
    goblet variant 88–89
    Hutchison's freckle 36–7
    melanoma of right arm 46–7
    neurovascular axis as basis for orientation 40
    omega variant 176–7
    squamous cell carcinoma in preauricular region 48–9
    squamous cell carcinoma of index finger joint 44–5
    ulcerative lesions of thigh 50–1
    Yin Yang variant 133
    see also planning a keystone island flap
dog ears 32, 34, 35, 88, 178
    clinical demonstrations 63, 66, 109, 127, 145
dorsum of foot flap elevation 150, 152
dorsum of hand and fingers 100–2
double flaps
    clinical demonstrations 21, 41
    indicating IVAC 166
    red dot signs 21, 133
drain tube
    closure over 34
    insertion 42
    removal 45
    U-shape for arm 47
DRAPE *see* delayed reconstruction after pathology evaluation
Dupuytren's contracture of hand 110–11

E

elbow cutaneous vascular territories 101
elbow reconstruction demonstration 103–5
elevation *see* keystone island flap elevation
Emergency Management of Severe Trauma (EMST) 199
    see also trauma
epidermis layers 10–11
eye region surgery 77–9

F

facial nerve 57
    landmarks 57
    paralysis 64
    preservation 57–8
    sacrifice 65
    see also head and neck reconstruction
fasciocutaneous angiotomes as island flaps 6–7
fasciocutaneous flap types 12
fasciocutaneous island flap versus skin graft 112–13
fasciocutaneous tissue anatomy 10
    arterial perforators 12
    arterioles 16
    basement membrane 11
    capillaries 16
    cutaneous microcirculation 16
    cutaneous neurovascularisation patterns 13–15
    cutaneous vascular physiology 16–17
    cutaneous vascularisation patterns 11–13
    dermatomal roadmap 14
    epidermis layers 10–11
    metarterioles 16
    skin circulation 11
    skin function 10

subcutaneous tissue 11
terminal arterioles 16
vascularisation patterns 11–16
venules 16
see also vascular regulation within keystone island flaps
fibula exposure following wound breakdown 218–19
flap see keystone island flap
foot reconstruction
    acral lentiginous melanoma 174–5
    ankle and dorsum of foot 141–2
    closure of defects in dorsum 152
    cutaneous vascular anatomy 141–3
    dorsum of foot defects 152
    flap elevation 150
    medial aspect of foot 142
    plantar surface of foot 143
    see also heel reconstruction; lower limb reconstruction
forearm 100
forearm cutaneous vascular territories 101
forehead flap 5
free-flap reconstruction 3–4
free-tissue transfer 3
French curve flap 6, 8

G

goblet variant 31, 32, 35, 88, 100, 121, 143
    clinical demonstration 88
grid pattern application 26
groin and thigh reconstruction
    cutaneous vascular anatomy of the thigh 136–7
    flap elevation 143
    melanoma in naevus of thigh 144–5
    see also lower limb reconstruction

H

haemodynamic changes during islanding 25–6
hand reconstruction
    blood supply to dorsum 101
    blood supply to volar aspect 102
    cutaneous perforators within hand 102
    dorsum of hand and fingers 100–2
    Dupuytren's contracture of hand 110–11
    injured palmar surface of hand with full-thickness tissue
        loss 216–17
    palm 102
    T1b melanoma of right hand 171
    trauma 201
    vascular anatomy 102
    volar aspect of hand 102
    see also see upper limb reconstruction
head and neck reconstruction 55–7, 97
    anatomical layers of the face 57–8
    blood supply summary 61
    cutaneous vessel network 58–60
    facial nerve landmarks 57
    facial nerve preservation 57–8
    multiple subunit 94–7
    neurovascular anatomy 58–60
    preserving neurovascular supply 73–4
    subcutaneous musculo-aponeurotic system (SMAS) 57–8

head and neck reconstruction demonstrations
    advanced basal cell carcinoma of nose 77–9
    atypical fibroxanthoma of vertex of scalp 88–9
    melanoma involving the parotid 56
    multiple basal cell carcinoma 74–6
    multiple squamous cell carcinoma of dorsum 90–1
    multiple subunit 94–7
    perioral defect 80–7
    secondary deposit of squamous cell carcinoma in neck
        92–3
    squamous cell carcinoma of oral commissure 83–7
head and neck reconstruction zones 60
    cheek 32–4, 77
    neck 91–4
    nose 90
    perioral 80–7
    periorbital 77–9
    scalp 88–9
    see also periauricular region
heel reconstruction 153–4
    see also foot reconstruction; lower limb reconstruction
hemming sutures 29, 40, 82, 126
Hutchinson's melanotic freckle 36–7, 167–9
hyperaemic flare 17, 18, 26, 35, 69
    clinical demonstrations 19, 197
    red dot sign 20
    see also vascular flare
hypogastric flap 5
    deep inferior epigastric artery perforator 6

I

immediate vascular augmentation concept (IVAC) 5, 25, 26,
        98, 127, 181, 182, 200
    clinical demonstrations 18, 21, 24, 65, 75, 154, 164,
        166, 172, 175, 177, 184–5, 187, 193
    see also red dot sign; vascular flare
inset and defect closure 31
islanding 15, 35, 38
    along axis of superficial temporal artery branches 40
    intercostal 41
    paraspinous 41
    perfusion during 25
    see also planning a keystone island flap
IVAC see immediate vascular augmentation concept

K

keystone design see design; design variation
keystone island flap
    angiosome concept 5–7
    angiotome concept 4–5, 7
    cadaveric studies 4, 6
    computerised tomographic (CT) angiography 6
    development 4, 8–9
    immediate vascular augmentation concept 5
    linkage vessels 4
    movement into the defect 35
    subdivision 35
    see also planning a keystone island flap
keystone island flap elevation 5–6
    abdomen 121

ankle 150–1
buttock 131
chest wall and breast 118
design 30
dorsum of foot 150
groin of thigh 143
in the back 115–16
knee 143
leg 148
lower limb 143
plantar foot 153
principles 33
procedure 18–20
upper limb 98–9
see also head and neck reconstruction; planning a
    keystone island flap
keystone origins v, xi, 3, 8
knee injury, trauma 205–8
knee reconstruction
    cutaneous vascular anatomy 137
    flap elevation 143
    infected prepatellar bursa 146–7
    trauma 205–8

L
leg reconstruction
    cross-sectional anatomy 141
    cutaneous vascular anatomy 137–41
    flap elevation 148
    mid-thigh transverse section 139
    peripatellar plexus 139
    posterior tibial artery 140
    trauma 201
    see also lower limb reconstruction; lower limb
        reconstruction demonstrations
linkage vessels 4
lip defects 80–7, 190
locoregional flaps 3, 55, 57
lower limb reconstruction 135–6, 155
    ankle and dorsum of foot 141–2
    ankle flap elevation 150
    ankle vessels 142
    anterior ankle region arteries 141
    cross-sectional anatomy of leg 141
    cutaneous perforators of lateral aspect of leg 140
    cutaneous perforators to medial aspect of foot 142
    cutaneous vascular perforators 138
    dorsum of foot flap elevation 150
    flap elevation 143
    groin and thigh flap elevation 143
    knee 137
    knee flap elevation 143
    leg 137–41
    leg flap elevation 148
    leg, lower third 201
    mid-thigh transverse section 139
    peripatellar plexus 139
    plantar foot flap elevation 153
    plantar surface of foot 143
    posterior tibial artery of medial aspect of leg 140
    skin territories 137

thigh 136–7
lower limb reconstruction demonstrations
    chronic calf ulcer 18–19
    dorsum of foot defects 152
    groin and thigh 143
    infected prepatellar bursa of knee 146–7
    knee 143
    melanoma in naevus of thigh 144–5
    melanoma of calf 163–5
    melanoma of posterior of calf 148–9
    posteromedial calf injury, trauma 202–4
    recurrent melanoma of calf 166–7
    sinus of lateral aspect of ankle 150–1
    ulcerated acral lentiginous melanoma of heel 153–4

M
mattress sutures 19, 26, 33
melanoma 159, 163
    management 159
    revisional surgery 178
    skin grafting 159
    surgical management of nodal metastases 160
melanoma — closure principles 160, 178
    AJCC guidelines for melanoma 161–2
    delayed reconstruction after pathology evaluation
        (DRAPE) 161–2
    pathology and staging 160
    quality of life with low morbidity 163
    sentinel lymph node biopsy 161–2
    timely adjuvant therapies 162–3
    see also melanoma; melanoma demonstrations
melanoma demonstrations
    acral lentiginous melanoma of the foot 174–5
    arm 46–7
    calf 163–5
    calf, posterior 148–9
    cheek 182–3
    Hutchinson's melanotic freckle 167–9
    metastatic melanoma 22–5
    naevus of thigh 144–5
    nodal metastases of the neck 172–3
    parotid 56
    recurrent desmoplastic melanoma of molar eminence
        169–70
    recurrent melanoma of calf 166–7
    right arm 46–7
    spindle cell tumour of the back 176–7
    T1b melanoma of right hand 171
    thigh 144–5
    ulcerated acral lentiginous melanoma of heel 153–4
metacarpal compound fracture 214–15
mid-thigh transverse section 139
    see also leg reconstruction
multiple facial skin cancers 20–2
multiple head and neck subunit reconstruction 94–7

N
neck reconstruction zone 91–4
    blood supply 61
    see also head and neck reconstruction

nerve territories 14
neural mediation of flap perfusion 20–5
    see also vascular regulation within keystone island flaps
neurocutaneous perforator zones 25
neurovascular anatomy 58–60
neurovascular axis as basis for orientation 40
neurovascular-based keystone island flap 15
nodal metastases of the neck 172–3
nomenclature 8
nose reconstruction 90, 77–9
    blood supply 61
    see also head and neck reconstruction
nuchal keystone island flap 72–3

O

omega variant 31, 32, 35, 88, 100, 116, 121, 143
    clinical demonstrations 63, 66, 72, 73, 109, 176–7, 189
orientation of keystone flaps 29
    see also planning a keystone island flap

P

palm anatomy 102
palmar surface of hand trauma 216–17
pectoralis major flap 55, 72, 91, 182, 186
    pedicled 181
perforators see cutaneous vascular perforators
perfusion during islanding 25
perianal reconstruction 131–4
periauricular region 60, 73
    anterior 64–6
    central 60–4
    infra-auricular 67–8
    postauricular 69–70
    supra-auricular 71–2
    see also head and neck reconstruction
perineum reconstruction 127–30
perioral defect 80–7
perioral reconstruction zone 80–7
    see also head and neck reconstruction
periorbital reconstruction zone 77–9
    see also head and neck reconstruction
peripatellar plexus 139
    see also leg reconstruction
peripheral nerve classification 14
placement of keystone flaps 29
planning a keystone island flap
    bipedicled flap similarities 28
    classification 31–2
    convex structures 32
    deep fascia/panniculus carnosus remnants 34
    de-epithelialisation 35
    dermatomal axes–perforator zones 29–30
    design 28
    design variations 34–5
    flap elevation 30
    flap inset and defect closure 31
    flap movement into the defect 35
    flap subdivision 35
    islanding 35
    pinch test 28, 44

placement, size, orientation 28–9
    preoperative imaging 28–9, 32
    skin incision shape 35–6
    technical refinements 32–4
    transverse mark-out 38
    type A, B, C flaps 12
    type I, II, III, IV flaps 31–2
    see also cervicosubmental (CSM) keystone island flap;
        design; design variations; omega variant; planning
        a keystone island flap; Yin Yang variant
platysma flap elevation 67
postauricular periauricular defect 69–70
posterior tibial artery of medial aspect of leg 140
posteromedial calf injury, trauma 202–4
preoperative imaging 28–9, 32, 136–7
previous scarring 37, 56, 58
procedure demonstration see clinical demonstration
pudendal vessels 127–8

Q

quadriceps keystone flap closure 174–5
quality of life 4, 9, 55, 135–6, 159–60, 163, 178–9, 199,
    201
    postoperative demonstrations 97, 212–13
quaternary response 18, 25, 27, 35
    clinical demonstrations 19, 21, 24, 47, 185, 211–12, 221
    see also vascular regulation within keystone island flaps

R

radionecrosis 195
    clinical demonstration 195–7
    see also radiotherapy
radio-recurrent squamous cell carcinoma of parotid 184–5
radiotherapy 179, 198
    defect management 8
    effects 179–80
    initial postoperative 181
    reconstruction of radionecrosis 195–7
    skin grafts and 181
    see also reconstruction in previously irradiated tissues
reconstruction in previously irradiated tissues 181–2
    carcinoma of parotid 190–2
    carcinoma of tongue postoperative radiotherapy 186–9
    carcinoma over mastoid 193–4
    immediate vascular augmentation concept (IVAC) 181,
        184–5
    melanoma of cheek 182–3
    radio-recurrent carcinoma of parotid 184–5
reconstructive surgery era 9
recurrent desmoplastic melanoma of molar eminence 169–70
recurrent melanoma of calf 166–7
red dot sign 18–19, 25–6, 35, 50
    anterior abdominal wall defect 126
    apex of flap 191
    both sides of suture line 188–9
    confirming hypervascularity 209
    continuous suturing with absorbable suture 130
    cyanotic 183
    cyanotic tinge due to tourniquet 206
    demonstrating IVAC 164

denervation 20
double 21, 133
double flap 21
double flaps indicating IVAC 166
during mattress suture insertion 96
extreme point of flap 166
flap side versus non-flap side 193
increased perfusion of flap side of wound 145
indicating reliable vascularity 219
infra-auricular defect closure 68
inner canthus and bridge of the nose 79
perioral defect of left oral commissure 85
posterior flap 24
right iliac fossa 122–3
SMS cheek flap 75
strategic point of mattress sutures 26
revisional surgery for melanoma 178
    see also melanoma

S
scalp blood supply 61
scalp flap 5
scalp reconstruction zone 88–9
    see also head and neck reconstruction
SCC see squamous cell carcinoma
sentinel lymph node biopsy (SLNBx) 161–2
septocutaneous nature of perforators 100
shape of keystone flap 28–9
    see also planning a keystone island flap
sinus of lateral aspect of ankle 150–1
size of keystone flaps 29
    see also planning a keystone island flap
skin anatomy see fasciocutaneous tissue anatomy
skin grafting 4
    and radiotherapy 181
    fasciocutaneous island flap versus 112–13
    for melanoma 159
skin incision shape 35–6
    see also planning a keystone island flap
skin territories 137
SMAS see subcutaneous musculo-aponeurotic system
spindle cell tumour of the back 176–7
squamous cell carcinoma (SCC)
    dorsum 90–1
    index finger joint 44–5
    lip, secondary carcinoma of parotid 190–2
    neck, secondary deposit 92–3
    oral commissure 83–7
    parietal region, despite radiotherapy 195–7
    parotid, radio-recurrent 184–5
    preauricular region 48–9
    thenar eminence, multifocal 108–9
    tongue 186–9
    tonsil, recurrence over mastoid 193–4
strategic mattress sutures 19, 38
    apposition of the flaps 133
    closure 40, 42, 126
    forehead flap 38
    lumbar region 116
    metacarpophalangeal joint of index finger 45
    posterior vaginal 130

red dot sign during insertion 96
right molar eminence 40
to effect flap positioning 68
to encourage skin creep 33
to provide approximation 82, 93
V–Y closure 104
subcutaneous musculo-aponeurotic system (SMAS) 57–8, 73
supra-auricular periauricular defect 71–2
surgical management of clinical nodal metastases 160
    see also melanoma
sutures
    bleeding 51
    bone anchoring 70
    circumferential 19
    continuous hemming 126
    continuous suturing with absorbable suture 130
    deep absorbable 116
    definitive continuous everting mattress 68
    forehead flap 38
    hemming 29, 40, 82
    horizontal everting mattress 43
    insertion red dot signs 96
    mattress 33, 42, 45, 68, 93, 96, 116, 126
    red dot sign 19, 26, 188–9
    right molar eminence 40
    tension 30, 85
    vertical mattress 19, 29–30
sympathetic vasoconstriction and red dot sign 20

T
T1b melanoma of right hand 171
temple defects 77
temporal island flap 5
temporoparietal region blood supply 61
tension in flap closure 26
    infra-auricular defect 67
    linear tension on perfusion within subdermal plexus 19
    see also wound tension
territories of cutaneous arterial supply for head and neck 60
thigh flap elevation 143
thigh melanoma 144–5
tibial compound fracture 208–11
tophaceous gout extruding through olecranon skin 103–5
total forehead flap 5
total scalp flap 5
trapezius blood supply 61
trauma 199–200, 220
    acute versus chronic 200–1
    EMST/ATLS principles 199
    hand 201
    isolated versus multi 200
    knee 205–8
    low-energy versus high-energy 200
    lower third of leg 201
    management of primary defect 201–2
    simple versus complex 200
trauma demonstrations
    chronic non-healing ulcer 212–13
    compound fracture to second metacarpal 214–15
    compound tibial fracture 208–11
    fibula exposure following wound breakdown 218–19

injured palmar surface of hand with full-thickness tissue
        loss 216–17
    knee injury 205–8
    posteromedial calf injury 202–4
trigeminal angiotomes as island flaps 6–7
trunk reconstruction 114, 134
    abdominal 120–6
    anterior trunk blood supply 117
    buttock and perianal 131–4
    chest wall and breast 116–19
    dorsal trunk blood supply 115
    lateral trunk blood supply 116
    perineum 127–30
    the back 114–16
trunk reconstruction demonstrations
    abdominal wall defect with paramedian stoma 124–7
    basal cell carcinoma of iliac fossa 121–3
    fungating spindle cell tumour of breast 118–20
    radio-recurrent carcinoma of vaginal wall 129–30
    recurrent abscesses in the buttock 132–4
type A, B, C flaps 12
type I, II, III, IV flaps 31–2
types of peripheral nerve vascular patterns 14

U

ulcer, distal forearm 105–7
ulcer, chronic non-healing 212–13
ulcerated acral lentiginous melanoma of heel 153–4
ulcerative lesions of thigh 50–1
undermining while preserving neurovascular supply 73–4
upper limb reconstruction 98, 113
    blood supply to dorsum of hand and fingers 101
    blood supply to volar aspect of hand 102
    cutaneous arterial anatomy of arm 99
    cutaneous perforators within hand 102
    deltoid region 99–100
    dorsum of hand and fingers 100–2
    elbow cutaneous vascular territories 101
    flap elevation 98–9
    forearm 100
    forearm cutaneous vascular territories 101
    hand trauma 201
    palm 102
    septocutaneous nature of perforators 100
upper limb reconstruction demonstrations
    Dupuytren's contracture of hand 110–11
    fasciocutaneous island flap versus skin graft 112–13
    multifocal squamous cell carcinoma of thenar eminence
        108–9
    tophaceous gout extruding through olecranon skin
        103–5
    ulcer on distal forearm 105–7

V

vascular anatomy
    anterior abdominal wall 120
    anterior trunk 117
    arm 99

basement membrane 11
    buttock 131
    deep fascia 11
    dorsal trunk 115
    dorsum of hand and fingers 101
    hand 102
    knee 136
    lateral aspect of leg 140
    lateral trunk 116
    lower limb 136
    medial aspect of foot 142
    perineum 127–8
    plexuses 11–12
    subcutaneous tissue 11
    thigh 136
    volar aspect of hand 102
vascular flare 18, 25
    clinical demonstration 24, 45, 47, 85, 96, 172, 177, 210
    double flap 21
    flap colour and 183
    previous radiotherapy and 191
    skin graft 219
    spread 104
    subsidence 97
    tourniquet release 104, 111, 207
vascular pattern of peripheral nerve classification 14
vascular regulation within keystone island flaps 17, 27
    chronic calf ulcer demonstration 18–19
    haemodynamic changes during islanding 25–6
    keystone island flap elevation 5–6, 18–20
    metastatic melanoma 22–4
    multiple facial skin cancers 20–2
    neural mediation of flap perfusion 20–5
    quaternary response 18
    red dot sign 18–19, 25–6
vascularisation patterns 11–16
    see also fasciocutaneous tissue anatomy; vascular
        anatomy
venules 16
    see also fasciocutaneous tissue anatomy
V–Y flap advancement and closure 5, 6, 8, 28–9, 32, 35,
        123, 143, 150, 178
    blunt dissection mobilisation 29
    clinical demonstrations 18, 25, 36, 89, 104, 110, 149,
        151, 152, 153
vertical mattress sutures 19, 29–30
    see also sutures

W

white lines of tensile closure 26
    clinical demonstrations 40, 46–7, 48, 85, 165, 166,
        177, 190
    see also tension in flap closure

Y

Yin Yang variant 31, 116, 121, 123, 131, 143
    buttock and perianal reconstruction 131
    clinical demonstrations 92, 133, 166

Learner Services

Please return on or before the last date stamped below

Tel: 01603 773114

CITY COLLEGE
NORWICH

A FINE WILL BE CHARGED FOR OVERDUE ITEMS

247 669

WOMEN IN SPORT

IOC MEDICAL COMMISSION

SUB-COMMISSION ON PUBLICATIONS

IN THE SPORT SCIENCES

Howard G. Knuttgen PhD (Co-ordinator)
Boston, Massachusetts, USA

Francesco Conconi MD
Ferrara, Italy

Harm Kuipers MD, PhD
Maastricht, The Netherlands

Per A.F.H. Renström MD, PhD
Stockholm, Sweden

Richard H. Strauss MD
Los Angeles, California, USA